A Brief History of Disease, Science and Medicine

A Brief History of Disease, Science and Medicine

From the ice age to the genome project

Michael Kennedy

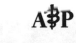

Asklepiad Press
Mission Viejo, California

A Brief History of Disease, Science and Medicine
From the ice age to the genome project
by Michael Kennedy

Copyright © 2004 Michael Kennedy

Library of Congress Cataloging-in-Publication Data

Kennedy, Michael, 1938-
  A brief history of disease, science and medicine : from the Ice Age to the Genome Project / by Michael Kennedy.
       p. ; cm.
Includes bibliographical references and index.
  ISBN 0-9749466-4-8 (alk. paper)
  1. Medicine--History. 2. Science--History. 3. Diseases--History.
  [DNLM: 1. History of Medicine. 2. Science--history. WZ 40 K36m
2003] I. Title.
  R131.K44 2003
  610'.9--dc21

                                        2003006852

Interior design by Jon Moore, Eyelevel Books
Cover design by Mayapriya Long, Bookwrights

Printed in the United States of America

Published by

Asklepiad Press
27525 Puerta Real
Suite 100 #481
Mission Viejo, CA 92691
949-756-2812

Acknowledgments

THIS BOOK BEGAN AS A SERIES OF LECTURES, REQUESTED BY MEDICAL students at USC. A number of them read an early draft of the manuscript, once I decided to turn the material into a book as well as a lecture series. They suggested corrections, both to make the material more understandable and to expand on areas of particular interest to students. One of them provided considerable encouragement by telling me she stayed up until two AM to finish reading the last chapter. This was during their Christmas vacation and I'm sure they had better things to do. A number of physician friends and acquaintances read the manuscript and suggested additions and corrections. Chief among these were Kenneth Janis, David Berman (who taught me pharmacology in 1962 and is still teaching pharmacology at USC), C. Rollins Hanlon, and Peter Lee.

My interest in medical history was stimulated by brief lectures in medical school given by a clinical faculty member named Robert McCallister, a pathologist from Children's Hospital of Los Angeles, and by six months I spent at the Massachusetts General Hospital during my senior year of medical school. It provided me with the opportunity to read medical journals from the nineteenth century and to research the history of cardiac surgery. During that few months I became acquainted with Benjamin Castleman and Oliver Cope, pioneers of medical care who stimulated my interest in history with anecdotes from their own lives. My surgical teachers, Clarence J. Berne and Leonard Rosoff, were both interested in the evolution of surgery and Dr. Berne had a collection of books, which included W.W. Keen's textbook of surgery from 1905. These men are gone now but I hope they would approve of my attempt here to pass along the stories of those who have gone before.

Michael Kennedy

About the Author

MICHAEL KENNEDY ATTENDED THE UNIVERSITY OF SOUTHERN California from 1956 to 1959, with a major in mechanical engineering, then worked for a year as an engineer at Douglas Aircraft Company while taking premedical courses at night.

After a two-year period in the Air Force, he returned to the USC School of Medicine, graduating in 1966. He spent the next six years completing an internship and residency in general surgery at Los Angles County Hospital, then another year in cardio-thoracic surgery at Children's Hospital of Los Angeles.

He practiced vascular surgery in a suburban community in southern California until 1994 when he retired from practice after back surgery.

Since 1972, he has been a member of the clinical faculty at USC in the department of surgery. After retiring from practice, he spent a year at Dartmouth Medical School, in New Hampshire, obtaining a graduate degree in medical outcomes research. Since 1996, he has taught first and second year medical students at USC in a program called Introduction to Clinical Medicine.

He is a fellow of the American College of Surgeons and of the Royal Society of Medicine. He has served as president of his county medical association, a delegate to the California Medical Association and to the American Medical Association and, in the 1970s and 1980s, on the Commission on Legislation of the CMA.

Table of Contents

Introduction

Fools say that they learn by experience. I prefer to profit by others' experience.
Bismarck

THIS BOOK IS WRITTEN FOR MEDICAL STUDENTS AND YOUNG PHYSICIANS most of whom receive little information on medical history in the curriculum. Certainly, the volume of medical knowledge has expanded exponentially in the past fifty years and their time is limited. On the other hand, there has always been a great deal of material that medical students were expected to learn in four years (or less). The difference is that much of what they learned in the past has now been shown to be in error. The 1892 edition of Osler's textbook of medicine spends seven pages of the chapter on typhoid fever on therapy. Not one item in this section is of any value in the treatment of the disease. Antibiotics were fifty years away, but once they arrived on the scene, all that the medical students of 1892 had learned was useless. It is unlikely that all or most of the information medical students work so hard to learn in 2003 is incorrect. It is, however, probable that fifty years from now most of it will be useless. Knowledge of history, where we came from and how we got here, gives perspective on these matters. Nurses and other medical professionals, and perhaps even the non-medical public, may be interested in the subject as well.

I have lived through forty years of medical history since I began my medical studies and over sixty years since I had scarlet fever, at the age of four, in the days before penicillin was available. My parents were frightened that I might develop rheumatic fever as a consequence of my scarlet fever episode (both are sequelae of streptococcal infection) and I remember how my mother, father, and sister were given the option of remaining in the house where I was to be quarantined, or leaving. Once the quarantine sign went up, no one but the doctor could enter or leave. My mother stayed; the others moved in with relatives for two weeks. I remember the fear of polio every summer until the Salk vaccine became available and I knew people who contracted the paralytic form of the disease. My mother had diphtheria as a two-year-old child in 1900 and the family doctor performed a tracheostomy on her, on her mother's kitchen table. For those of us in the older generation the last fifty years does not seem like "history" but it is.

I have always been interested in history and the book that first stimulated my interest in medicine was titled *Century of the Surgeon*, describing the discovery of anesthesia and antisepsis. The same author, Jurgen Thorwald, also wrote *The Triumph of Surgery*, an account of the early experience in surgery once the two major barriers were conquered. I read them in high school and college. Over the years I have collected books, old ones and reprints of classics like Osler's *The Principles and Practice of Medicine* and Withering's book, *An Account of the Foxglove*. I have also collected medical biographies and reread favorites many times. For the past five years I have taught first and second year medical students in a program called "Introduction to Clinical Medicine" at the University of Southern California, my alma mater. The students interview patients, beginning the second week of medical school, and, in the second semester, begin to perform physical examinations on them. We spend a considerable amount of time discussing the patients' diseases and all the ethical and humanitarian issues that arise. Inevitably, given my interests, the students have heard a lot about medical history. In the annual (anonymous) evaluations of the faculty, among the favorite items the students list are my stories about medical history.

The reader will immediately discover that my concept of medical history includes subjects other than those in a "classical" account. I am interested in how infectious diseases evolved and think it important to understand this aspect of science to make sense of the story of smallpox in the New World and syphilis in the old. There is also some anthropology, especially in the first chapter. I think that medicine and science, especially chemistry, developed in parallel; most early (prior to the seventeenth century) chemists were physicians. This is also true of physics, to a lesser degree, and understanding the developments of the nineteenth and twentieth century requires some review of that subject.

The emphasis, in some places, varies from what is usually found in the classical "medical history." Physicians and nurses, for example, should know that Florence Nightingale, generally regarded as the founder of the nursing profession, is also a towering figure in the conquest of infection. Ignaz Semmelweiss, a tragic figure of the early nineteenth century, realized that physicians' and medical students' hands were the source of puerperal (childbed) fever. He could not convince anyone else of the importance of hand washing. Florence Nightingale succeeded where Semmelweiss failed. She also revolutionized military medical care in

Britain almost single handedly. Her influence lasted for sixty years and her work is being re-discovered in epidemiology. My students know far more molecular biology than I do but I am trying to catch up by studying the subject. I try not to get too far into this part of the story lest my ignorance become too obvious.

I have spent the last thirty years practicing surgery and teaching surgery residents and medical students. I am not a historian. History is a hobby but students have been asking me for several years to provide lectures on the history of medicine. Here they are in book form. The first third of the book is what the historians write about in minute detail. The last two-thirds are about the development of modern medicine. Some of this material I had to dig out of primary sources. Some of it gains perspective from one who was there and lived through it.

The reader is not expected to be either an expert in medical history or knowledgeable about medicine, itself. The target reader is a first year medical student, a nurse, a premed student or someone with an interest and a bit of science education. This is not a book for experts.

Foreword

by Peter V. Lee, MD

Why study the history of medicine?

"Those who compare the age in which their lot has fallen with a golden age which exists only in imagination, may talk of degeneracy and decay; but no man who is correctly informed as to the past will be disposed to take a morose or desponding view of the present."

(Macaulay, History of England, v. 1, ch. 1, 1848.)

"If I have seen further (than you and Descartes) it is by standing on the shoulders of giants."

(Isaac Newton, Letter to Robert Hooke, February 5, 1675.)

THE MEDICAL STUDENT OR YOUNG PHYSICIAN WHO READS THIS FOREWORD will hope to find answers to the following questions: For whom is it written? What sort of a History is it? Should I read it?

First of all, it is written primarily for medical students and young physicians who are curious about the evolution of their profession. Although the book is well documented and historically sound, It is not primarily a reference work: it has been written to be read, rather than studied.

It is written by a surgeon with years of experience teaching the history of medicine as an aside, as a bonus, for the medical students whom he has been helping to gain clinical competence. The need for the book arose from Dr. Kennedy's bedside teaching of medical students, (who have little time in their crowded curriculum for history) not from a library-based seminar for graduate students or a survey course for undergraduates.

In recent years in our medical schools there has been an increased interest in helping students to understand the concept of professionalism in medicine – what are the attributes of the professional person, and how are these best fostered? A study of our heritage – our historical roots - helps us to understand how some of the attributes and components of the profession arose, and how they have changed and evolved over the centuries.

Reading about the scientists and clinicians of the past allows us to perceive the many kinds of contributions that have resulted in the body of knowledge that we utilize today. And having access to publications of original work that have changed the direction of medicine adds a human dimension – reminding us that medical progress is not simply a steady, "upward" accretion of knowledge, technology and wisdom, but has been the result of the individual insights, observations, hypotheses and errors of many men and women, often working independently, and not infrequently introducing ideas at variance with accepted theory.

My own interest in the history of medicine was stimulated at an early age by turning the large pages and marveling at the anatomical plates in a large, leather bound 16th Century folio anatomy in my father's library, (the gift of a grateful patient, a bibliophile.) The illustrations showed the subjects accommodatingly holding open large incisions to expose their internal organs; skeletons stood, conversing in groups, displaying different views of the bones. I was attracted more by the artistic poses, the composition and meticulous detail of the engravings, than by the anatomical content. Our library also contained biographies, Cushing's *Life of Sir William Osler*, and Vallery-Radot's *Life of Pasteur*, and books on the history of some diseases, such as Hans Zinsser's *Rats, Lice and History*. Sinclair Lewis's novel, *Arrowsmith*, gave to a scientifically unsophisticated adolescent a sense of the excitement of scientific discovery.

In my second year of medical school, as we were learning physical diagnosis from the brilliant, taciturn George Barnett, we were introduced to R. H. Major's *Classic Descriptions of Disease*, (as well as to Voltaire's *Zadig*.) In the clinical years, we were inspired by two clinician-scholars, Arthur Bloomfield, Professor of Medicine, and Frederick Reichert, Professor of Surgery, who introduced almost every topic they discussed, even on bedside rounds, with references to the original descriptions of the patient's disease, or to the contributions the "great men" of medicine and surgery had made to the growth of our knowledge and understanding.

So my approach to this book is that of a doctor and teacher with fifty years of commitment to the professional growth of my students, and an even longer interest in the history of my profession. This interest, largely stimulated by the examples of my own clinical teachers, is not that of the historian or specialist in the history of science and medicine, who examines medicine and its history from the "outside." I am part of this three-thousand-year tradition, and am reminded almost daily of the ways in which it has shaped me as a physician. It is my hope that this book, written from "within" the profession, will help to convey to medical students and other readers some of this sense of belonging to (and contributing to) this ancient and still-evolving profession.

Dr Kennedy has done especially well in describing many of the experiments and studies on which medical and scientific advances have been based; he gives the reader a sense of the actual work, the process involved, in making a "discovery." By recounting the stories of the achievements and failures of scholars, clinicians and scientists of each era in the context of the contemporary knowledge of science, Dr. Kennedy allows each contribution to be seen in perspective – as a part of the growth of scientific knowledge generally, and not just as a free-standing work of genius. In contrast to most of the standard surveys of medical history his chapters covering the past 150 years are replete with references to the original papers in which the scientists and clinicians recorded and published their findings. Students can read for themselves, rather than accept a historian's interpretation of what the original author wrote. Today's medical students are accustomed to reading the current medical literature and evaluating the quality of the data upon which conclusions are based. But most of their textbooks of necessity emphasize the most recent literature, not the original works in the field. We are grateful for Dr. Kennedy's meticulous pursuit of original sources.

I hope and believe that this scholarly and well-written book will serve its primary purposes – both to inform and to stimulate further exploration of original sources. Dr. Kennedy shows his skills as a master teacher, letting his own personality and point of view shine through his treatment of the issues that interest him, and letting the investigators speak for themselves.

There are other excellent surveys of the history of medicine. Unlike most books on medical history this one is designed and written primarily for the medical student, not like Roy Porter's masterly survey, for the general reader, or like Lois Magner's excellent text, for students in a college course. Another difference is that Dr. Kennedy gives much more attention to recent history, while the historians devote more attention to earlier periods.

Dr Kennedy has followed his own interests in emphasizing some areas, especially surgery. But this is not an idiosyncratic book, with the author riding his own hobby-horse. It is a wise, readable, scholarly selection from the mass of historical data; it provides, in a volume of readable size, a view of the origins and development of our profession. It has a personal touch. You know it's his book.

In summary, then, this is not primarily a reference book – it is a sharing of knowledge and experience, and in some cases a story of Dr. Kennedy's own pursuit of knowledge, fueled by his curiosity and nurtured by his infectious enthusiasm and meticulous scholarship.

Peter V. Lee, MD
Professor and Chair, Emeritus
Deparment of Family Medicine
Keck School of Medicine
University of Southern California

1
In the Beginning

On September 18, 1991, a pair of hikers in the Tyrolean Alps, at the 11,000-foot level, found a frozen corpse in the Niederjochferner glacier. At first, they, and the others they directed to the scene, thought this was a modern climber who had fallen into a crevasse. Such frozen corpses are found from time to time, and five other bodies had been found in the glacier that season. It had been an unusually warm summer and the glaciers have been retreating for years, perhaps due to global warming. Soon, it became apparent that this body was very old after an axe and other implements found near the body were examined. Eventually, the axe was recognized as a Bronze Age (actually Copper Age, slightly earlier, before the use of tin to harden the copper) tool and the age of the "Iceman" was estimated at 5,000 years (3350BCE by current best dating) or more.

Paleopathology is the study of the diseases of antiquity. Most examinations involve excavation of ancient cemeteries or other burial sites. The remains in these sites are almost invariably skeletal. Much can be learned from skeletal remains, but many diseases leave no skeletal signs. Discovery of an intact frozen corpse is incredibly rare. The practice of embalming by the Egyptians provides another source of information about ancient disease. Occasionally, intact bodies are found in peat bogs, where an anaerobic condition prevents decay. About 1,800 such "peat bog corpses" have been found, but few have been carefully studied and most of the bodies' organs have deteriorated into "grave wax" or adipocere, a soap-like decomposition product of body fat. Another source of information is the study of a few small populations living today, or in the recent past, in "stone age" cultures. These groups have been found in Africa and New Guinea, but the small populations may occupy ecological niches that are different from the conditions of the Paleolithic (Stone Age) and Neolithic (agriculture and bronze) periods in most of the world.

During the lengthy investigation that followed (and continues) the discovery and recovery of the "Iceman," called "Otzi" by the Austrians, a pouch was found containing mushrooms strung on a leather thong. The initial theory was that they were a type of tinder fungus used to start fires and known to have been used by other prehistoric people. However the fungus, not tinder after all, was identified as *Piptoporus botulinus*, a mushroom that grows on birch trees and has antibiotic properties. Perhaps, this was a first aid kit. In addition, tattooing of his skin was present in locations suggesting medical practice, possibly for relief of pain due to arthritis. X-rays of the bones show signs of arthritis in the spine and hip. The tattoos were along his lumbar spine, his left ankle, and right knee, areas not visible when the man was clothed and sites of arthritic changes on x-ray.[1]

Recently, after CT scans of the entire corpse revealed evidence of fecal material in his colon, an incision was made in his abdomen and a tiny sample was removed using an endoscope. The material in his colon indicates that he ate a meal including unleavened bread made from einkorn wheat and an unknown herb about eight hours before his death. Also present were fragments of meat and bone, most likely coming from an ibex, an alpine goat. Pollen in the sample indicates that he died in the spring, during the blooming of the hop hornbeam tree, contradicting the theory of an early fall snowstorm as a cause of death and preservation. He must have come from the south side of the mountain, since that tree grows only in areas warmer than the high-altitude site where he was found or the high valleys to the north of it. Thus, his last day can be partially reconstructed through paleopathology. In fact, the pollen contains its sperm, which degenerates within hours, suggesting that he ingested fresh pollen at the lower elevation less than eight hours before his death. The nearest valley where the pollen might be found is the Schnals Valley in northern Italy. Also present in his colon were eggs of the whipworm, *Trichuris trichuria*, a human parasite. The wheat had been ground and baked: excess bran and charcoal particles were present, both evidence of baked bread.[2]

Einkorn wheat is not native to Europe and provides evidence that agriculture and the importation of cereal crops had begun in the culture of the Iceman.[3] His copper axe, apparently constructed at least 1,000 years before the accepted date of the "Bronze Age," and the presence of copper and arsenic in his hair, suggesting that he was engaged in the smelting of copper (his axe was cast in a mold), have brought some reassessment of that period of prehistory.

Keeping in mind some reservations about using the study of present-day and recent-past "Stone Age" people to understand paleopathology, trends can be identified. Hunter-gatherer societies, because the family or tribal groups were small and isolated from large populations, were afflicted only with those few infectious diseases acquired from game animals.[4] Trauma and starvation were the most likely fatal events in these societies. Trauma occurred as an occupational hazard during the hunt and inter-tribal warfare resulting in massacres has been documented. The image of the noble savage living in peace with his environment is a concept introduced by French Romantics like Rousseau and has little application to the world of the Stone Age.[5] Dental abscess, another potentially fatal illness, has been identified in a number of skeletons from this era.[6] The Iceman had no dental caries, although his molars were heavily worn, giving some information about his diet.

Malnutrition exists in some present-day New Guinea tribes, especially in children, due to the limited sources of nutrition, some of which lack essential amino acids. Meat eating was the source of many of these micronutrients in hunter-gatherer societies. Most cereal grain, the diet of agricultural societies (especially those without domestic food animals), is deficient in protein and, if meat is not available, legumes must be mixed with cereals to provide adequate protein. Legumes are twenty-five percent to thirty-eight percent (with soybeans the highest) protein. Only with modern nutritional knowledge (or thousands of years of trial-and-error) is a healthy vegetarian life possible.

The invention of agriculture marks the transition to the Neolithic, or "new stone age," period. With it came the development of larger social groups and the advent of infectious disease. The earliest cultivation of crops occurred in the Fertile Crescent near the Tigris and Euphrates rivers about 10,500 years ago. The area has mild weather, abundant water and was the origin of ten of the fourteen species of grass suitable for cultivation. These grass species had heavy seeds and tended to grow in large clusters making them attractive for the gatherers of edible plants. The earliest domesticated plant species were wheat (one of which was einkorn), barley (both cereals), peas (a legume), and olives (a source of oil). The domestication of cereal crops may have been stimulated by climate changes at the end of the last ice age. Wheat and barley became abundant and the local population of hunter-gatherers found that collection of the heavy seeds was easy enough to justify the development of threshing technology and of grain storage, requiring defense of community grain stores. Huge herds of gazelles had previously supported a large population but were being over-hunted. The decline of these herds added another stimulus to the development of agriculture.[7]

The same geographic area was home to the majority of large mammal species that were amenable to domestication. These included the aurochs, ancestor to the cow, the pig, the sheep, and the goat. One theory of the desertification of the Middle East is the extensive domestication of the goat, which is particularly destructive of plant life. Horses were domesticated in the Ukraine, known in early history as Scythia. The combination of abundant grass, with its useful seed, and animals that could be tamed to assist in cultivation and for food purposes made the Fertile Crescent the birthplace of agriculture.

The fact that Europe and Asia are geographically oriented with an east-west axis, rather than the north-south axis of sub-Saharan Africa and the Americas, permitted the rapid (by pre-historic standards) spread of the new technology along latitude lines sharing the same climate and seasons. The north-south long axis of the Americas (especially the Isthmus of Panama) and Africa results in changing seasons and climates along the path of migration, and this retarded the progress of agriculture in those continents. In North America, herds of horses and camels, present at the end of the last ice age, became rapidly extinct, possibly as a result of the arrival of man. The early humans who reached North America as a result of the land bridge across the Bering Strait appear not to have had experience with agriculture and did not consider large mammals candidates for potential domestication. They rapidly hunted them to extinction. In the Fertile Crescent, huge herds of gazelles sustained the population until agriculture led to domestication of the suitable species.

In sub-Saharan Africa, enormous herds of large mammals persist to this day, but none is suitable, because of temperament, for domestication. The zebra, for example, looks like a horse with stripes, but the adult zebra is vicious and has never been successfully tamed. The African elephant is similarly unsuitable for domestication, while the Indian elephant has been used as a beast of burden for thousands of years. In South America, the llama, a relative of the extinct camel, became the only large domestic animal in the Americas before the coming of the Spaniards. The potato, a discovery of the Incas, is an American vegetable eventually imported to Europe after Columbus. It was not found north of the Isthmus of Panama. A dearth of suitable species of grass for agricultural use led to the cultivation of Mexican corn, or maize as it is called in Europe, as the principle cereal crop of North America. Even then, the great Southwestern deserts inhibited migration of the cultivation of corn from the Aztecs to northern tribes of Indians, especially to the California tribes who subsisted on fish, game, and acorns. The Isthmus of Panama provided a bidirectional barrier to the sort of evolutionary adoption of agriculture and cereal grain that occurred in Europe and Asia. Civilizations, the Aztec on the north and the

Maya and Inca to the south, developed on either side of the isthmus, but there was little or no exchange of crops (maize or the potato) or domestic animals as occurred in Europe and Asia.[8]

AGRICULTURE AND SOCIAL CHANGE

As the cultivation of food sources, rather than the seeking of wild edible plant material and hunting, became the basis of society, several major changes occurred. There was a transition period when agriculture alone was not capable of sustaining a family or tribe. This is still observed with Australian aborigines and New Guinea tribes who plant some crops then leave them to grow without further cultivation for months. The aboriginal group returns from "walkabout," a period of hunting and gathering of wild plants and other edible materials, at a point when the crop is ready for harvest. The arid climate of Australia, not to mention the appropriation of more fertile areas by European settlers in the eightenth century, seems to have limited the further development of agriculture. The climate and topography of New Guinea limit agriculture to high mountain valleys only recently discovered by whites. Hunters, more primitive than the highland residents, occupy the coastal lowlands and are beset by malaria and other diseases.

Eventually, the cultivated crops and domesticated animals provided an adequate food source and the agricultural society adopted a less migratory life style. The necessity for continued cultivation plus protection from scavenging animals and depredations from other tribes required that the people remain close to the fields. As agriculture became more productive, a population explosion occurred. Women of hunter-gatherer societies have a child about every four years, birth spacing probably maintained by lactational amenorrhea (women usually do not ovulate while nursing). Women in agricultural societies have annual births since there is no need to carry (literally) the immature child as the clan moves from place to place. There is some evidence that the early farming societies were not as well nourished as the hunters, however, suggesting that population growth may outstrip food production. For example, Neolithic skeletons average less height than Paleolithic skeletons.[9] Still, the trend continued as farming techniques and domestication of animals improved. More labor increased the output of the fields and the increasing food supply ensured the survival of the enlarging population. The cereal grains themselves evolved, with larger yields and less wastage from the harvest. Seed heads of cereals and seedpods of legumes began to retain the seeds rather than opening spontaneously as the wild varieties did. The proto-farmers planted the desired variety reinforcing the evolving characteristic. Eventually, increasing population led to increased complexity in the relationships of family groups. Close proximity between humans and animals allowed cross-species transmission of organisms and the introduction of groups larger than the hunter-gatherer family unit allowed human to human transmission of disease when unrelated groups came in contact with each other.[10]

Infectious Disease

Tuberculosis and Malaria are diseases closely connected with agriculture, the former coming from domesticated cattle, especially their milk, and the latter related to the presence of standing water and mosquito proliferation.[11] Malaria profoundly influenced the evolution of the African population. 50,000 years ago the Sahara Desert did not exist. It was a zone of Mediterranean climate and vegetation that, as recently as 4,000 years ago, had extensive cultivation. The end of the last Ice Age began the progression of the desert, which eventually separated the continent into two areas whose populations had little communication. *Plasmodium vivax* is thought to be the oldest malaria organism and ninety-five percent of sub-Saharan Africans lack the red cell Duffy antigen, which the *P. vivax* parasite requires to produce infection. The absence of the antigen is likely the result of tremendous evolutionary pressure south of the Sahara desert, a nearly impassible barrier. The sickle cell trait and Thalassemia, both of which increase resistance to malaria infection, are also found in areas where the organism is prevalent. Falciparum malaria, thought to be a later form of the disease that does not require the Duffy antigen for infection, resumed the evolutionary pressure on a population now mostly immune to the *Plasmodium vivax* form. This probably increased the incidence of sickle cell trait south of the Sahara. Sickle cell anemia will be discussed in the chapter on blood, but is a disease in which red blood cells become "sickle-shaped" due to an abnormal hemoglobin molecule. Anemia and painful crises, caused by obstruction of small blood vessels by clumps of abnormal red cells, occur as a result. Sickle cell anemia is a lethal disease, caused by the presence of two genes for the S hemoglobin (rather than one S gene and one normal gene as in the trait), and the fact that the trait has survived in spite of the lethal consequences of the homozygous state suggests the enormous pressure of malaria on the population. Thalassemia, another inherited disease with abnormal hemoglobin, is found chiefly north and east of the Sahara and may represent another evolutionary change after separation of the two populations. Thalassemia also produces anemia in homozygous individuals, although it is less severe than the sickle cell anemia, and it appears to be due to a similar evolutionary mechanism.

Influenza and measles undoubtedly appeared with the domestication of their natural hosts, the pig and the dog. Measles may actually be a descendent of rinderpest, a disease of cattle rather than dogs, but both the dog distemper virus and rinderpest are closely related to measles.[12] Possibly the transition was from cattle to humans to dogs. Dogs arrived in New Guinea, and eventually in Australia and Polynesia, from Asia thousands of years ago. Measles and distemper were unknown in the Polynesian islands until the arrival of European explorers.[13] The disease nearly wiped out the native Polynesian population who had no natural resistance, suggesting no previous contact with distemper or measles. The arrival of the dog may have occurred before the evolution of the virus from rinderpest to distemper and measles. We have little evidence from ancient remains to confirm these theories about the viral diseases, although smallpox has been identified in mummies including that of Rhamses V.[14]

Tuberculosis has definitely been identified in skeletal remains dating back to the early Neolithic period and in Egyptian mummies, but it has not been identified in human skeletal remains prior to the agricultural period and the domestication of cattle. The origin of tuberculosis could have been with elephants, which carried the organism as far back as 2000 BC.[15] Possibly, the elephant was the original host and the auroch, or domestic cow, acquired the disease later. The earliest evidence of human tuberculosis is found in the spine, the common site of infection when the source is milk from infected cattle. The pulmonary form is passed from human to human and leaves less skeletal evidence but the organism is the same and both probably existed at the time. Parasitic diseases are very old (the Iceman had intestinal worms) and schistosomiasis is documented in Egyptian mummies that contain calcified eggs in liver and kidneys.

Another consequence of the Neolithic adoption of agriculture is an increase in the frequency of dental caries (cavities) in the skulls from the period. Prior to agriculture, with few carbohydrates in the diet, the incidence of caries was about one percent in skeletal remains (and none are found in the Iceman). In the Neolithic period, with a diet including cereals and other carbohydrates, this incidence rose about five fold, still far below the incidence after the introduction of sucrose in the seventeenth century.[16]

Microorganisms evolve just as their multicellular hosts do and the jump from the original host species to humans may have taken some time. We still see many animal infectious diseases that do not cross the species barrier, but AIDS, and possibly Tularemia which was unknown prior to the last century, may be examples of such an evolution in our own time. The major infectious diseases all seem to have originated in animal hosts. Smallpox is thought to have come from cattle as cowpox or other similar pox producing diseases in animals. Smallpox may be an example of the changing virulence of an infective organism with passage from one host to another. Cowpox retained its antigenic similarity to smallpox and four thousand years later that relationship provided the source of immunity by vaccination, inoculation with vaccinia, the cowpox virus (*vaca* is Spanish for cow). Malaria may have originated in birds and, if so, the domestication of chickens brought the parasite into proximity with humans. The anopheles mosquito provided the means of transmission from one species to another. Influenza infects pigs and ducks, and may have originated in these species. Pertussis (whooping cough) infects pigs and dogs and probably originated in these domestic animals. Interestingly enough the *Mycobacterium*, which produces tuberculosis (*m. tuberculosis*) and leprosy (*m. leprae*) also infects birds and cold-blooded animals, but those varieties do not infect humans. In fact, tuberculosis may have originated as a saprophyte, a non-virulent scavenger, feeding on decaying carcasses.

The evolution of these disease-causing organisms continues in the present time. Typhus can be identified in the fifteenth century in Spain during the wars of Ferdinand and Isabella with the Moors, but more ancient descriptions of the typical rash cannot be found. The Plague of Cyprian in 250CE may have been typhus, because the seasonal nature, beginning in the autumn and subsiding during the summer, is similar, although no rash was mentioned in contemporary descriptions. It raged for sixteen years and contributed to the fall of Rome. The typhus organism, a rickettsia, seems to have originated as an infection of mice and rats transmitted by the bite of fleas. Rats, while not intentionally domesticated, have adopted the agricultural and urban lifestyles as they developed. Rats were unknown in Europe prior to about 1000CE although mice were plentiful. The disease in man was transmitted by the flea at a time when personal hygiene and the presence of an abundant mouse population produced favorable circumstances. The typhus organism seems to have adopted another host, the human body louse, when other circumstances made this alternative more favorable. The two varieties are referred to as "murine" (mouse) typhus and "endemic" typhus. The organism has demonstrated further evolutionary activity as it has adopted the flying squirrel (and its flea) as a host. Cases have been identified in which transmission was from squirrels nesting in the attics of homes in the eastern U.S. Body lice and mice have become less successful routes of transmission to humans with changing concepts of personal hygiene and the organism has adapted accordingly.[17]

PREHISTORIC SURGERY

There are skeletal remains which show evidence of surgical procedures, the most interesting being examples of trephination of the skull. In 1865, E. George Squier, who had served as American *charge'-d'affaires* for Central America and in other diplomatic posts, was shown a Peruvian skull showing clear evidence of trepanning before death. Trepan and trephine are synonyms and come from the early term for an auger, a tool that bores holes. Squier was an experienced amateur archeologist having written several books on American Indian mounds in Ohio and the Mississippi valley. He obtained the skull and brought it back to New York where examination by members of the New York Academy of Medicine demonstrated that there were signs of healing indicating that the skull's owner had survived the operation. It created a sensation.[18] A few previous skulls with similar openings had been found but they were attributed to fatal injuries. None had shown signs of healing. Trephination, the sawing of holes in the skull, was very frequent in prehistoric times and has been observed in recent times in Melanesia. There has been much speculation about the reason for this procedure with its considerable pain and risk of death from meningitis. It is difficult to believe that these cases all involved magical rituals since many have been found in association with other pathology such as depressed skull fracture and sinusitis. The most astounding part of this practice is the number of skulls showing definite evidence of healing, indicating the survival of the subject. In one study of Peruvian skulls with evidence of trephination, over fifty percent show healing.[19] The fact that many of them survived and healed their incisions suggests that the surgeon may have been skillful enough or lucky enough to avoid fatal complications like meningitis. It is unlikely that any of the intracranial problems we see would be amenable to Stone Age surgeons but there is one skull that may represent a successful neurosurgical operation. The skull contains a depressed fracture, undoubtedly from trauma of some sort, and evidence of partial removal of some of the depressed area. There is healing of the fracture edges, which leads us to believe that the surgeon opened and partially elevated a depressed skull fracture, and the patient recovered, or at least survived. There has been speculation that cocaine, well known in South America, could have been used as a local anesthetic.

Another skeletal finding suggestive of ancient surgical practice is amputation of limbs. Most such examples show no evidence of healing and are assumed to represent evidence of a fatal attack by predatory animals or other humans. A few do show evidence of healing and several show signs of saw marks on the bone indicating amputation by other humans.

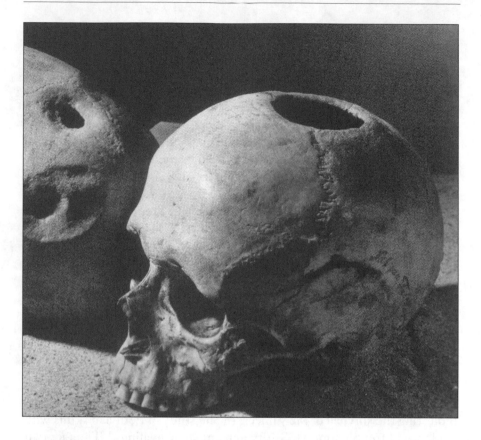

Figure 1 – These examples of trephination show evidence of healing with smooth edges of the defects.

MEDICINAL PLANTS

Some very primitive societies have discovered medicinal properties in plants and applied these remedies to treat diseases. The bark of the Cinchona tree is a well-known example of this practice. Quinine, the extract of this bark, is effective in treating malaria and has been known for hundreds of years. When was quinine discovered? Indians in Central and South America were using this remedy when European explorers arrived. There are few examples of effective medical remedies dating from primitive cultures other than quinine and cocaine, both of which were unknown outside of America. The earliest examples of effective pharmacology are poisons. One can imagine that these substances, most of them plant extracts, would be discovered through accidental consumption and the knowledge preserved to avoid further contact and, also, to use the substance as a weapon against enemies. Curare, now widely used in anesthesia for muscle paralysis, was used by Indians of Central America as arrow poison. Opium was an early discovery and rhubarb was introduced as a laxative in late Roman times. The ancient Chinese developed an extensive pharmacology and this will be covered in that chapter.

1   Brenda Fowler. *Iceman.* p 205, Random House (2000).

2   Dickson, J. et al. "The omnivorous Tyrolean Iceman: colon contents (meat, cereals, pollen, moss, and whipworm) and stable isotope analysis," *Philosophical Transactions of the Royal Society of London* 355, 1843 - 1849 (2000).

3   Jared Diamond, *Guns, Germs and Steel*, p 133 and 141, Norton (1999).

4   Charlotte Roberts and Keith Manchester. The Archeology of Disease. Cornell University Press. Second Edition. Pp 11-12 (1997).

5   Steven Pinker, *The Blank Slate*, Ch 17, Viking Penguin (2002).

6   Roberts and Manchester, p 50.

7   Jared Diamond. Chapter 10.

8   Jared Diamond, pp 187-188. Chapter 10 covers this topic thoroughly.

9   M. N. Cohen, *Health and the Rise of Civilization*, Yale University Press, New York (1989).

10   M.S. Bartlett, "Measles periodicity and community size," *Journal of the Royal Statistical Society, Series A,* 120:48-70 (1957). The classical study of minimum population size for epidemic diseases.

11   Diamond, p 207.

12   John M. Adams and David T. Imagawa, "Immunological Relationship Between Measles and Distemper Viruses," *Proceedings of the Society For Experimental Biology and Medicine,* 96:240 (1957).

13   Diamond, p 308.

14   Albert S. Lyons MD and R. Joseph Petrocelli II MD, Medicine, *An Illustrated History,* p 92, Harry N Abrams, New York (1978).

15   Roberts and Manchester, pp 136-137.

16   Roberts and Manchester, pp 47-50.

17   DH Walker and DB Fishbein, "Epidemiology of rickettsial diseases," *European Journal of Epidemiology* 3:237-245 (1991).

18   Stanley Finger and Hiran R. Fernando, "E. George Squier and the Discovery of Cranial Trepanation: A Landmark in the History of Surgery and Ancient Medicine," *Journal of the History of Medicine,* 56:353-381 (2001.)

19   Stewart, TD. *Stone Age Skull Surgery.* Smithsonian Institution Annual Report (1957).

2
The Beginning of History

WE KNOW THAT THE BABYLONIANS USED CHEMISTRY BECAUSE THE invention of perfume occurred at this time.[20] The written record, in cuneiform (*cuneus* is Latin for wedge), is very terse and consists mostly of the accounting of stores and records of taxes and other transactions. Tablets from about 2000BCE, written in Akkadian (the language of the people ruled by Sargon) script, show the development of numbers and arithmetic. Interestingly, the mathematics uses the base sixty instead of the base ten we use. From this we get, via the astronomer Ptolemy, our convention used to describe curves and circles in degrees. It is thought that the base sixty was derived from still earlier peoples, one of which used a base five (probably derived from fingers and toes) and another which used a base twelve, like the early English. Combining the two systems would give many common factors if sixty is the base.[21] There is even a primitive form of algebra (disproving the theory of its invention by Arab mathematicians although several did contribute). History, in the form of recording the deeds of others, appears with the Hittites, but no record of medical information exists.

Assyrian medical texts on clay tablets exist and clearly describe gonorrhea in the second millennium BCE. A bronze tube is recommended for relief of urethral obstruction, the first example of a urinary catheter procedure.[22] The relief carving of an Assyrian priest-physician, made during the reign of Sargon II, shows a plant thought to be the poppy. Much of what we know as the Egyptian pharmacopoeia is first described in laboriously deciphered Assyrian tablets. One Assyrian drug of considerable potency, not used by the Egyptians, was belladonna, "the deadly nightshade," the source of atropine. There is some evidence that the Assyrians used it for bladder symptoms, cough, asthma and to dilate the pupil of the eye. The name belladonna means "beautiful woman" in Italian and modern psychology experiments have shown that men choose photographs of women with dilated pupils as more attractive than those with small pupils. It is known that the Mesopotamians, like the Assyrians, used prisoners and slaves as guinea pigs in medical experiments. *Quunabu* was the Assyrian name for

Indian hemp, the source of cannabis. (Most young readers will recognize this as the active ingredient of marijuana.) It was used for insomnia, among other purposes. Most of the medical remedies of the Assyrians were mixtures of magical potions and charms, but a few contained other biochemically useful items such as licorice for stomach ailments.

The Egyptians recorded diseases and remedies and, again, magic and religion are heavily intertwined with practical advice. The practice of embalming the dead exposed the Egyptians to anatomy and they were capable of sophisticated chemistry in the preparation of embalming spices and preservatives. The Egyptians recognized sanitary principles and their houses contained water closets with wastewater being carried to the street in copper pipes. They used mosquito nets on their beds, suggesting some awareness of disease carrying by mosquitoes.

EPIDEMICS

Epidemics of infectious diseases began with the development of cities in Babylon and Egypt. Malaria and tuberculosis do not require high concentrations of people as they are transmitted from animal to human. In the absence of human hosts, malaria is maintained in the bird population and tuberculosis infects herds of cattle. Both are called endemic diseases because they occur at a steady rate in the presence of the animal host and, in the case of malaria, the vector mosquito. Epidemics involve transmission from person to person and high population density is required. Epidemiological study shows that smallpox requires more than 250,000 people to perpetuate itself since the initial infection kills or immunizes all the cases. Since it is highly contagious, in the absence of new susceptible populations, it would quickly die out in small societies.[23] Large populations, or those with a high mobility (a recent development), provide enough new susceptible hosts to perpetuate the virus. Some infectious diseases involve an arthropod (insect) vector, like typhus, but spread as epidemics in crowded populations like armies. Bubonic plague occurs in epidemics in spite of the fact that susceptible hosts, rats and their fleas, are present in the environment continuously. The epidemic may represent a wave of more virulent bacteria appearing in the rat-flea population. The fleas prefer the rats as hosts and seem to seek human hosts only when there is a high mortality in the rat population. Ancient cities were so unhealthy that, until the nineteenth century, the mortality rate of the city-dwellers exceeded their birth rate and the population was only maintained by an influx of rural immigrants.[24] Rome was an exception because of the high quality of sanitary facilities but other factors intervened, as we shall see.

THE FIRST MEDICAL RECORDS

The earliest Mesopotamian medical text comes from the library of Assurbanipal in the seventh century BCE, but represents older Assyrian practices. *The Treatise of Medical Diagnosis and Prognosis* describes a case in which the patient coughs continuously producing bloody sputum. The description is identifiable as tuberculosis. The Code of Hammurabi prescribes fees for physicians, including fees for bleeding with a lancet. Two documents from the second millennium BCE describe Egyptian medicine. The Smith Papyrus has been called the "Book of Wounds" and describes forty-eight cases, including a method of reducing a dislocated jaw. It also describes reduction and splinting of fractures using ox-bone splints with resin-soaked bandages. Sutures and cautery are mentioned and mummies have sutured abdominal incisions, which were used to remove viscera during embalming. The Ebers Papyrus, written about 1550 BCE but listing information much older in origin, is extremely lengthy, over twenty meters long, and hundreds of medical remedies are listed. Most are magical potions using exotic ingredients like the testicles of a black ass and black lizards. A few are potentially effective, such as fried ox liver (liver is a rich source of vitamin A) for the treatment of night blindness. Castor oil was prescribed for a laxative, and opium and cannabis (the active ingredient of marijuana) are mentioned. Leprosy is not described.[25]

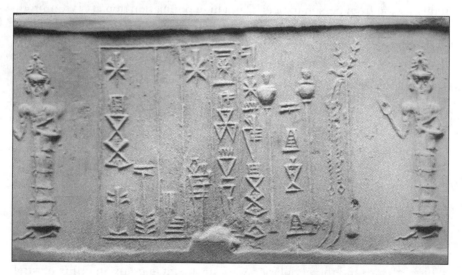

Figure 2 – The cylinder seal of Urlugaledena

Some have concluded that a remedy for wounds, the "yeast of sweet beer," described in the papyrus, is the first instance of the use of antibiotic properties of yeasts.[26] Imhotep, an Egyptian physician in the archaic period and vizier to Pharaoh Zozer about 2600BCE, became a revered and, finally, god-like figure in later dynasties, establishing a following somewhat like that of Asclepius in Greek medicine. By the sixth century BCE he had replaced Thoth as god of healing. A few other Egyptian physicians' names are recorded including Iri, "Keeper of the Royal Rectum," presumably an enema expert. A cylinder seal belonging to a Sumerian physician named Urlugaledina was found in the ruins of the Sumerian city of Lagash. The seal, from approximately 2000BCE is perfectly preserved and depicts surgical instruments, jars for medicines and a pestle for grinding drugs. The inscription in Sumerian reads, "O god Edinmugi, vizier of the god Gir, who attends mother animals when they drop their young! Urlugaledina the doctor is your servant."

SCIENCE AND THE EARLY GREEKS

The beginning of science as we recognize it occurred in classical Greece in the sixth century BCE. The Babylonians and Egyptians were capable of scientific discovery; the Babylonians studied the stars and invented astrology and astronomy; and the Egyptians, possibly due to the necessity of calculating the timing of the Nile floods, developed mathematics. When the floods receded, it was necessary to re-survey land boundaries leading to knowledge of geometry. Most of the knowledge derived from these early civilizations, however, became enmeshed in religious practices, as astrology in particular did, and the knowledge itself was confined to priestly castes. The Greeks, perhaps because their gods' behavior did not inspire awe and the priestly caste was weak, were free to apply scientific thought to non-theological subjects. Additionally, Greek political division as a consequence of geography resulted in small city-states. The absence of a strong central government permitted a revolution in science and philosophy unconstrained by theology or despotism. The earliest budding of science, as we know it, occurred in Miletus, an Ionian city-state located in modern Turkey. Ionia was a collection of Greek colonies established on or near the coast of Persia which began the period of classical Greek civilization. Unfortunately, the Persian kings conquered these small states one by one later in the sixth century BCE extinguishing the early flowering of classical Greek learning, but setting off an Ionian diaspora that included Simonides, the poet who composed the epitaph for the Spartans at Thermopyle, and Pythagoras, who derived the formula for the hypotenuse of a right triangle.

THALES OF MILETUS

Thales of Miletus is considered the first Greek philosopher. He was walking one day in the hills above the city when he noticed fossilized sea shells in rocks along the path. This observation led him to conclude that the world was once composed entirely of water. The combination of observation and arriving at a conclusion based on evidence makes him sound almost modern to us. He is also said to have predicted the solar eclipse of 585BCE. Eventually he was reproached by critics asking, if he was so wise, why wasn't he rich? His response, unlike most modern scientists and intellectuals, was to use his knowledge of science, particularly concerning weather, to do just that. He quietly concluded that the coming olive harvest would be unusually good and hired all the local olive presses before this fact became apparent to others. When the harvest came in as he predicted, he made a fortune from his monopoly of the presses. With his fortune, he founded a school of philosophy called the "Milesian School" that continued his work. He calculated the height of the pyramids by measuring the length of their shadow and that of a stick standing on end. Using the concept of similar triangles, he made the calculation and also determined the distance of a ship offshore by the same method. He may have discovered the attractive power of magnets and static electricity.

One of his students, Anaximenes, extended Thales' theory of matter to conclude that the fundamental element was air. As air descended to the Earth's surface, it was compressed to water. As the element came still closer to the center of the Earth it was compressed to stone. This theory is interesting for several reasons. It anticipated the concept of gravity and it shows an attempt to explain natural phenomena with evidence and logic. Thales' death was reported to Pythagoras, another of his pupils who had already left Miletus, in a letter from Anaximenes. The letter told how Thales, by now an old man, was gazing at the stars in the company of a maidservant when he forgot where he was and stepped off a steep slope. In another letter to Pythagoras, Anaximenes warned of the coming conquest of Miletus by Persia. In 494BCE Miletus was overrun by the Persia army and the Milesian School came to an end. Anaximenes fate is unknown.[27] Four years after the fall of Miletus, the Greeks stopped the Persian invasion at Marathon and prevented a premature end to the development of philosophy.

PYTHAGORAS

The next steps in the development of science took place in Sicily, near the sanctuary sought by Pythagoras before the fall of Miletus. Pythagoras was one of the great mathematicians of all time. He recognized that the number pi was incommensurable making it what we now call an irrational number. This was part of his work on the abstract character of numbers. To the Egyptians, a line was no more than the side of a field and a rectangle was the boundary of a field. Pythagoras' students concluded that all objects were composed of whole numbers, what we call atoms. Incommensurable means that, no matter how many places to which the number is calculated, it never becomes a whole number and does not repeat. It cannot be divided by another whole number with a whole number quotient. They called this result *alogos*– inexpressible. This discovery probably came from the study of right triangles and calculation of the hypotenuse. The hypotenuse of a right triangle, with sides valued at one, is the square root of two, an irrational number. Earlier civilizations had estimated pi (at approximately three) in calculating the area of a circle, but Pythagoras went far beyond those early efforts in accuracy. The Greek mathematicians of this early period used whole numbers and the use of fractions was restricted to commerce.

Whole numbers occupied a central position in the religious beliefs of the Pythagoreans and the irrational numbers, like pi (π) and $\sqrt{2}$, challenged their entire philosophy. It was said that the discoverer of this concept, Hippasus of Metapontum, was thrown overboard from a ship when he told his fellow Pythagoreans of his conclusion. Some of the number theory of the Pythagoreans derived from the notation used by the Greeks to write numbers. We use the Arabic system (imported by them from India) of number symbols but the Greeks used dots arranged in patterns of squares, triangles, and rectangles.[28] They used symbols based on the first letter of the word for larger units such as H for *Hekaton* (hundred) and arrayed these symbols in a similar pattern to show multiples, such as "HHH" for three hundred. It was very difficult to depict non-whole numbers and fractions. The basis of Euclid's geometry was the work of Pythagoras and his school.[29]

EMPEDOCLES

Empedocles was a student of Pythagoras who lived in Sicily during the fifth century BCE. He expanded upon the theories of Thales and Anaximenes adding a fourth element, fire, to the concept of matter. In addition, he concluded that matter could not be created or destroyed, a surprisingly modern idea that was to be lost again for centuries during the Dark Ages. Empedocles described a theory of evolution concluding that form followed function and that the best fitted survived. This concept of evolution was also lost for another 2,000 years. Empedocles, unfortunately, became convinced of his own immortality and eventually, to convince skeptical students, leaped into the crater of the volcano Mt. Etna. After a few years, when Empedocles failed to reappear, his students concluded that he had been mistaken about his mortality, but the theory of four elements survived into the Middle Ages. Empedocles left other concepts that were central to Greek medicine. One was "innate heat" as the source of living processes including digestion. Like several others he attributed a cooling function to breathing which we will see again with Hippocrates. He also considered the liver as the central organ making blood and the heart as the center of sensation.

A contemporary, and fellow Pythagorean, was Alcmaeon of Croton (the city in southern Italy founded by Pythagoras) who believed that the brain was the center of sensory function. He used experimental data to arrive at this conclusion, discovering and dissecting the optic nerves. He also concluded that smell and hearing were brain functions, since the nose and ears provide passages into the skull. These early Greeks established principles later prominent in the teachings of Hippocrates, although no direct connection can be demonstrated.

20   Roy Porter, *The Greatest Benefit to Mankind*, Norton (1997) page 46 where he describes their discovery of distillation and the use of volatile oils for their scent.

21   Morris Kline, *Mathematical Thought From Ancient to Modern Times*, Oxford Press (1972) Volume I Chapter 1, page 3-14.

22   R. Campbell Thompson, *Assyrian Medical Texts from the Originals in the British Museum*, (1923).

23   JA Yorke, N. Nathanson, G. Pianigiani and J. Martin, "Seasonality and the Requirements for Perpetuation and Eradication of Viruses in Populations," *American Journal of Epidemiology* 109:103-123 (1979).

24   Jared Diamond, *Guns, Germs and Steel*, W. W. Norton & Co. (1997), page 205.

25   George S. El-Assal, "Ancient Egyptian Medicine," *Lancet*, (August 5, 1972) pages 272-274.

26   F Marti-Ibanez, "Historical perspectives of antibiotics; past and present" In; *Antibiotics Annual* 1953-54, New York, Medical Encyclopedia, Inc. (1953).

27   Paul Strathern. *Mendeleyev's Dream. The Quest for the Elements*. pp 12-15, St. Martin's Press. (2000).

28   Georges Ifrah, *The Universal History of Numbers,* pages 182-187, John Wiley and Sons, (2000).

29   Morris Kline, *Mathematical Thought From Ancient to Modern Times*. Pp 28-34. Oxford University Press. (1972).

3
Classical Greece and Rome

DISCOVERY OF BENEFICIAL DRUGS OR OTHER THERAPY REQUIRES SOME capability for scientific analysis, studying the effects of administration to sick patients and recognizing evidence of improvement. Before such analysis is possible, the natural history of disease and the diagnosis of different maladies must be known. Greek physicians were capable of scientific observation and ancient medicine was mostly a matter of diagnosis and prognostication since useful remedies were few. The physician who was successful was a good observer and able to predict the outcome of the illness. He often took credit for successful outcomes that he had nothing to do with, a characteristic that makes him seem only more modern.

SOCRATES, PLATO, AND ARISTOTLE

We have a few records from this early era that survived the destruction of the library at Alexandria in 391CE and some of these contain Greek medical concepts. Most of our knowledge of these times comes from Arabic translations that preserved Greek science for posterity. It is apparent that the history of medicine paralleled that of science and philosophy. Socrates, born in 469BCE, began the Athenian school of philosophy (called the Academy) that, under his student Plato and succeeding students, was to last for a thousand years. Socrates taught his students in the open air and charged no fees. He supported himself as a sculptor and was scolded by his wife for wasting his time. He was chiefly concerned with ethics and politics, an interest that ultimately cost him his life, but his rules of logic and open debate were to have a profound effect on science.

Plato had more interest in health and disease, but he scorned experimentation and emphasized deductive reasoning. His work *Timaeus* linked form and function, medicine and human nature, in a teleological explanation of anatomy and health. Temperance, wisdom, and self-control were the keys to health. Aristotle, Plato's pupil, a physician and the tutor of Alexander the Great, returned to experimentation and observation. He acquired a vast knowledge of natural history and created the scientific method with his observations. His studies of biology emphasized teleology again and his methodology persisted for nearly two thousand years. He used animal dissection to study anatomy, dissected living eggs, and described the beating heart. Unfortunately, he did not differentiate between veins and arteries and his observation of the heart was flawed as he inexplicably described it as having three chambers, not four. Of course, amphibian hearts do have three chambers, but Aristotle did not mention the species of animal he dissected and his conclusions were applied to humans. Alexander the Great, during his conquest of Persia, sent specimens back to Athens for his teacher Aristotle's collection.

Aristotle returned to Empidocles' theory of the nature of matter and recorded volumes of material from observation of plants and animals. Still, infected with Plato's concepts, Aristotle decided that the nature of these elements (arrived at by deduction, not experiment) governs their behavior and expanded this concept to include astronomy. Since a pebble, dropped into water, sinks and bubbles rise, he concluded that earth is the lowest or heaviest element in nature, next comes water, then air and finally fire because it rises in air. To explain the motion and suspension of heavenly bodies he deduced a fifth element, "aether," that fills the space above the earth and between the celestial spheres to which the stars are attached. His belief in the nature of the elements led to a conclusion that the earth must be the center of the universe, even though earlier Greek philosophers had measured the motion of the planets and Eratosthenes later calculated the circumference of the earth by measuring the elevation of the sun at noon from the bottoms of two wells a known distance apart. Aristarchos of Samos even proposed a "heliocentric universe" with the stars fixed in the heavens and the earth revolving around the sun.[30]

Aristotle's pupil, Theophrastus, took over as head of the Peripatetic School of Athens in third century BCE and established a scientific basis for botany and *materia medica*. He classified 550 varieties and species of plants, including specimens sent back from India by Alexander's expedition. His work would be rediscovered during the Renaissance and would lead to the revival of medical botany and botanical gardens. Unfortunately, the use of plant and animal material in Greek and Roman remedies became progressively more enmeshed with magical potions and Galen's "medicines" include enormous numbers of worthless concoctions many of which continued in use for centuries.

HIPPOCRATES

The state of medicine in this era of great scientific awakening can be judged from the writings of Hippocrates. These writings, referred to as the *Corpus*, are known only through the accounts of others. They were collected in 250BCE, more than a century after his death in 377BCE. Not all sections have proven to be his writing and the author of the *Corpus* is, like Homer with the *Iliad* and the *Odyssey*, subject to the interpretations of later writers. There are several sections; *The Epidemics* is a series of case histories that are so clear and well described that the diseases can be recognized. Unfortunately, dissection was prohibited and anatomy was limited to surface anatomy which led to theorizing that offered little in the explanation of the pathology of disease and its cause. The origin of *On the Nature of Man* as a genuine work of Hippocrates has been disputed, but it is the source of the "Four Humours" theory of disease that persisted until recent times.

The Humours were Blood, obviously necessary to life in animals and analogous to the sap of plants, Phlegm, seen only in illness, Bile, a component of diarrhea, and Black Bile, a late addition to the theory. The analogy to the four elements of matter, air, water, earth and fire, is implied and the pattern of four elements is seen again in other topics such as the "primary qualities" of Hot, Cold, Dry and Wet, a staple of Pythagorean theory of illness. The physician is advised to spend time at the bedside and adopt an "expectant" therapeutic stance. This consisted of waiting and watching their patients relying on the "healing powers of nature," which was emphasized in *On Ancient Medicine*. In this treatise, Hippocrates begins by attacking the Pythagorean concept of "Opposites," which uses the qualities of Hot, Cold, Wet, Dry to describe the origin of illness. He spends most of the treatise discussing diet and the use of juices in therapeutics. Surgery is never mentioned in these sections of his writings and the Oath specifically prohibits "cutting for stone." The treatment of bladder stone will be discussed later and the prohibition will be seen to be reasonable in the practice of a humane physician.

There are several treatises which do discuss surgery and one, *On the Surgery*, is devoted to the placement of bandages and details about the position of the operator but mentions no actual surgical procedures.[31] The treatise *On Fractures* describes the reduction of fractures advising traction to restore the length of the femur and tibia in particular. Splints and bandages were treated with wax for stiffness (quick-drying plaster would be first described by the Arabs) and the large bones of the leg would heal in about forty days according to Hippocrates.

HIPPOCRATIC SURGERY

Two surgery treatises are very astute and the therapy should have been effective, predating current practice by nearly 2,500 years. A fistula in ano is described accurately in *On Fistulae* and the physician is advised to drain a perirectal abscess promptly. Perirectal abscess and anal fistula are related disorders. The entire GI tract is lined with a mucus-secreting layer called endothelium (or endoderm in embryology). This wet layer begins at the vermilion border of the lips where dry skin, which protects the body from dehydration and from foreign invaders like bacteria, gives way to a soft moist lining that participates in digestion by secreting various enzyme-containing fluids and absorbing nutrients. At the other end of the GI tract, the transition from the wet to dry layer is abrupt and the anal skin layer downstream sometimes overlaps the upstream wet mucous layer. This creates a condition called an "anal crypt" in which the fecal stream undermines the overlapping skin and burrows under it to create pockets where fecal material may collect. The crypt, if it gets deep enough, may give rise to a pocket of infection and then an abscess.

Abscesses always burrow from areas of higher pressure to those with lower pressure to drain. The pressure inside the anus is higher than atmospheric pressure (or else we would absorb water sitting in a bathtub or swimming) and the abscess seeks to drain to the outside. As it burrows its way to the outside it becomes a "perirectal abscess" and presents a red, hot, tender mass beside the anus. If neglected, it will eventually drain itself by eroding a hole in the skin, but the pain is severe and it is not surprising that drainage of this condition was advised in ancient times. Once the abscess is drained the potential exists for a false passage around the anal sphincter as the abscess track persists in many cases. The abscess begins with a crypt inside the anus and the residual passage (if it persists) may continue to drain fecal material to the outside. If the fistula track (the medical definition of fistula is an abnormal connection between a hollow viscus and another hollow viscus or the outside world) gets plugged by a bit of fecal material another abscess forms. The condition, once established, persists and causes recurring pain, fever, and intermittent drainage of fecal material (as the plug is pushed out by pressure) and pus into the underclothes. It is a very uncomfortable condition.

One method of treating an established fistula, recommended by Hippocrates, involves placement of a thread through the fistula track into the rectum using a probe. The inner end of the thread is pulled back out the anal canal and tied to the external end, making a loop. This description is identical to the Seton method of treatment introduced in the seventeenth century and used up to the current time. It is an effective method and suggests considerable clinical competence. The ends of the thread, or Seton, are retied every few days as the thread is slowly tightened. It gradually cuts through the bridge of tissue between fistula track and anus without damaging the sphincter, which is kept in continuity by a band of scar as the thread cuts through. The essence of successful treatment to this day is to cut the bridge of tissue between the false passage of the fistula track and the anal canal without damaging the sphincter muscle. Today, this may be accomplished under anesthesia directly, repairing the sphincter if necessary, but the Seton method is still used.

Another surgical treatise, *On the Hemorrhoid*, recommends the use of hooks to pull an internal hemorrhoid outside of the anus where it is cauterized with a hot iron. This would also be effective and is similar to modern therapy. Hemorrhoids are ano-rectal veins that become dilated by straining to pass constipated stools (or by increased pelvic vein pressure during pregnancy). They are, in essence, varicose veins of the rectum. When the patient strains again, the vein bulges out and may bleed. Cauterizing the vein will obliterate it because the bulging distended vein clots off and atrophies. Another treatise, *Articulations*, describes the diagnosis of dislocation of the shoulder and recommends a method of therapy still used and called by many "The Hippocratic Method." It is also called "the dirty sock method" and involves placing the physician's foot in the patient's axilla while the wrist is grasped with both of the physician's hands and traction is placed on the arm. The humeral head is pushed up as the arm is pulled down and the dislocation reduced with the physician's foot. This is an effective method for reducing the most common type of shoulder dislocation and is still in use.

This treatise also contains a discussion of gibbous deformity of the spine, hunchback, and associates it with lung disease, a sign that Hippocrates connected tuberculosis of the spine with the pulmonary form. In the *Aphorisms* he mentions opening the chest to drain an empyema (a collection of infected fluid in the chest). Aphorism number forty-four states, "When empyema is treated either by the cautery or incision, if pure white pus flow from the wound, the patients recover; but if mixed with blood, slimy and fetid, they die." This observation anticipates the modern therapy of empyema that would only be established in the 1920s by Evarts Graham and the Empyema Commission, which studied the influenza epidemic after World War I. Hippocrates was absolutely correct, but it would take 2,500 years to understand why. The matter is discussed in Chapter 12.

INFECTIOUS DISEASE

The treatise *Air, Waters, Places* discusses the significance of weather and the incidence of fever. Rainfall in the fall and winter predicted a healthy year, but rain falling heavily in the spring would lead to fever in the summer. With no knowledge of the role of the mosquito, the Hippocratic physicians noted the relationship of wet conditions and malaria. The Humours were related to the seasons with Phlegm being the dominant Humour of winter, when colds, bronchitis, and pneumonia were more common. Blood was the Humour of spring when dysentery, nose bleeds, and tertian malaria (three day) fevers were more common. Summer was hot with Yellow Bile the predominant Humour, leading to more severe fevers from quartan malaria (four day fever) and diarrhea. Fall saw the decline of Yellow Bile, but an increase in Black Bile. Black Bile was concentrated in the spleen and spleens are enlarged in patients recovering from quartan malaria. In one of the cases in Epidemics I, that of Philiscus, the patient was clearly suffering from falciparum malaria with black urine ("black water fever" from hemolysis of red cells) and an enlarged spleen. The spleen and its relationship to Black Bile (and depression) has been incorporated in the "splenic rage" concept of literature and was in common usage as an explanation for behavior up to the very recent past.

Other than the few surgical procedures described above, therapy was mostly dietary and prognosis was more important. The "Hippocratic Facies" was the appearance of one about to die: "a protrusive nose, hollow eyes, sunken temples, cold ears that are drawn in with lobes turned outward, the forehead's skin rough and tense, like parchment, and the whole face greenish or black or blue-grey or leaden." *The Aphorisms* contain most of the experience in prognostics and contain brief elements like: "When sleep puts an end to delirium, it is a good sign."[32] The Hippocratic Oath was developed at the same time, although some of its provisions represent sentiments uncommon in classical Greece. Its prohibition of abortion, for example, is in contrast to the common practice of infanticide that was approved of by Plato and Aristotle. Some of the aphorisms may be more representative of the Pythagorean philosophy of healing and reincarnation (and which opposed abortion). The first Aphorism "Life is short, the Art long, opportunity fleeting, experience fallacious, judgment difficult" suggests the need for humility and the Oath establishes the Art as a noble calling.

THE ALEXANDRINE SCHOOL

The city of Alexandria was founded by Alexander before his death in 323BCE. Ptolemy, Alexander's half brother and heir to the Egyptian portion of his empire, established an enormous library at Alexandria, his capital. The library existed until it was destroyed by Christians in 391CE. A modern version has just opened in Alexandria. During its existence, a prominent school of medicine, the Alexandrine School, existed alongside the other disciplines of physics and mathematics. Archimedes, Euclid, and the astronomer Ptolemy, namesake of the king, taught there. A 1901 discovery has prompted some rethinking of Greek technological achievement. A sunken ship, found near Crete, contained an astronomical computing machine of incredible complexity. It has been reconstructed and is an analog computer capable of calculating planet and star positions. [33]

Two prominent members of the Alexandrine School were Herophilus of Chalcedon and Erasistratus of Chios, both of whom lived during the third century BCE. Herophilus distinguished between arteries and veins, improving upon Aristotle's anatomy. Praxagoras, another member of the school and teacher of Herophilus, had concluded that arteries are filled with air and conduct air from the lungs to nourish the body. This may have followed the observation that, in the dead, arteries (because of their elastic recoil) are usually empty while veins are filled with clotted blood. Praxagoras believed that veins arise in the liver to carry digested food, converted to blood, to the body. The combination of air (pneuma) and blood generated the heat necessary for life. This theory would persist until Harvey in 1615.

HEROPHILUS

Herophilus practiced medicine in Alexandria and was said to have dissected human bodies, in contrast to earlier Greeks who knew only surface anatomy. He discovered the duodenum, which he named using the Greek for "twelve fingers," the length of the bowel segment. He also identified the prostate gland. Herophilus, unlike Praxagoras his teacher, believed that the arteries were filled with blood and noted the difference in wall thickness between arteries and veins. Even more impressive, he discovered the peripheral nerves and identified the dorsal and ventral roots. His identification of the nervous system confirmed the importance of the brain as the seat of intelligence and he differentiated the cerebellum from the cerebrum. He took up the subject of the pulse from his teacher Praxagoras and concluded that the heart was its source.

ERASISTRATUS

Erasistratus dissected human bodies, some of which may have been living subjects. He identified the cerebral ventricles and distinguished between motor and sensory nerves. He returned to the earlier belief of Praxagoras that arteries contained air and concluded that "spirit," a gas transmitted in motor nerves, stimulated muscles to contract.

As the years went by, medicine split into sects divided by the argument between the "Theorists," also called "Rationalists," and the "Empirics." The Theorists believed in Hippocrates' concept of Humours, and the Empirics rejected all theory and relied on case histories and remedies.

THE ROMANS

The contributions of the Romans to science are sparse and it is often written that the only Roman to appear in the history of mathematics is the one who slew Archimedes during the sack of Syracuse. Roman inventions tended to be of a practical nature. For example, the water wheel, used to turn flour mills, was first described by Philo of Byzantium in the third century BCE. The Romans were less interested in theoretical matters, like mathematics or basic science including biology. The Romans considered healing of the sick to be a family duty and did not employ physicians even while other parts of the Roman world continued the traditions of Greek medicine. An exception was Pliny the Elder, not a physician, but a skilled observer, who recorded a considerable volume of data including his obser-vation of the eruption of Vesuvius. Pliny did write a *materia medica*, in 77CE, based on his studies of botany, but he deplored the recent influx of luxury and worthless Greek physicians. He died in the Vesuvius eruption on August 24, 79CE (he drew too close to the volcano while observing). An inscription attributed to Alexander the Great appeared on Roman monu-ments: "It was the crowd of physicians who killed me." As a result of this prejudice professional doctors (*medici*) were all immigrants to Rome for many years. Medical practice in the Roman world did not require medical degrees or any sort of license. Swarms of healers and midwives competed with physicians, many of whom were slaves. In fact, prior to the reign of Julius Caesar, all physicians were slaves and Caesar freed them.

The Romans set great store on stoic behavior and a number of traditions, including resistance to torture, determined their response to illness. Cato was an enemy of all doctors, accusing them of poisoning Roman youth and he believed that doctors, all Greeks in his time, hated the Romans who had conquered Greece. He advocated cabbage as a universal remedy, including using it as a poultice for wounds, as well as eating it. He even provided a charm that was supposed to reduce dislocations; no randomized clinical trial of his method has come down to us.[34]

CELSUS

The first medical work in Latin was written by Celsus, a wealthy landowner, not a physician, and was part of a larger treatise on the natural sciences. Celsus wrote during the reign of Tiberius (14-37CE), and his book included a history of medicine going back to the Trojan Wars. He lamented the division between Empiricists and the Theorists and his books presented a synthesis of reason and experience. Several of his books, there were eight in all, discussed surgery and his description of the signs of infection in a surgical wound has survived to this day. The four signs were described by Celsus as, *calor*, Latin for heat, *rubor*, redness, *dolor*, pain and *tumor*, swelling. A few other Roman physicians left valuable works.

ARETAEUS

Aretaeus of Cappadocia (140CE) left some of the most accurate descriptions of diseases in ancient times, writing in Greek. He described diabetes as "a liquefaction of the flesh and bones into urine" so much that "the kidneys and bladder do not cease emitting urine." *Diabetes*, in Greek means, "I pass through," suggested by his theory of dissolution of tissue into urine. The Romans later added the term "mellitus," which means sweet or honey, to distinguish the condition from diabetes insipidus, related to pituitary disease. His description of tetanus shows considerable clinical experience and he coined the terms *tetanus* and *opisthotonus*, the hyper-extended posture of full-blown tetanus.

SORANOS

Soranos of Ephasos (98-138CE) began the study of gynecology and conception with his book *Gynecology*. The text was lost until 1838.[35] He described the anatomy of the female organs and described the ovaries using the term *didymos*, meaning "twin" gonads. We use the term *epididymus* to describe the structure attached to, and above, the testis. He also invented the vaginal speculum, lost again until Sims in the nineteenth century. He described the use of pessaries for contraception and noted the most favorable time for conception during the menstrual cycle. There were other prominent Roman physicians, but they were eclipsed, at least in history, by Galen.

GALEN

Galen was the most prolific writer on medical subjects of ancient times and his fame has survived, at least partly, because his writings survived, unlike those of most of the Greeks. He was born in Pergamon, now Bergama, Turkey to a wealthy father who was an architect. He enjoyed a liberal education and, after his father had a dream in which Asclepius appeared to him, was sent to Alexandria for a medical education. In 157CE he was appointed physician to the gladiators in Pergamon and consequently learned a good deal about wounds and anatomy.

Five years later, he moved to Rome and, after some self-promotion, developed a successful practice (There is nothing new under the sun). Like many other physicians of the time, he dissected animals, but not human cadavers. This led to errors in anatomy, and he used Hippocratic theory to speculate about the cause of disease. His errors were perpetuated by his fame and inhibited further progress for a thousand years. He advocated energetic blood letting even to the point of unconsciousness. Some of his enthusiasm for bloodletting was based on his observation that women, who bleed monthly with menses, have fewer diseases (for example gout) than men. Like the earlier Greeks, he was convinced that blood was formed in the liver and carried nutrients to the body via the veins. He concluded that some blood was carried to the heart from the liver and split into two streams, one going to the lungs, the other passing through "pores" in the ventricular septum and mixing with air in the left ventricle from where it was carried to the body in the arteries. The pulse did not represent the circulation as we conceive it but a pulsation of heart and arteries. He wrote a number of books on the pulse and his enthusiasm for the subject carried on until nearly modern times. He believed that nerves were hollow ducts and carried *pneuma* or vital spirits to the muscles.

PUBLIC HEALTH AND CIVIL ENGINEERING

The great contribution of the Romans to medicine was in the area of public health and civil engineering. Roman public health and sanitation were more advanced in 300CE than any country's would be again until the nineteenth century. The only hospitals constructed by the Roman government were for the military and a good example has been excavated in Scotland. There was a long corridor with individual small rooms or cells arranged along it. There was a top-lit hall, perhaps a dining hall, and latrines and baths. The city of Rome was the first, with the possible exception of the Labyrinth of Knossus in Crete (before 1450BCE), to have running water, sewers and water closets in homes. Fourteen great aqueducts carried millions of gallons of water into the city each day. Some of those aqueducts are still in use. The first was constructed in 312BCE and in 100CE 250 million gallons of water per day traveled through ten aqueducts to the city.

Half the water was used for public baths and the other half provided fifty gallons per day for each of the two million residents, the same volume used today by residents of New York City and London.

The Cloaca Maxima is the great sewer opening into the Tiber River and its ruins may still be seen today. Vitruvius, author of "On Architecture" in 27BCE, set out sanitary standards for towns stressing the need for good water supplies. He also described an improvement on the water wheel using gears to turn the grind stone.[36] Roman construction and Roman roads confirmed their expertise as the greatest civil engineers of antiquity, notwithstanding the pyramids of the Egyptians or the temples of the Greeks. Pompeii and Herculaneum, covered in volcanic ash (preserving the towns as time capsules) in an eruption of Vesuvius in 79CE, each have an elaborate system of waterworks with flushing water closets. In 70CE a public building with marble urinals was erected by Vespasian. In England, similar public lavatories were constructed for the Great Exhibition of 1851. In spite of a small fee and significant distance from the location of the Exhibition, the public lavatories raised four times the cost of construction in five months use. They were the first to be built in Europe since Rome.

After the fire of 64CE (during which Nero fiddled) the city was rebuilt with wide straight streets and large squares. The streets were cleaned by officials called *aediles* who also supervised the food supply to ensure freshness and quality of perishables. Burial within the city walls was prohibited, which increased the healthy practice of cremation until the Christian preaching of resurrection prompted a return to burial. The state of public health in Rome exceeded that of the large cities of Europe until modern times.

THE PLAGUES

The Roman sanitary systems reduced the incidence of endemic diseases, but the roads, and the armies that marched across the Roman Empire, brought great epidemics to the city. Greek cities, in contrast, were small and travel was much more difficult and less common. With the exception of the great plague of Athens in 430BCE, epidemics were rare. That Athenian plague has been the subject of much speculation in the medical literature. It was carefully described by Thucydides in his history of the Peloponnesian War. Athens was crowded at the time because much of the rural population had entered the city walls to escape the raiding Spartans. It seemed to come from Ethiopia, through Egypt and Libya, and entered Greece at the seaport of Piraeus. Victims were struck suddenly with a severe headache and reddened eyes. Inflammation of the mouth and throat was followed by cough then intestinal symptoms developed with vomiting and diarrhea. Delirium was common and death occurred at seven to ten days. At the height of the fever, a rash occurred which was red and became ulcerated. Some of the victims who survived lost fingers and toes. The plague had a profound effect on the war and Greek history.

Modern writers have tried to identify the disease; some attributing it to typhus and others to smallpox. Because of the combination of sore throat and red rash, a virulent form of scarlet fever has also been considered. It may be that time has caused changes in the behavior of the organism, similar to the profound evolution of syphilis which has occurred since its introduction to Europe in 1495. An epidemic attacked a Carthaginian army besieging Syracuse in Sicily in 396BCE, thirty-four years after the Plague of Athens, and was described by Diodorus Siculus. His description is very similar to that of Thucydides and the same disease may be responsible. This epidemic caused a very high death rate and forced the Carthaginians to raise the siege and disperse their army. Had Carthage succeeded in conquering all of Sicily 100 years before the first Punic War with Rome the outcome of that conflict, and the two subsequent Punic Wars, might have been very different. Instead of a Roman Empire, the Carthaginians, colonists from semitic Phoenicia with a merchant and trading tradition rather than a military culture like Rome, might have become the dominant civilization in Europe. These two epidemics could represent smallpox with somewhat different clinical manifestations from the modern disease. Smallpox is reported to have occurred in China about 1700BCE and the epidemics did seem to originate in the East.

THE DECLINE OF ROME

In the first century BCE, a new and much more severe variety of malaria appeared in the marshy districts around Rome and produced a great epidemic in 79CE, shortly after the Vesuvius eruption. The epidemic severely affected the Campagna, the market garden of Rome, and the whole area went out of cultivation for centuries. It remained a notorious malarial district until the end of the nineteenth century. The endemic malaria caused a fall in the birth rate and weakened the city, perhaps beginning its long decline. There has been another theory of this decline, namely that a new fashion in pottery led to the extensive use of blue pigment containing lead. Daily use could have caused a gradual leaching of the lead from the pottery glaze producing chronic lead poisoning of the population. Lead was also used in Roman plumbing just as it was until very recently in Europe and America. At the peak of the Roman Empire lead production was 80,000 tons per year and it has been written that lead intake in Rome varied with the socio-economic class of the citizen. The aristocracy may have consumed as much as 1 mg. /day, but contemporary accounts of illness attributable to lead poisoning are rare. Archeologists have measured the lead content of bones and found that ancient Peruvians, who did not use lead in any form, had the least lead exposure detectable. Ancient Romans, according to some accounts, had lead levels approximately the same as those of modern Europeans and Americans, 1,000 times the lead levels of the ancient Peruvians. Another, quite sophisticated, study has partially contradicted this finding and, using the Peruvians as a "physiologic zero point," present day Germans are reported to have a lead "burden" twenty times that of the Peruvians and the Romans had about forty-six percent of the present lead content. Thus, the lead theory of Rome's decline is not proven. The malaria theory has more support although later epidemics contributed nearly as much to the problems of ancient Roman society.

THE ANTONINE PLAGUE

The first great epidemic attributable to the Roman Empire was called the Antonine Plague and slew five million people between 165 and 180CE. It began among legions at the eastern border of the Empire in 164CE. It caused havoc among troops dispatched to Syria to suppress a revolt. It reached Rome with returning soldiers in 166CE and caused the first retrenchment of the previously expanding Empire. In 169, the army threw back German invaders, but the epidemic, transmitted to the German barbarians by sick prisoners or clothing, may have been as effective as the legions. The plague raged until 180CE and finally claimed the life of emperor Marcus Aurelius, one of the last to die. He sent his son, Commodus, out of the city during the plague and the son did not smother him as depicted in the movie *Gladiator*. Commodus was a monster as emperor and, after an assassination attempt organized by his sister, Lucilla (she recruited the assassins from her numerous lovers), in 183, grew even worse. He did act as a gladiator, as depicted in the movie, but died by a combination of poison administered by his favorite concubine, Marcia, and smothering in 192.[37]

Galen was reported to have fled the plague, but he left a description that sounds similar to the plague of Athens. The mention of a skin eruption similar to that of smallpox, and the eastern origin of the epidemic has caused this to be labeled the first smallpox epidemic. At its peak, it killed 2,000 people a day in Rome but after 180CE it subsided and no further epidemics were reported for seventy years. In 250, a new epidemic appeared which was called the Plague of Cyprian. It did not have a skin eruption and, for the next sixteen years, it recurred on a seasonal basis with new cases appearing in the fall and fading out in the hot summer. Thousands fled the cities carrying the disease to the countryside. The seasonal fluctuation of the epidemic suggests typhus, but nothing can be confirmed. Typhus is seasonal because it is carried by the body louse, which dwells in unclean clothing. Fall and winter are associated with more clothing and less frequent bathing, hence the seasonal trend. The recurring outbreaks suggest a developing immunity as the virulence seems to decrease with time but this is typical of all epidemics.

THE PLAGUE OF JUSTINIAN

As Rome declined under the combined threats of disease and barbarian invasion, Byzantium, the eastern capital of Constantine, flourished. In the sixth century CE Justinian, the greatest of the Byzantine rulers, attempted to reestablish the Western Roman Empire. By 540, he had conquered all of North Africa and Italy and was planning a further campaign into Gaul. Unfortunately for Justinian, the Goths counterattacked and recaptured most of Italy. During a siege of Rome, the Goths cut the aqueducts and Rome descended into squalor, which was to continue until the Renaissance. The same year of his greatest success saw the first outbreak of bubonic plague in Egypt. By 542, it had reached Byzantium and, during the summer peak of the epidemic, 10,000 people died every day in the capital. From contemporary descriptions, the disease was clearly bubonic plague and it killed forty percent of the population of the capital.

Procopius, an archivist not a physician, provided an exact record of the spread of the disease from the coast to the interior. He also noted that the physicians and attendants who cared for the victims were not themselves infected. This is consistent with bubonic plague since it is contracted from rat fleas, not victims. Pneumonic plague (transmitted by coughing), of course, is another matter. Recent research, in the era of DNA analysis, has been able to recover *Yersinia* DNA from the teeth of plague victims buried in cemeteries during the later Black Death. The organisms produce such an overwhelming bacteremia that bacterial DNA can be recovered from the pulp of teeth in skeletal remains.[38] Thus far, the DNA recovery has been successful in victims from as early as 1348 and there are plans to attempt recovery from victims of the Plague of Justinian. Gibbon, in his history of Rome, states that entire countries were depopulated and Procopius describes a wave of licentiousness and depravity during the height of the epidemic. Thucydides observed the same phenomenon during the Plague of Athens. Both authors suggested that the honorable and law-abiding, perhaps because they refused to steal from their neighbors, died in the epidemic and the wicked seemed to survive.

There has been speculation that the great plagues of the first three centuries of the Christian Era might have had some role in the success of the new religion. The Gospel of St. Luke, himself a physician, describes twenty miracles. All but three of these miracles were of a medical nature, raising the dead or curing disease. St. Luke further has Christ giving his twelve disciples "power and authority over all devils, and to cure diseases." The dichotomy between the religious and the scientific aspects of healing in the Bible is illustrated by two other passages in the Gospel of St. Luke. The parable of the Good Samaritan has the Samaritan washing the wounds of the traveler with wine, an example of Greek medical practice. In another instance, Luke has Jesus healing a blind man by forgiving his sins. Thus, illness is a consequence of sin and not a physical malady to be studied and analyzed as the Greeks did.

The Christian religion may have been more attractive to a population terrorized by epidemics. As the Church increased in power, healing the sick became a role of priests and religion assumed a dominant role in science. The Roman goddess of fever, *Febris*, became Saint Febronia of the Christian Church. Saint Sebastian, an early Christian convert and martyr, became the patron of epidemic sickness. For a thousand years sickness was a matter for prayer and votive offerings. For reasons that are not clear, Galen became the source of Christian orthodoxy on medical matters. He was not a Christian, although he seems to have been a monotheist.

As Rome declined and the long darkness of learning characteristic of the Middle Ages began in Europe, the Church assumed a role in healing, especially with the construction of almshouses, and hospitals. Basil of Cappadocia built a great "hospital city" in 375CE and Chrysostomos built several hospitals in Constantinople. The *Pantokrater* was a large monastery whose public hospital was called the *Xenon*. In Constantinople, several large hospitals were built and, by 650CE, the Pantokrator had teaching facilities and a medical staff of sorts. The Byzantine ruler Joannes II Comnenos endowed it in 1136CE and the facility continued in operation until the fall of the Byzantine Empire. The hospital for the monks was called the *triclinon* and the Xenon would not accept monks as it was devoted to the sick poor of the city. A third facility, called the *Gerocomeion* was devoted to the care of the aged, including those disabled. If any of its residents became ill, they were transferred to the hospital.

There were still some centers of new knowledge, mostly in the Middle East, and Paul of Aegina, in 640, wrote medical works that included mention of tracheostomy. He recommended colchicine for gout, an effective remedy still in use. His *Epitome* was highly regarded by Islamic physicians who carried on the tradition of scientific medicine. In the West, all was darkness but a few tiny flickering lamps in monasteries.

30   T. Heath, *Aristarchos of Samos: The Ancient Copernicus*, Oxford Press (1918).

31   Hippocrates, *The Genuine Works of Hippocrates*, Francis Adams translation, Syndenham Society, London (1849).

32   Hippocrates, *The Aphorisms of Hippocrates,* Thomas Coar translation, AJ Valpy, London (1822).

33   Derek J. de Solla Price, "An Ancient Greek Computer," *Scientific American* (June 1959) pages 60-67.

34   Florence Dupont, *Daily Life in Ancient Rome,* Chapter 14 "The Body: Moral and Physical Aspects," Blackwell. (1989).

35   NE Himes, *"Medical History of Contraception,"* Gamut Press, New York (1936).

36   Vitruvius, *De Architectura*; quoted in Joel Mokyr, *The Lever of Riches*, Oxford (1990).

37   Edward Gibbon, *Decline and Fall of the Roman Empire. Vol. I*, John Murray, Albemarle Street, London (1862).

38   Michel Drancourt, Gérard Aboudharam, Michel Signoli, Olivier Dutour, and Didier Raoult. "Detection of 400-year-old *Yersinia pestis* DNA in human dental pulp: An approach to the diagnosis of ancient septicemia," *Proceedings of the National Academy of Sciences* 95, Issue 21, 12637-12640, (October 13, 1998).

4
India and China

THE INDUS RIVER CIVILIZATION

THE NEOLITHIC REVOLUTION IN AGRICULTURE OCCURRED AT ABOUT the same time in India and China as in Mesopotamia. All three areas progressed at a more rapid pace, if the evolution from hunter-gatherer to farmer can be referred to as rapid, than in Europe. The use of cereal grains and construction of mud-brick houses appeared in eastern Rajasthan about 7000BCE. Evidence of domestication of cattle, sheep, and goats is found from the same era, as well. In about 3000BCE (Some say as early as 4600BCE), an elaborate civilization developed in the Indus River region, an area now mostly in Pakistan. The river flowed through a desert country, similar to Egypt and Mesopotamia, and nearby trading communities provided contact with other developing civilizations. Great cities have been excavated that show evidence of complex societies, including great public water tanks suggesting public bathing and sanitation similar to that of Rome. They cultivated cotton, wheat, barley, and sesame. They raised zebras, water buffalo, swine, horses, and donkeys. They domesticated elephants. All of this occurred in the fourth millennium BCE. A pictographic writing, called Harappan script, was developed, but the materials used for writing, perhaps based on cotton cloth or paper, have not survived and the script is still undeciphered. Indian goods and writing have been found in Bahrain, the island in the Persian Gulf, which at the time was a trading center called Dilmun. By 1500BCE, this Indus River civilization was declining, possibly because of changes in the course of the rivers and of the climate, perhaps a consequence of deforestation.

At the time of the decline of the Indus River society, Indo-European peoples migrated into south Asia bringing a brotherhood of hereditary priests, the *Brahmana*. They called themselves Aryans and, later, *Sindhu* or Hindu. There is evidence of great destruction in the Indus River valley cities' ruins from the time of the invasion. The city of Mohenjo-daro, northeast of modern Karachi, when excavated, showed evidence of a violent sack and destruction by the invaders. Skeletons of slaughtered inhabitants filled the streets, many of which showed fatal sword wounds. The cities of the Indus River civilization showed more advanced water and sanitation systems than any found in Mesopotamia or Egypt. Not until Rome would such an advanced society appear again. Nothing like it would exist in India again until modern times. This evidence of sophisticated sanitation systems suggests advanced medical knowledge but no records have survived. The cities of the Indus River civilization rivaled Rome in their sanitation and water systems and existed a thousand years before Rome was founded.[39]

THE HINDU INVASION

The invaders created a caste system to separate themselves from the earlier, darker skinned, inhabitants. Five castes resulted: the *Brahmans* or priests, the *Kshatriyas* or kings and soldiers, the *Vaisyas* peasants and traders, the *Sudras*, lower caste workers and the *Pariahs*, the outcasts. The principle god was *Brahma* and reincarnation became part of the religion. The fact that references to *karma* (fate in the Hindu religion) and reincarnation appear in Plato's work suggests some contact between the Greek and Indian civilization prior to Alexander's expedition. The three classes of Plato's ideal state, in *The Republic*, are soldiers, philosophers, and laborers, another similarity to the Hindu caste system. Sanskrit religious teachings called *Veda* (the knowledge) show some evidence of contemporary beliefs about health and healing. The Veda was an oral tradition memorized by the brahmana priests through millennia before it was preserved in writing. Illness and healing became intertwined with religious and magical beliefs similar to those of Egypt.

Distinctive healing powers were attributed to certain deities and evil spirits could produce diseases. The deities were to be propitiated by rites involving *mantra* (incantations), supplications, and expiation. Herbs were valued for therapeutic power, but recognizable diseases, *yaksma* which was possibly tuberculosis and *takman*, a fever of monsoon season (malaria?), were thought to be signs of demonic powers. There was limited knowledge of anatomy, although hollow reeds were used as catheters to relieve urinary retention, and the Veda showed little interest in science. Around 1000BCE the Veda was the basis of the principle religion of the north of India, but other groups were appearing. In the sixth century BCE, Gautama Sakyamuni, the Buddha, was born, and he established an alternative to the Hindu religion, which he judged to be flawed by the caste system and the role of the powerful Brahmins.

BUDDHISM IN INDIA

By the time of the invasion of Alexander in 326BCE, India was rent by dissention between the two religious groups. After Alexander's invasion, King Chandragupta Maurya seized power in the north and established the Mauryan Empire, which lasted 150 years. Megasthenes, the Greek ambassador from the Seleucid kingdom, successor to Alexander's Eastern Empire, left accounts of this Indian empire that have survived. The empire became more splendid and rich over the years and the *Kama Sutra*, a well-known erotic book (out in a new translation this year), was written there at the time. The third Mauryan emperor, Ashoka, was, himself, converted to Buddhism and encouraged the medical activities of the new religion. By the fourth century CE, Buddhist monasteries contained sick-rooms and a large pharmacopoeia had been assembled. Buddhist monks used five basic medicines: clarified butter, fresh butter, oil, honey, and molasses. Hospitals run by Buddhists appeared around the same time as those in the Middle East, although monastery sick-rooms are found as early as 300BCE. The Buddhist community may have developed the principle system of Indian medicine, called *Ayurveda*, although there are other traditions. The early works, described below, may have originated in a more objective and scientific tradition, perhaps by the Indus River people, only to be modified by later religious additions.

THE BEGINNING OF AYURVEDIC MEDICINE

In 1300BCE, according to tradition, a terrible epidemic was ravaging India. Millions died horribly. Charaka, the great sage (of whom more later), chronicled the epidemic. The great sages, he wrote, gathered at the foot of the Himalayas to decide what to do. They deputized *Rishi* (sage) Bharadwaja, one of their number, to go to Indra, King of the Gods in Heaven, for medical knowledge. He succeeded and brought back the knowledge for long life. He taught another sage, Rishi Atreya, the healing art of Ayurveda and Atreya founded the first college of Ayurvedic Medicine at Taxila. Atreya is considered the Father of Indian Medicine. His six most learned disciples wrote texts of medicine; that of Agnivesha was the only one to survive, or so it was thought until another, written by Bhela, was found in Tanjore Library in South India in this century. The *Bhela Samhita* has not been critically edited and translated. It exists only in a single, damaged manuscript. Rishi Dhanvantari founded a school of surgery at Benares around the same era and his most learned disciple, Susrutha, wrote a textbook of surgery. Susrutha is considered the Father of Indian Surgery. His text was preserved by a chemist named Nagarjuna during the "Buddhist period" and survived.

THE AYURVEDA

The word in Sanskrit means the knowledge needed for longevity and it included a code of life and practical advice including diet, washing, exercise, and a regimen. The theoretical beliefs include a three-humour system of wind (*Vatha*), bile (*Pitta*), and phlegm (*Kapha*). There are also seven fundamental bodily constituents (or *dhatus*): chyle (*Rasa*), blood (*Raktha*), flesh (*Mansa* also translated as muscle), fat (*Medas*), bone (*Asthi*), marrow (*Majja*) and semen (*Sukra* described by Susrutha as being present in the child from birth but only becoming visible at puberty. Perhaps *Sukra* is a concept of sexual hormones or maturation). The Ayurvedic pharmacopoeia includes ointments, enemas, douches, massage, sweating, and surgery. There are few useful drugs, opium being introduced from Islamic sources. The earliest written texts date from the Christian Era, although practitioners claim much more ancient origins. The Ayurveda, itself, has been lost and its contents are known only, like the writings of Hippocrates, from the works of others.

The era of Buddha (or an earlier period) is more likely the source of the Ayurveda. Hindu beliefs led to extensive use of dung and urine, especially cow dung, in many remedies as it was considered a disinfectant. King Ashoka, a convert to Buddhism, brought the empire to its peak but after his death it went into decline. His own soldiers assassinated the last king of the dynasty in 183CE and warlords overthrew the empire. India broke up into mutually hostile kingdoms. Eventually, the Hindu Gupta Kings defeated the Buddhists and they left India almost completely. By 480CE, the White Huns were attacking India in the north. In 977, the armies of Islam invaded from Afghanistan and the Muslim conquest of India began.

THE ATHARVAVEDA

The *Atharvaveda*, a medical text which dates after the Aryan invasion and after the Ayurveda, gives descriptions of rheumatism, gout, epilepsy, dropsy (called "water in the belly"), jaundice, elephantiasis, and mentions a connection between dropsy and cardiac complaints. Treatments were of a magical or religious nature, along the lines of exorcism, although a few drugs are prominently mentioned. One was called "soma" and was derived from a plant of the same name. The plant and the nature of the drug are unknown, but the name survives as a soothing, pain relief remedy. Two great textbooks of medicine survive from the early Vedic age. The *Charaka Samhita* is the older and is attributed to the sage Charaka in a city of northwest India and the ancient university of Taksasila (or Taxila). The city and university did not survive, but the text is dated to 100CE or earlier. It contains much philosophic discussion of the causes of disease, a *materia medica*, and praises the Brahmin healer. Prominent in its proposed remedies are dung and urine. An oath, similar to the Hippocratic Oath although it includes a promise of vegetarian life, is provided. It proposes a three humour (wind, bile, and phlegm) system of physiology and disease. The English translation of this text runs 1,000 pages.

The Susrutha Samhita includes medical remedies similar to Atharvaveda and the Charaka Samhita, some with similarities to Hippocrates works. Susruta (or Susrutha) was a physician who lived in Benares, a holy city of the Brahmins that has survived, and the remarkable book he wrote contains, unlike Charaka's book, a discussion of anatomy, including instructions for dissection of a human cadaver. The explanations for disease and of normal physiology were no more accurate than those of Hippocrates and there was even an argument at one time that Susrutha was another name for Hippocrates. This has since been disproved but the book contains references to four humours and breath, or air, serves a similar function in both men's works. The English translation of the Susrutha Samhita is 1,700 pages long.

THE SUSRUTHA *SAMHITA*

The first description of leprosy, called *kustha*, is in the Susrutha Samhita and dates to about 600BCE, rather late in the development of infectious diseases. The account of loss of sensation, the loss of fingers, deformity, and ulceration of limbs and the sinking in of the nose provide a clear description of the disease.[40] An account in China about 300BCE is also thought to describe leprosy. There is no evidence of the typical skeletal changes of leprosy in Mesopotamia, Persia, or Egypt prior to the expedition of Alexander in 336BCE and it is possible that this disease, which was to become a scourge in biblical times up to the present, was brought back to the Greek world by returning soldiers or their camp followers. If true, this would be the first example of transmission of a plague from an area where it was endemic to a susceptible population with no prior exposure. The slow progression of the disease, four to five years after infection before the symptoms appear, may explain how it was transported in the era prior to the Roman roads. The first evidence in the Middle East is in Coptic mummies from 300CE[41] and in Europe, the first skeletal findings are in Roman Britain and in Scandinavia about 400CE. This suggests that the Romans may have transported the disease from Egypt to Europe after the Greeks brought it from India.[42]

One of the drugs mentioned in the Indian medical works is the plant later named *Rauwolfia*, after a German physician and botanist (Rauwolf who traveled widely in the sixteenth century) who described it in 1558. The Indians used it as a sedative and it has several powerful effects. It was one of the first effective drugs for hypertension and it has a side effect of causing depression. Another drug, thought to date to the early Vedic Age, is a preparation of the powdered seeds of the Cowhage plant, *Mucuna pruriens*. A condition which resembles the modern disease described by Parkinson in 1817 is called *kampavata*: tremors *(Kampa)* in the psychomotor system called *vata*, or "wind" in the *Ayurveda*. It has been treated with the drug and a modern study, published in an Indian neurology journal, reported significant improvement in symptoms.[43] The plant seeds contain L-dopa.

The most remarkable section of the Susrutha Samhita is the discussion of surgery. Many surgical instruments are described and special tables for "major operations" are mentioned. An accurate description of a cataract treatment called "couching," (the lens was displaced out of the visual axis by a knife through the edge of the cornea) is included and, while the translation has been controversial, there is no question about the procedure. The Code of Hammurabi also mentions the procedure, in the second millennium BCE, but its origin is pretty clearly in India.

RESTORATION OF THE NOSE

A procedure with no precedent outside of India is the restoration of a mutilated nose. Amputation of the nose was a common punishment of the early Vedic Age and the number of such cases no doubt stimulated interest in the procedure. In the early Hindu myths Prince Rama, a virtuous model prince, and the Demon King, Ravana, are rivals. The Demon King sends his sister, the Lady Supanakha, to tempt Prince Rama. Rama's brother, Lakshan, recognizes her intent and, to reveal her evil nature, cuts off her nose. The procedure, called *nacta* in the Hindu language, is still practiced at times and cases of unfaithful wives, who have had their noses cut off by husbands, are still seen in modern British emergency rooms, as well as in India. The reconstruction of the nose was successfully performed in spite of the lack of asepsis or anesthesia, although opium might have been used to relieve pain. The earliest method described by Susrutha used a cheek flap to reconstruct the nose. Later, the practice still called the "Indian Method" raised a flap of skin on the forehead and transfered it, attached to the point of origin at one end, to the site of the missing nose. If raised on the forehead, the flap was left attached just above the nasal defect and was rotated 180 degrees as it was turned down to cover the open nasal cavity. Once the skin flap had healed to the new location, the attachment between nose and forehead was divided. The forehead defect left by the flap was repaired by pulling together the sides. An illustration (Figure 3) shows the results.

Another variant, described by Gasparo Tagliacozzi, an Italian surgeon around 1550, was to raise the flap on the arm, but this required immobilization of the arm across the face for weeks until the healing had established a new blood supply. It is uncertain if he learned the technique from Indian sources, but trade routes had established communication between Italian cities and India by then, and it seems likely that the information came this way. There is no other European history of the method. The European knowledge of the operation was lost again until a newspaper article from India in 1794 reintroduced the procedure to

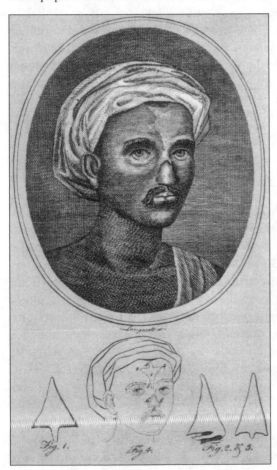

European surgeons. The forces of Tipoo Sultan captured a bullock driver for the English army and cut off his nose as punishment for his treason. A man of the bricklayers', or potters', caste performed the transfer flap to repair the man's nose. English surgeons witnessed this previously unknown procedure and published their account in England. The account, by "B.L.," was published in the *Gentleman's Magazine* in 1794 and included this illustration, Figure 3.

The operation was common in India for centuries, practiced by itinerant surgeons, before it was imported to Europe again. One family, the Kanghiaras, practiced the art of nose reconstruction for centuries keeping the technique a family secret.

Figure 3- Illustration from 1794 article in Gentleman's Magazine.

A woman of the family, often a daughter-in-law, assisted the surgeon. The secret was never conveyed to an unmarried daughter, lest she marry and disclose the method to her husband and new family.[44] The caste system in India limited the development of surgery, since touching another person became taboo and, while the knowledge obviously survived, the higher caste physicians limited themselves to examination of the pulse and tongue. Surgery survived in lower caste practitioners, while Indian physicians shared their European (and modern) colleagues' distaste for surgeons.

Treatment of bladder stone was another surgical procedure that originated in India and, while not described in the Vedic medicine texts after the Susrutha Samhita, was being performed by lower caste practitioners until modern times. The incidence of such stones may have been higher in tropical countries with hot climates and inadequate safe water supplies. Hippocrates requires the physician taking his oath to foreswear performing the procedure. Celsus, in the fourth century CE mentions removing bladder stones with a knife, but provides no other details. The procedure was described in medieval times in Europe but the account in the Susrutha Samhita is identical and suggests the origin of the procedure.

The procedure, as described about 800BCE in the Susrutha Samhita, requires the lithotomist to lubricate the second and third fingers of his left hand with fat and insert them into the patient's anus. The fingers are used to reach the stone, palpable in the bladder through the anterior wall of the rectum, and pull it down as close to the perineum as possible. The knife in his right hand is inserted into the perineum between the anus and scrotum and plunged deep upward, through the prostate, to reach the stone. When the knife had entered the bladder, the stone could be pressed down and out the hole with the left hand. No effort was made to repair the incision and, if the wound did not heal, a urine fistula resulted. There is no description of the procedure in women, which would require a vaginal approach since the uterus would block access to the bladder from the rectum. Perhaps bladder stone did not affect women as frequently since small stones might pass through the shorter female urethra. The procedure, while disdained by physicians (*vaidya*) and the domain of poorly educated lithotomists, persisted until recent times. In spite of the Hippocratic Oath, it was carried to Europe and persisted in the absence of an alternative. The invention of the lithotripter in 1822 by Civiale, and the electrically lighted cystoscope late in the nineteenth century finally provided an alternative treatment.

Sutures, which included needles of bone and bronze and thread made of hair and animal material (similar to our catgut, which comes from sheep intestine "*kitgut*" in Swedish), were used in the Susrutha Samhita. More unusual was the use of large Bengali black ants for suturing intestine. The text describes using the ants to bite the edges of the wound; then, after the edges were approximated by the ants' mandibles, the ant bodies were removed leaving the head and clamped mandibles attached. The ants were used to repair intestine and then the abdomen was closed with sutures. There has been considerable skepticism about the success of such operations in 800BCE since peritonitis complicated almost all such attempts until the development of asepsis late in the nineteenth century. The book does include a description of intussusception, which he called *Baddha Gudodera,* and describes surgical repair including using the ants for intestinal anastomosis. Since the anatomy of the condition is provided it is difficult to refute the claim that abdominal surgery was performed. Pregnancy, conception, and women's diseases are described, including tubal pregnancy. For the performance of surgery he advocated cleanliness even to requiring that surgeons shave their heads.

The early Indian physicians believed that conception resulted from mingling of semen and menstrual blood. The menses represented the release of that blood which had been contained in the uterus during the month (not that far from the truth). Their concept of the function of the uterus was vague and mention was made of a "child's bed" in the female abdomen during pregnancy, but labor was not understood and the Susrutha Samhita attributed the expulsion of the child at the end of pregnancy to "the wind." Fetal development was accurately described and complications of childbirth were considered including a description of manual extraction of a breech birth. In the event of the death of the mother a procedure, later known as "Caesarian Section" because Shakespeare supposed Julius Caesar to have been a product of one, was recommended to save the fetus.

YOGA

Critics of these accounts of advanced medical developments have questioned how "the absolutely pessimistic, inactive, passively enduring religion of Hinduism" could have produced such pioneering achievements. There were several alternatives to the Brahmin dominated Hindu religion, which emphasized passive suffering and karma in hopes of a better life in another incarnation. One alternative emphasized breathing exercises and mind control that resonates with the emphasis on "wind" in early physiological theories of Indian physicians. It is called *yoga* and tablets illustrating typical yoga positions have been found in Mohenjo-daro, the city of the Indus River civilization from the third millennium BCE. The other candidate for the source of medical progress and experimentation was Buddhism and it is clear that, by 300BCE, Buddhist monks and nuns were constructing and staffing hospitals. The Tamils of southern India and Ceylon had their own medical traditions and King Duttha Gamani, on his deathbed in 151BCE, listed among his achievements the building of eighteen hospitals for the poor in Ceylon. The Tamils' practices differed from the Atharvaveda, particularly in the use of metals, such as mercury, in therapy. The legendary founders of *Siddha* (Tamil) medicine were Bogar, who was said to have visited China, and Ramadevar, who was supposed to have visited Mecca and taught the Arabs alchemy. When Buddha died in 483BCE (most likely of a bleeding duodenal ulcer from the description), he left a number of disciples who were physicians, among them Kasyapa who left a list of prescriptions for children's diseases. One of the remedies in his list was garlic and its properties were extensively discussed. The Bower manuscript, discovered in Turkestan in 1890 by an English officer, has been dated to 400CE and lists the prescriptions of Kasyapa.

Rules of behavior for Indian physicians were written down and included many of the same precepts contained in the Hippocratic Oath. An additional precept not contained in the Oath was, "Treat no woman except in the presence of her husband," an indication of Hindu social practices of the time. Students were obligated to swear obedience to the oath just as the students of Hippocrates were said to be. The origins of the great advances of Indian medicine are still obscure, possibly because of the loss of the written records of the Indus River civilization. Still, the great antiquity of the Ayurveda and the later Atharvaveda of Indian medicine, and the surgery of the Susrutha Samhita, are indisputable. Some of the concepts attributed to the Greeks may have had their origin in India.

The Muslim invasion of India brought Arabic medicine and, through the Muslims, the traditions of the Greeks and of Galen. In the eleventh century CE, invasion from Afghanistan and the Turkic speaking region now called Turkmenistan brought medical practices called *Yunani*, an Indian word meaning "Ionian." *Yunani* medicine is derived from Galenical medicine and continues to flourish in India today. Physicians are referred to as *hakims* in rural areas and Persian- and Arabic-speaking people embrace their practices. *Yunani* physicians treat Muslim patients and Ayurvedic physicians treat Hindu patients. The British rule brought western medicine and support for traditional Ayurvedic medical education declined. Indian independence and nationalistic instincts revived the traditional practices, but most Ayurvedic physicians in India today use modern drugs, especially antibiotics. Research on Ayurvedic herbal remedies has been limited, but a RAND Corporation study has suggested that a number of these therapies are effective in lowering the blood sugar in diabetics.[45]

CHINA

Chinese medicine is marked by a profound conservatism that persisted until the nineteenth century when it was forced to confront western medicine and science. Bloodletting evolved into acupuncture and elements were added from other cultures over the centuries. Buddhism brought Indian medicine and the construction of hospitals. The concept of "hot" and "cold" in Chinese medicine may represent transplants from Ayurvedic theories of disease, and drugs were imported from many other cultures.

THE DYNASTIES

The development of early China can be traced to the Shang Dynasty when written language using characters similar to modern ideograms is found. This began as pictographic writing, much as hieroglyphics began, and progressed to ideograms. Neolithic sites are found near the junction of the Wei and Yellow rivers that date back to about 6000BCE. The dynasty is thought to have begun about 1765BCE and traditions basic to Chinese civilization, such as ancestor worship, appear. Astronomy, the calendar, arithmetic and writing all seem to have developed independently during this period. The forces of *yin* and *yang* and the *Tao*, the world spirit, all appear in writing from the Shang Dynasty period. The dynasty was overthrown in 1027BCE by the succeeding Chou (or Tzou) Dynasty, which introduced a feudal system. The last Shang emperor, Chou Sin, was said to have invented chopsticks and his wife Ta-ki was a "model of licentiousness and cruelty."

The new Chou Dynasty rulers seem to have been monotheist or worshipers of nature, recognizing their king as a "Son of Heaven." They retained the Shang priests and raised them to the status of "scholars" or sages. The first books of ancient China were written during this period and the concept of humours, or elements, appear here. They were five in number and consisted of wood, fire, earth, metal and water. In addition to this variation on the theme of classical Greece and the nature of matter, the Chinese added a series of five element systems. There were five directions, five planets, five seasons, five times of day, five colors and tones, five flavors, and five human relationships: father to son, man to woman, older to younger brother, official to prince, and friend to friend. An effort to reduce mysteries of the world to fixed systems is reminiscent of some Greek theorizing, but it became more rigid in China. The Chou Dynasty descended into civil war between feudal princes (the number of feudal principalities declined from 1,700 to fifty-five during this period, mostly because of conquest) and society became less secure. In 551BCE the scholar K'ung Fu-tsu, known to the West as Confucius, was born. He spent his life trying to restore order by teaching a life of virtue, especially to rulers. He credited Kuan Chung, the chief minister of Ts' I (the greatest of the principalities) with making civilized people of the Chinese (still not known by that term). The population of China about this time was large enough to support several armies of one million men (the "Warring States Period" 421 to 401 BCE).

Another group from the same period were disciples of a man called Lao~Tse (that is not his real name, it means "Old Master") who emphasized a turning away from squabbles and disorder by submission to an active spirit world. Taoism emphasized a submission to fate that persisted in Chinese civilization. These doctrines, while perhaps providing comfort to their disciples, did nothing to stabilize the Chou Dynasty, which was swept away by the Prince of Chin in 221BCE. He established many standards, such as language, weights and measures, and the gauge of wagon wheels, and destroyed the feudal system. The caravan routes to India were established about this time. Merchants supplanted the nobles at court and *Shih Huang Ti*, "The Sublime Emperor of China"- the title he assumed, rejected the philosophy of Confucius ordering the burning of all books except those about agriculture, medicine and soothsaying. He began the Great Wall, but his Empire lasted only five years after his death in 210BCE.

Civil war resumed until the peasant General Kao Tsu defeated his rivals and began the Han Dynasty. The bourgeois upper class derived from the merchants of the Chin period retained their status and, for four centuries, stability survived. This is the era of the movie *Crouching Tiger, Hidden Dragon*. The rule of China was extended over areas that comprise modern China including Korea, Manchuria, Annam (Vietnam) and Turkestan. The great emperor Wu Ti is credited with much of this expansion during his long reign from 140 to 87BCE. During the Han Dynasty, the casting of iron was accomplished, a technological feat that would not appear in Europe until the fourteenth century. The iron plow, made with wrought iron that does not require the high temperatures needed for casting, was in use in China in the sixth century BCE. Other advanced technology appeared in China at this time, including the draw loom, capable of weaving complicated patterns in silk and cotton. In 100CE, Tsai Lun is credited with the invention of paper, using tree bark as his raw material. There is more recent evidence that paper was in use at an even earlier time.[46] The horse collar, which would revolutionize European agriculture in the Middle Ages was invented in China about 250BCE, although improvement in rice culture would gradually move the population south and reduce the use of animal power in agriculture.[47]

A combination of official corruption, high taxes, and hostile invaders from the steppes, which the Great Wall could not keep out, brought about the fall of the Han Dynasty in 221CE. A medical text and autobiography of a physician exists from this period, written by Ko Hung (*pao-p'u tzu wai p'ien*)[48] The author is a follower of Confucius, uses the term *tao* as a synonym for God, and writes of "five chords" on a lute and "six breaths" in nature. *Yin* and *yang* are discussed and the uses of medicine and alchemy are included. This era was the end of ancient China and 580 years of turmoil followed. The great written works of ancient China, those that escaped the wrath of Shih Huang Ti, give us the portrait of this ancient dynastic period. The population of China actually declined after the fall of the Han Dynasty from a high of about sixty million. There is a school of thought that epidemics, like those that afflicted Rome, contributed to the downfall of the Han Dynasty. Like Rome, China had developed an active trading economy and may have paid the price for being a pioneer.[49] The more immediate cause was the invasion by Tatars that devastated the northern and western areas for centuries.

CHINESE SCIENCE

In spite of this turmoil, scientific progress continued. Rice cultivation expanded and fed the rapidly increasing population, although wet field methods resulted in serious problems with parasite infestations, especially schistosomiasis. The rice culture was enabled by great advances in hydraulic engineering. Between the tenth and fifteenth centuries, water control projects increased seven-fold while population doubled.[50] Wang Chen published a massive *Treatise on Agriculture* in 1313 and included 300 detailed illustrations of implements and techniques. The Chinese were making cast iron bells, a method that eluded Western science until the last century. The spinning wheel arrived in China at the same time as it did in Europe (about the thirteenth century), but progressed more rapidly in China. The vertical water-wheel was in use in 1280. The Chinese never did develop mechanical clocks but a sophisticated water-clock was constructed by Su Sung in 1086 that surpassed anything available in Europe. The compass was invented in China about 960CE, and Chinese ships were built using the carvel planking method (planked side-to-side on frames and caulked to make water-tight). The rudder was a Chinese invention and their ships had water-tight compartments to prevent sinking. Chinese ships explored the sea and there have been recent reports that they discovered America in the 1400s.[51]

THE END OF INNOVATION

The rise of the Ming Dynasty, which overthrew the Mongol Empire in 1368, put an end to Chinese progress in science and exploration. Shipyards were closed and ships with more than two masts were banned in 1430. Progress in textile manufacture stopped and nothing like the English spinning jenny, that created the modern industrial revolution in England, was developed. By the mid-nineteenth century thirty-five percent of silk exported from China was in the form of raw silk, not fabric. Movable type was invented in 1045 by Pi Shêng but wooden block printing continued until modern times. The Chinese invented gunpowder, but never constructed guns. Even after Portugese traders introduced muskets in the fourteenth century, the Chinese purchased them from westerners and did not develop an arms industry as the Japanese did. China adopted some new crops from North America, like the sweet potato and the peanut, but dry land staples like corn and potatoes were ignored for the most part. The original pioneers of metallurgy, by 1700, were unable to construct simple devices introduced by Europeans because of the cost of metal. A great technical encyclopedia, *Thien Kung Khai Wu* (Exploitation of the Works of Nature), written by Sung Ying Hsing in 1637, was destroyed because of official displeasure and is known only through a Japanese reprint. The most popular theory is that China was ruled by very conservative dynasties after the fourteenth century which prized stability over innovation. Europe suffered religious wars and similar levels of intolerance from rulers, but was divided into small states that competed with one another and offered refuge for persecuted rabble rousers. The emigration of the Huguenots to England, after the revocation of the Edict of Nantes in 1685, sent thousands of Protestant potential inventers to England. There was no equivalent refuge for Chinese.[52]

CHINESE MEDICAL WRITINGS

The oldest medical work dates from the Chou period and consists of a long list of useful herbs called the *Shen Nung Pen Tsao*. The earliest copy of this huge work (fifty-two volumes and 1,892 drugs) was published in 1597CE but it was compiled in ancient times. Han Dynasty documents refer to it and it probably dates from the Chou period. Another ancient work dates from about 2600BCE and consists of a dialogue between the Emperor

Huang Ti (2698 to 2598BCE, long before the Shang dynasty) and his minister, Ch'i Po. Its title translates to *"Huang Ti's Teachings Concerning the Insides"*. It is also referred to as *The Yellow Emperor's Inner Canon of Medicine,* its more common title.[53] Other information comes from the Shang Dynasty where flat pieces of bone, oracle bones resembling the Greek pottery shards called ostrakon, are found with inscriptions that appear to be prayers to gods for relief from illness (and for other reasons). Some diseases are recognizable and malaria, leprosy, typhoid fever, cholera, and plague all seem to be present in these ancient prayers for relief. Eastern Mongolia has always been a location of plague and may be the original site of this disease's jump to the human species.[54] The existence of these oracular bones suggests that disease was attributed to gods and relief was sought by prayer. There are a few accounts of physicians in the Chou and Han Dynasties and one document describes the consequences of failure, at least in the case of failed treatment of a high official. The physician was executed. A physician of the Han Dynasty, T'ai I Ling, was described as chief physician of the court and received a salary of 600 to 1,000 bearer loads of rice per year. One early remedy, soy flour poultices, may represent an early use of the antibiotic properties of yeast.[55]

The early objective accounts of anatomy and disease give way in later years to very stylized and inaccurate descriptions, many of which seem influenced by cosmological speculations and a lack of observation. Dissection of a human body is not described until 1145CE and anatomy seemed to be ignored until very recent times. It is possible that ancestor worship prohibited violation of the corpse of dead patients. The only account of dissection was that of a prisoner put to death and perhaps without family. An example of the cosmological speculations influencing Chinese medicine is the five-element theory. Since the world was composed of five elements, there were five chief organs, the yin organs: the heart, liver, lung, kidney and spleen. Then there were five auxiliary organs, the yang organs: the large intestine, small intestine, gall bladder, stomach, and bladder. The relationship of these organs between each other was influenced by the relationship of the elements. The kidney, as the organ of water, must be antagonistic to the heart since that was the organ of fire. Each organ had a specific planet and season. The heart had a relationship with summer. The interplay between *yin* and *yang*, concepts going back to the Shang Dynasty, were important as was the role of Tao, the world spirit. The world spirit entered the body with air, through the lungs, and earth, through food taken into the intestines. It moved through a system of arteries and nerves that do not correspond to human anatomy. Note the absence of the brain in the list of important organs. When the sympathetic and parasympathetic nervous systems were discovered in the nineteenth century some speculated that the forces of *yin* and *yang* had correlated with these pathways.

An early Chinese medical text was attributed to Pien Ch'io, a famous physician of the fifth or sixth century BCE. He traveled extensively and was very successful treating diseases of women and children. His book, *Nan Ching*, survived even though he was assassinated by a jealous rival. Professional jealousy began early. Examination of the pulse was given great weight in diagnosing illness, much as the Romans did, and external signs of internal disease eventually became so fantastic that the ear was thought to indicate kidney disease and the lips, disease of the spleen. Skin color was thought to be a reliable source of information about internal disease, as it is in some cases, and the pulse became so important to physicians that the sex of a fetus was predicted by the quality of the mother's pulse in the left wrist. The pulse of the left wrist was divided into segments from proximal to distal and each segment indicated another organ.

The same was true of the other wrist and other parts of the body. The cause of any disease indicated by the nature of the pulse was, of course, due to an excess of *yin* or *yang*. These sites of interest began with pulses but later physicians adopted them as sites for acupuncture. The cosmology continued to influence the practice of acupuncture as certain days were unsatisfactory for treatment. For example, it was forbidden to acupuncture the thigh on the third day of the month and, on the sixteenth day, the chest. The Inner Canon described the "Eight Rubrics," which are the theoretical model of etiology of disease. There are four sets of polar opposites: inner-outer, cold-hot, depletion-repletion, and *yin-yang*. There is some similarity here to the Pythagorean concept of opposites in disease.

There were other ancient texts. The Inner Canon was the first and remained the most important for centuries, already described. *The Canon of Problems* is a later work that addresses eighty-one difficult "issues" from the earlier writing, mostly concerning needling treatment and diagnosis. It was considered an adjunct to the Inner Canon although after the Song Dynasty (960-1279CE) conflicts were generally resolved by adhering to the older work. The teachings of the Inner Canon were divided by core subject: the circulation of *qi*, a concept somewhat like the Greek *pneuma*, dominated the physiological constitution of the body It translates as "air," "vapors," or "energy." A buildup of *qi* results in life, its dissipation leads to death. Within the body, *qi* has two components: the *yang* element represents the capacity for action and transformation and is referred to as *yang qi*. The *yin* component, called *xue* (literally blood), represents the capacity

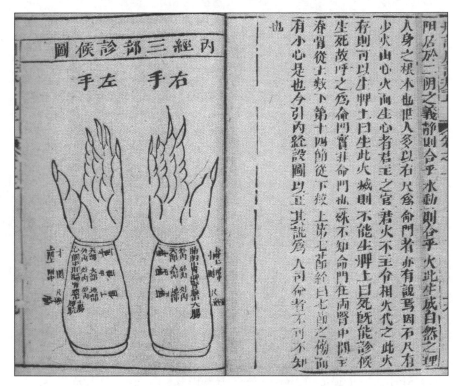

Figure 4 – Pulse chart from 6th century BCE by Pien Ch'iao.

for circulation, nourishment, and growth. Another vital substance called *jing* (essence) includes the nourishment from food plus the reproductive powers and substances, including semen, necessary for procreation.

The *Treatise on Cold-Damage Disorders* deals with the diagnosis and remedy of diseases caused by external cold factors (*shanghan bing*), what western medicine would call infectious fevers. The theory of disease contained in this work is known as the "Six Warps Theory," and treatment is by medication, not needling. In the twelfth century CE Chinese physicians began to distinguish another cause of these diseases and called it *wenre bing*, "heat-factor disorders." A series of epidemics in the seventeenth century CE led to dissatisfaction with the cold-damage theory and the heat-damage theory gained adherents. A later work on this subject was *Wenre lun*, by Ye Tianshi which proposed a "triple burner" system (*san jiao*) to classify the heat-damage diseases. The cold-damage theory postulated pathogenic *qi* which entered the body through nose and mouth and which, in some cases like smallpox and tuberculosis, could be communicated by contact. Here at least, even though burdened with cosmological speculation and clumsy theory, was a concept of infectious disease. In Europe up to the Renaissance "malaria" meant "bad air" and "consumption" was caused by mysterious elements not transmitted from others.

Chinese concepts of anatomy were stylized and did not correspond to human anatomy, as we know it. The "triple burner," for example, was a supposed anatomical structure that has no equivalent in human anatomy. The absence of dissection or any experimental analysis allowed these theoretical speculations to become more and more convoluted until the original grains of real knowledge in Chinese medicine were submerged by traditions that had no basis in science.

Early Chinese pharmacology begins with the *Shen Nung Pen Tsao*, which dates from the Chou Dynasty. A copy of this ancient work is found in a collection of drug recipes published in 1597CE by Li Shih~chen, a government official who spent twenty-six years cataloging the traditional knowledge of herbs and drugs. His work is titled *Pen Tsao Kang Mu*, ("Classification of Roots and Herbs"). Even here, Chinese cosmology influenced classification with drugs being divided into five categories. Red medicine is like fire and was therefore used to treat the heart, which is also fiery. The upper parts of plants are used to treat the upper parts of the body (A somewhat similar theory persisted in European medicine and is called the "doctrine of signatures." It will be discussed later). In spite of these fantastic speculations about theoretical functions, a number of the drugs listed have important pharmacological effects and were even used appropriately in illness. The dichotomy is reminiscent of the divide between the Theorists and the Empiricists of Alexandrine medicine.

In the second millennium BCE, a physician named Ma Hung recommended a drug derived from the Chinese joint fir, *Ephedra sinica*, as a remedy for cough and lung ailments. In 1887, the Japanese scientist Nagai extracted the drug ephedrine from this herbal remedy. Ephedrine, of course, is a widely used drug in respiratory diseases today and is a very common component of many herbal remedies. The Chinese used metallic mercury in the treatment of ulcers and copper sulfate solution to treat eye infection. Treatment of malaria used a plant alkaloid, *Dichroa fibrifuga*, which has been found to have some effect on the organism although it is not as effective as quinine. *Pien hsu*, an extract of knotgrass, was used as a remedy for lung diseases and it has been found to contain silicic acid, an active pharmacological agent. Chaulmoogra oil was used as a remedy for leprosy and this drug has been found to be effective against the mycobacterium responsible. The ginseng root was probably the most popular Chinese drug until recent times and was especially prized for effects on sexual function and fatigue. Modern analysis has identified many active ingredients of this substance, which continues to be used in herbal remedies. Randomized clinical trials have not shown significant beneficial effect, although there is some evidence of male sexual effects. The name is a derivation of *gin*, the Chinese term for "man" and *seng*, the term for "essence". There is a serious "ginseng abuse syndrome," among users of herbal medicines, involving hypertension, sleeplessness, and agitation.

SMALLPOX AND SURGERY

Smallpox was present in ancient China and was called the "flower of heaven." It seems to have arrived after the earliest suspected epidemics in the West, so the origin may have been somewhere between Greece and China. Epidemiology studies of viral diseases suggest that smallpox, having no animal reservoir, required the dense population of India and China. Its appearance in Europe followed the increase in population needed to provide an adequate number of susceptible subjects.[56] Several paintings depict the disease and a form of immunization was practiced. Court physicians recognized that the disease did not occur again in those who had survived one episode. There is some evidence that, by the tenth century CE, physicians, anticipating Jenner by seven centuries, induced immunity by having patients inhale the dust from a pulverized scab taken from a smallpox lesion.[57] We now know that the smallpox virus is transmitted this way in the disease. Thus, in spite of an irrational theoretical understanding of disease, China developed effective therapy for a few conditions.[58] Certainly, variolation, similar to that introduced to Europe by Paracelsus, was being performed by the sixteenth century CE.[59]

No similar development of surgery occurred and the sophisticated understanding of surgical procedures present in India seems not to have crossed the borders with the Buddhists. The only surgeon found in early Chinese history was Hua To who performed an operation to remove an arrow from the arm of General Kuan Yun. The same surgeon is later described in another incident. A prince named Tsao Tsao was suffering from severe headaches and called upon Hua To for relief. The surgeon recommended trephination of the skull to relieve the headaches. Just as he was about to proceed, his patient, Tsao Tsao, was seized with suspicion and accused the surgeon of conspiring to murder him in league with enemies. The luckless surgeon was arrested and, in 265CE, executed at the prince's order. This surgeon, who is unique in Chinese history, had authored many works on medicine and surgery. He requested that they be destroyed before his execution and this was done. The Chinese opposition to "mutilation" of the body seems to have prevented any development of surgery similar to that in India and this surgeon is the only one to appear in nearly two thousand years of Chinese history. Possibly, he was not Chinese in origin and may have been an Indian surgeon who came to China with the Buddhists.

ACUPUNCTURE

The oldest existing catalogue of insertion points for acupuncture needles, the *Ling shu* in the Inner Canon, dates from 100BCE but the points are named in earlier works. By the second century CE, there were 365 points and the number grew. The needles, once inserted, are twirled and vibrated. The basis of the practice, which may have developed from bloodletting, is the Taoist doctrine of *qi* and its circulation. The points are located on fourteen invisible lines or meridians running the length of the body. Points on those meridians control certain physical conditions. All disease is an imbalance in energy flow and the needles restore and balance *qi*. Moxibustion is a technique, related to acupuncture, of burning small pellets of dried wormwood at points on the skin. Physical contact between physician and patient was kept to a minimum and female patients might be concealed behind a screen communicating with the physician through servants or a husband. Carved figurines were often used, especially with females, to indicate the location of symptoms. These ivory figurines, often anatomically correct, can be found in museums and antique shops. Physical examination was minimal except for the pulse and often the eyes and tongue.

The physician could be a Confucian healer, known as *ruyi*, who studied medical arts as a scholar and was respected as such. Another tradition was that of a hereditary physician or *shiyi* who came from a family of physicians and whose training included apprenticeship as well as book learning. There was no profession as we know it although the state did give examinations for state medical officers. Women served as midwives and wet nurses, but were of low status. Religious healing was very prominent up to the present time in China in spite of the People's Republic's attitude towards religion. The earliest hospitals were established by Buddhist monasteries and, in the ninth century, the Tang Dynasty nationalized them and thereafter assumed the responsibility of maintaining them. The Song and Yuan Dynasties continued state interest in medical matters and the compilation of a *materia medica* and government pharmacies and clinics were developed.

Chinese medicine continued virtually unchanged from the Han Dynasty until the nineteenth century. The reasons for this have been the subject of speculation. One clue may be found in the Inner Canon. The Yellow

Emperor tells his minister: "The human body is the counterpart of a state...The spirit [the body's governing vitalities, *shen*] is like the monarch; the blood *xue* is like the ministers; the *que* is like the people. Thus, we know that one who keeps his own body in order can keep a state in order." This mixing of health and philosophy is seen in Hippocrates but remains a dominant force in Chinese society. The Chinese emperors kept Europeans away from Chinese people and there was almost no contact with western science.

Japan had more contact with westerners and Dutch scholarship which, after the eighteenth century, introduced western medicine. Smallpox vaccination was introduced to Japan in 1824 and schools of western medicine appeared. The Japanese Meiji government adopted the German system of medical education in 1869 and western style medical schools were common in Japan by 1900. China was exposed to western medicine by missionaries after 1860 and the Chinese Medical Missionary Association, founded in 1886, tried to introduce western medicine. The weak Quing Dynasty was unable to control the situation as the Meiji rulers did in Japan. By 1913, there were still only 500 Chinese students studying western medicine. The Communist government in the 1950s was very short of western-style medical practitioners and a renewed emphasis on traditional Chinese healing resulted. "Barefoot doctors" were encouraged to practice acupuncture and use traditional *materia medica*.

39   Recent developments in Hindu nationalism have led to revision of history books in India. The Indus River civilization is now being called the "Indus-Saraswati civilization" and this seems to be an attempt to include the Vedic civilization as part of the older culture. The Saraswati River is an ancient river important in Hindu myth. See the New York Times, December 30, 2002.

     See also: Akshaya Mukul, "Jagmohan announces team of experts to trace Saraswati river," *The Times of India*, June 15, 2002.

40   Dharmendra, "Leprosy in Ancient Indian Medicine," *International Journal of Leprology* 15:424-430 (1947).

41   Samuel Mark has recently pointed out that leprous changes in bone have been discovered in Egypt from about 200 BCE. "Alexander the Great, Seafaring, and the Spread of Leprosy," *Journal of the History of Medicine* 57:285 (2002).

42   E.V. Hulse, "Leprosy and Ancient Egypt," *The Lancet* (September 23, 1972) page 659.

43   AB Vaidya, TG Rajagopalan, et al., "Treatment of Parkinson's Disease with the Cowhage plant – *Mucuna pruriens* Bak," *Neurology (India)* 26:171-6 (1978).

44   David J Brain, "The Indian contribution to rhinoplasty," *The Journal of Laryngology and Otology* 102:689-693 (1988). This article includes an example of a modern case of nose amputation and the text of the letter of 1794 that alerted the European world to the method.

45   *Ayurvedic Interventions for Diabetes Mellitus: A Systematic Review.* Summary, Evidence Report/Technology Assessment: Number 41. AHRQ Publication No. 01-E039 (June 2001).

46   Tsien Tsuen-Hsuin, *Paper and Printing.* In *Science and Civilization in China* Volume 5, Ed. Joseph Needham, Cambridge University Press (1985).

47   Joel Mokyr, *The Lever of Riches,* pages 209-218, Oxford Press (1990).

48   James R Ware translation, *Alchemy, Medicine, and Religion in the China of A.D. 320,* The MIT Press (1966).

49   William H. McNeil, *Plagues and Peoples,* New York (1976).

50   Dwight H. Perkins, *Agricultural Development in China, 1368-1968,* University of Chicago Press (1969).

51   Gavin Menzies, 1421: *The Year China Discovered the World,* Bantam/Transworld (2002). Menzies is a retired Royal Navy officer and his book has been discredited by scholars who point out that the voyage was possible but no mention of America can be found in original Chinese records.

52   Joel Mokyr, pages 220-231.

53   Ilza Veith Translation, *Huang Ti Nei Ching Su Wên* (The Yellow Emperor's Classic of Internal Medicine), The Williams and Wilkins Company (1949).

54   Achtman M, Zurth K, Morelli G, Torrea G, Guiyole A, Carniel E *"Yersinia pestis,* the cause of plague, is a recently emerged clone of *Yersinia pseudotuberculosis" Proceedings of the National. Academy of Sciences.* USA 96:14043-14048(1999).

55   F Marti-Ibanez, See Chapter 2.

56   Donald A. Henderson, "The Eradication of Smallpox," *Scientific American,* (October 1976), page 25.

57   Frederick F Cartwright & Michael Biddiss, *Disease & History,* page 71, Sutton Publishing (1972).

58   Jurgen Thorwald, *Science and Secrets of Early Medicine,* p 245 , Harcourt, Brace and World (1962).

59   K.C. Leung, *Guoshi shilun* ("Collection of essays on Chinese history"), quoted in Kiple, the *Cambridge World History of Human Disease,* p359 (1993).

5
The Rise of Islam and Arabic Medicine

THE EMPIRE OF JUSTINIAN WAS BESET BY TWO HUNDRED YEARS OF bubonic plague, which destroyed the confidence of the Greek civilization, and then a new religion appeared when the Byzantine Empire was at its weakest. Muhammad was born a poor orphan in 570CE, a member of the Quraysh tribe of Mecca. He became a successful merchant, however, and when he was forty the *Qur'an* was revealed to him in a series of visions. He assumed the mantle of prophet in a line going back to Adam and Noah. In 622, he fled an assassination plot and took up residence in Medina. By the time of his death in 632, all of Arabia had adopted the faith of Islam. A century later, Islam had spread to all of North Africa, Persia, and southern Spain. The Jews and Christians were tolerated as "people of the book" *(ahl al-Kitab)* until the Crusades ended the era of amity.

Greek and Galenical medicine were the basis of pre-Islamic medical beliefs, although animist spirits and magical forces were also important. The *jinn*, an evil spirit, and *al-'ayn*, the evil eye, were important sources of illness. The *jinn* (plural *jinni* as in "genie") were lesser spirits and could be bargained with or even killed. They could bring good luck, as genies often did in the "Arabian Nights" of Scheherazade, but they were often to blame for fevers and children's diseases. The *Qur'an* has almost nothing to say about medicine except for attributing healing power to honey.[60] The indigenous medicine of the people, including the magical origins of illness, persisted under Islam. In the seventh and eighth centuries, the developing orthodoxy of Islam began to conflict with traditional medicine. The *hadith*, the "Sayings of the Prophet" began to acquire traditions concerning the powers of the evil eye and the healing powers of water from the well of Zamzam in Mecca.[61] The continuing epidemics of plague constituted a problem since the teachings of Islam asserted that "God sends down no malady without also sending down with it a cure." The traditional attribution of epidemics to *jinni* conflicted with this teaching and some folk practices were suppressed.

ARABIC MEDICINE

The origin of the distinctive Arab-Islamic medicine occurred in the ninth century with the establishment by the Abbasid caliphs, in 832CE, of the *Bayt al-Hikma*, a center of scholarship where ancient texts were translated into Arabic. The death of Muhammad had been followed by the reign of several companions, whose usurpation over his son-in-law Ali led to the great schism in Islam between the Shï'a and the Sunni. The Meccan clan of Umayya held the caliphate from 644 to 747CE. In that year a revolution led by a freed Persian slave, Abu Muslim, overthrew the Umayyids. The Abbasids who succeeded to the caliphate were Persian and moved the capital from Syria, where the Arabs had placed it, to Iraq. The new capital was named *Madinat al-Salim* (City of Peace), but was called Baghdad after the ancient village on which the new city was built.

The "age of translations," (800 to 833) was one manifestation of the flowering of scholarship and the cosmopolitan atmosphere of Harun al Rashid's new capital of Baghdad. Most of the translations were performed by Christians who were skilled in Greek and Syriac. The main figure was Hunayn ibn Ishaq, a Nestorian Christian known in the West as Johannitius. He was born in Iraq in the town of al-Hira and traveled to the Byzantine Empire in search of Galen's works. He was said to walk the streets of Baghdad reciting Homer in Greek and was prolific in his scholarship. With his students, he translated 129 works of Galen into Arabic providing more copies in Arabic than survive in Greek. With official support from Harun al-Rashid and his son al-Ma'mum, who ruled until 833, hundreds of Greek texts were translated into elegant and accurate Arabic preserving most of the Greek literature for posterity. Galen became the father figure for Arabic medicine, but Hippocrates' works were also translated and preserved in commentaries. The translation movement continued into the eleventh century and revived learned medicine. The Greek works to be translated included medicine, mathematics, astronomy, pharmacology, geography, and agronomy. History, poetry and drama were not deemed worthy of preservation being the works of pagans and of no interest to Islam; thus these treasures were lost. Hunayn authored his own text on diseases of the eye, *Kitah al-'ashr maqalat fi l-'ayn*, ("Book of the Ten Treatises on the Eye"). The supreme achievement of Arab-Islamic medicine was the medical compendia, a synthesis of ancient and more recent work. The first of the great compendia was *Firdaws al-hikma* ("Paradise of Wisdom" c. 850) by Rabban al-Tabari, an Islamic convert who wrote for the Caliph al-Muttawakkil, summarizing not only Persian and Arabic translations of ancient Greek classics, but Indian work as well. Later compendia tended to ignore the Indian works, and the Greek tradition dominated.

ARABS AND MATHEMATICS

Mohammed ibn-Musa al-Khwarizmi (Khwarizm, his birthplace, is modern Khiva in central Asia) was born before 800CE. He was a mathematician and astronomer in Baghdad's "House of Wisdom." He is credited with the introduction of the Indian numerals and the decimal system. The Latin translation of his book, *De numero indorum* ("Concerning the Hindu Art of Reckoning") erroneously attributed the numerals to him, hence our term "Arabic numbers." The notation also became known as "al-Khwarizmi" and then "algorismi," leading to our modern term "algorithm," although the current meaning, a rule of procedure or operation, as in computer programming, is different from the original meaning which was simply the use of the new numerals. In 830CE he wrote *al-Kitab al-mukhtasar fi hisab al-jabir wa'l-muqabalah* ("The Compendious Book on Calculation by Completion and Balancing"). The section on what we now call "algebra" was titled *al-jabr wa'l muqabala*, (*al-jabr* means "completion" or "restoration" and *muqabalah* means "balancing" suggesting that simplification by canceling like terms on both sides of the equal sign is the practice intended). For this reason he is credited with the invention of algebra, although similar mathematical practices can be identified back to the Babylonians. The name of the mathematical system does take its name from his book. He also contributed some simple calculus and a trigonometric table of sine functions. He died in 847CE.[62]

AL-RAZI

One of the greatest Muslim physicians was a Persian named Muhammad ibn Zakariya al-Razi who was known in the West as Rhazes. He lived from 865 to 925 and was author of 200 treatises on medicine. He developed a medical philosophy and his book *al-Tibb al-ruhani* asserted that reason was the ultimate authority and should govern medical thinking. Another book, *Fi'l Shukuk 'ala Jalinius* (which translates as "Doubts about Galen") contains criticism of Galen, although he still declares himself to be Galen's disciple. Still, in another of his books, he states, "he who studies the works of the ancients, gains the experience of their labor," but, in another passage, he writes, "All that is written in books is worth much less than the experience of a wise doctor." Al-Razi was the first to describe the differences between exanthems in *al-Jadari wa'l-hasha* (Smallpox and Measles). He wrote, "physical signs of measles are nearly the same as those of smallpox, but nausea and inflammation are more severe, though the pains in the back are less." He considered measles to be a more severe disease, possibly indicating that changes in the behavior of the two diseases have occurred since then. He described the use of Plaster of Paris (heated gypsum powder that is mixed with water and rapidly hardens without shrinking) for immobilization of fractures and gave its formula. His great book was translated into Latin in 1279 as *Liber Continens* and became a reference work in the West for centuries. No copy of his work survives in Arabic, a commentary on the decline to come.

Al-Razi became famous especially in the Latin West. His fame derived from more than his medical writings. He is known to have written an encyclopedia on music and he was a poet, as were many Arabic writers. He was the second great Arabic mathematician and chemist, after Jabir ibn-Hayyan. Al-Razi described the glassware and instruments of alchemy, which would remain the standard equipment of chemists until the nineteenth century. He described the processes of distillation, sublimation (solid to vapor), calcination (powdering of solids), and solution. He classified substances and was the first to use the categories of animal, vegetable, and mineral in describing matter. He described the use of sal ammoniac (ammonium chloride) and conducted sophisticated experiments, which have been duplicated in modern times so thorough are his descriptions. Having become famous in his home city of Rayy, near Teheran, Al-Razi was invited to Baghdad to head the new hospital, *al-Mu'tadidi* where he became embroiled in a misadventure concerning alchemy. He wrote a treatise on the transmutation of base metals to gold and presented it to the Emir of Khorassan. The Emir was intrigued and summoned al-Razi to conduct a public demonstration of his procedure. Al-Razi hedged, telling the Emir that the apparatus would cost a fortune. The Emir provided a thousand pieces of gold and demanded a demonstration. On the appointed day the Emir arrived with his copy of the book so that he could follow the procedure exactly. After hours of fumbling produced nothing that even resembled gold, the Emir became enraged and beat al-Razi over the head with the book. This is said to have caused the blindness that left him in poverty during his declining years although glaucoma is also a possibility. He died in his seventies and, in spite of his failure as an alchemist; he was one of the great scientists of the Arab world.

AVICENNA

Fifty years after the death of al-Razi the greatest medical figure of the Arab world was born in Persia. Abu Ali al-Husayn ibn 'Abdallah ibn Sina (known to the West as Avicenna) was born the son of a Persian tax collector. He was said to have memorized the *Qur'an* at the age of ten and was practicing medicine at sixteen. In his active life, he held positions as a jurist, a teacher of philosophy, an administrator and a physician. In his autobiography, he boasts that his writing was done on horseback during military campaigns, in hiding, in prison, and even after drinking bouts. The result was two hundred and seventy titles with two huge works, one on science (*Kitab al-Shifa*) and the other on medicine (*Kitab al-Qanun*). *Kitab al-Qanun* (the "Medical Code") has chapters on the legacies of Hippocrates and Galen, plus later additions from the Alexandrine schools and earlier Arab physicians. It begins with the theory of the elements and goes on to discuss physiology and diseases. The *materia medica* portion lists 760 drugs along with their preparation and use. A third section covers specific diseases and includes some discussion of anatomy. Other sections describe generalized diseases, fevers, poisons, and even obesity.

The *Qanun* became the authoritative medical text for centuries and remains influential in Islam today. His status in the West was described by Dante who ranked him with Hippocrates and Galen. Avicenna made significant contributions to science aside from medicine. One, which won him few friends, was his skepticism about alchemy. He also proposed that a body remains in the same place, or continues to move at the same speed, unless acted upon by an outside force. This is Newton's First Law of Motion six hundred years before Newton's birth. Avicenna also wrote that, without motion, time had no meaning. If everything was at rest or moving at the same speed, time was meaningless. Albert Einstein was to arrive at the same conclusion in 1905. Avicenna's life was influenced by the political events of his time. He fell from favor as vizier to the Shah of Persia and was forced to flee for his life. When the Shah became ill and court physicians despaired, Avicenna was recalled and the Shah recovered (for which recovery, of course, Avicenna claimed credit). Later, the Shah was defeated in war and Avicenna was considered by the victors to be booty in spite of the fact that he had been directing the Shah's war effort. He died in 1037, probably by poison, but his works became progressively more famous and his pharmacopoeia was the most influential medical text in Europe until the nineteenth century.

ALBUCASIS

These two bodies of work, that of al-Razi and that of Avicenna, dominated medicine and science until almost modern times. Neither reached beyond Galen in theory and other Arabic writers criticized the lack of anatomy.

Abu'l-Qasim Khalaf ibn Abbas al Zahrawi, born in Cordova in 936, (and known in the West as Albucasis) wrote a compendium title *The Recourse of Him Who Cannot Compose a Medical Work of His Own* (a play on Avicenna's works) which covered surgery, neglected by al-Razi and Avicenna. He described cauterization, widely practiced in Islamic countries, surgery (cutting) for stone, and setting fractures. Al-Zahrawi also described and provided drawings of 200 surgical instruments, many of which he designed. He is the only Arabic author who seems to have had any practical experience with surgery.

MAIMONIDES

Rabbi Moshe ben Maimun (1135-1204), known as Moses Maimonides, was another prominent Spanish Arabic writer, although a Jew. A fanatical Muslim ruling group, the Almohads, Berber zealots, forced him into exile in 1148. He settled in Fez, but then moved on to Egypt where, in 1174, he was appointed court physician to Saladin, sultan of Egypt and Syria (and conqueror of the Crusaders). Maimonides was a polymath like al-Razi and wrote a major religious work, *Mishneh Torah*, plus ten medical works in Arabic. He commented on Hippocrates and Galen and was critical of Galen on biblical grounds. His most famous work was *Regimen of Health* which contained many bits of advice on such topics as constipation.

IBN AL-NAFÎS

Ala-al-Din Abu al-Hasan Ali Ibn Abi al-Hazm al-Qarshi al-Dimashqi (known as Ibn Al-Nafis) was born in 1213CE in Damascus. He was educated at the Medical College Hospital (*Bimaristan Al-Noori*) founded by Noor al-Din Al-Zanki. In 1236 Ibn Nafis moved to Egypt and worked in Al-Nassri Hospital then in Al-Mansouri Hospital where he became chief of physicians and the Sultan's personal physician. When he died in 1288CE he donated his house, library, and clinic to the Mansuriya Hospital. He was childless and the last of the great Arabic physicians. His principle contribution was the correct description of the pulmonary circulation.[63]

In 1924 an Egyptian physician, Dr. Muhyo Al-Deen Altawi, discovered a script titled, *Commentary on the Anatomy of Canon of Avicenna* in the Prussian state library in Berlin while studying the history of Arab Medicine at the medical faculty of Albert Ludwig's University in Germany. In this book is found the following: "...The blood from the right chamber of the heart must arrive at the left chamber, but there is no direct pathway between them. The thick septum of the heart is not perforated and does not have visible pores as some people thought or invisible pores as Galen thought. The blood from the right chamber must flow through the vena arteriosa (pulmonary artery) to the lungs, spread through its substances, be mingled there with air, pass through the arteria venosa (pulmonary vein) to reach the left chamber of the heart, and there form the vital spirit." This is the first description of the pulmonary circulation and was discovered by Spanish physician and scholar Michael Servetus (1511-1553) and transmitted by him to Realdo Colombo, a professor of anatomy at Padua, who is usually credited with the concept.[64] Colombo will be discussed in Chapter 7.

Servetus, also known as Miguel Serveto, probably learned of al-Nafis through the writings of a Syrian scholar and translator of Arabic works named Andrea Alpago, who died about 1520. Servetus was arrested in Geneva by Protestant (Calvinist) authorities, charged with heresy and, when he refused to renounce his Catholic religion, burned at the stake on October 27, 1553. Fortunately for science, his work and writings survived. Al-Nafis' writings had no effect on science (other than through Servetus) and were only discovered in 1924. They exist as an example of what might have been in the world of Islam.

Other than al-Nafis, Arabic medicine contributed little original, being based on the Greek models, but they made huge contributions in pharmacology, discovering and cataloging thousands of new drugs. The word "drug" is Arabic as are alcohol, alkali, syrup, jujube, and spinach. New drugs introduced by Arabs include benzoin, camphor, myrrh, musk, laudanum (the alcohol solution of opium), naphtha, senna, and alcohol itself. Both al-Razi and Avicenna emphasized reason and suggested that mineral or chemical remedies would be superior to the magical potions and herbs of folk medicine. The great value of Arab contributions to medicine lies in the thoroughness of their preservation and systematic organization of knowledge. Aside from pharmacology, they contributed little that was new and the influence of Avicenna, like that of Aristotle, finally became a barrier to new learning. By the thirteenth century, Islam was in retreat and the great teachers and writers would not be replaced. Some of this resistance to innovation, which developed after the early period, was related to a negative concept of imitating the infidel. In Islamic tradition, *bidaa* (innovation) is similar to heresy in western tradition. The printing press was not adopted and the first book in Arabic script was printed in Istanbul in 1759. The *Qu'ran* was not printed until the twentieth century.

THE FALL OF THE ARAB EMPIRE

The caliph al-Mu'tasim had begun importing Turkish slaves in the ninth century. The slaves ultimately gained power as military officers. In 960, the Turks were converted to Islam and, in the tenth century, the Seljuk Turks migrated into what is modern Turkey from the steppes of Central Asia. In 1055, the Turks seized Baghdad and their leader, Tughrul, adopted the title "Sultan." The Turkish Sultans were much less interested in the arts and translations and, thus, the Islamic era of medicine declined. In 1206, Jenghiz Khan formed an empire from the tribes of Mongolia, conquered China, and moved west, conquering as he went. In 1258, the Mongols, ruled by Jenghiz Khan's descendents (he died in 1227), sacked Baghdad killing all the members of the Abbasid family who could be found. The empire of the Arabs and Islamic culture never recovered.

Islam did build hospitals and the *Qur'an* advocated humane treatment of the mentally ill. The first European mental hospital was built in Granada in 1365 following the expulsion of the Muslims. The great hospital of Cairo, built in 1283 by al-Mansur Qalawan, had chapels for Christians as well as a mosque and continued in existence until Napoleon invaded Egypt 500 years later. After Cordova fell to the Christians in 1236 and Baghdad was sacked by the Mongols in 1258, Arab civilization began its decline. The Ottoman Turk Empire, which succeeded it, did not inspire the same intellectual effort but the Islamic medical system continues in India and Pakistan as *Yunani* medicine.

TAQÏ AL-DÏN

The Turks had one more chance to catch up to the western world in science. Taqï al-Dïn (1526-1585), author of books on astronomy, optics and mechanical clocks, moved to Istanbul in 1571 to become astronomer (and astrologer) in-chief to the Sultan Selim II. He persuaded the next Sultan, Murad III, to build a huge observatory in Galata, in Istanbul. The observatory was constructed in 1577 and was comparable to Tycho Brahe's observatory in Denmark, built about the same time. He might have made a major contribution to science, comparable to that of Brahe whose observatory marked the beginning of Renaissance science in Europe. Instead, al-Dïn fell victim to the fate of the scientist who lives in a pre-scientific society. After observing a new comet in the sky, Taqi al-Dïn told the Sultan that he was going to win many battles. Unfortunately Taqi al-Dïn was wrong (the Sultan lost his next battle) and his observatory was demolished after only five years. A squad of Janissaries razed it to the ground on the order of the Chief Mufti. There had been other observatories in Islamic countries before al-Din's but there would be no more. Primitives executed scientists in the West, as well, but there were others to take their place. Servetus was burned at the stake by Calvinists in Geneva and Lavoisier was executed by the French Revolution in 1789 but Islam could not afford to lose these few pioneers.[65] The next example of Islamic interest in western science came after Napoleon's conquest of Egypt in 1798 when the Turks sought military hardware from the Europeans.

60   The sale of honey to Muslim fundamentalists is today one source of funding for the *al qaeda* organization of *Usama bin Laden.*

61   The name of that well is used as the name of an Iranian-made soft drink in the Middle East. Islamic countries, which bar the sale of alcoholic beverages and are nearly all in warm climate zones, are the greatest market for carbonated soft drinks in the world.

62   Morris Kline, *Mathematical Thought From Ancient to Modern Times,* pages 190-197, Oxford Press (1972).

63   Haddad, S.E. & Khairallah A.A., "A Forgotten Chapter in the Circulation of the Blood," *Annals of Surgery*; 104:1-8. (1936).

64   Coppola, E.D., "The Discovery of the Pulmonary Circulation: A New Approach," *Bulletin of the History of Medicine* ; 31:44-77. (1957).

65   Bernard Lewis, *What Went Wrong: Western Impact and Middle Eastern Response,* Oxford University Press (2001) Lewis recounts the stories of al-Nafis and Taqi al-Din and the consequences on pp 78-81.

6
The Middle Ages

THE FALL OF THE WESTERN ROMAN EMPIRE MEANT DISASTER FOR civilization and its amenities, including the teaching and practice of learned medicine. City life collapsed and society retreated to a feudal world of castles and peasant labor. Life became, in Thomas Hobbes' words, "nasty, brutish, and short." Literate men and women were confined to monasteries and convents where medical manuscripts were preserved and studied but the application of medical knowledge withered. The first stirring of medical revival was in Salerno around 1100 when Greek and Islamic texts were brought from Constantinople by the archbishop Alphansus, a Benedictine monk from nearby Monte Cassino. In 530CE, St. Benedict had written the Benedictine Rule that stated, "To labor is to pray." He has been called "the pivotal figure in the history of labor."[66] The Benedictine order would help to turn the Church away from mysticism and anti-science to practical subjects and worldly mechanical matters.

A medical school was founded and the Latin speaking world was reintroduced to Galen and Hippocrates. Arabic medicine reached the West through Constantinus Africanus, a native of Carthage who became a monk at Monte Cassino. He Latinized many Arabic translations of Greek texts and his translations were crucial for the survival of Greek and Arab medicine as the Arab Empire began to recede. Constantinus was born a Muslim and his journey to Monte Cassino was somewhat mysterious. He smuggled a copy of Avicenna's works to Italy and this may have been the key to his acceptance by the monks. The body of translations at Salerno became a new Latin canon titled *Articella*, "Little Art of Medicine," also referred to as *Ars medicinae*, and marked a turning point in Western medicine. The canon was based on Galen and all medical thought for centuries after was Galenical. After 1140, more translations appeared from Spain when Arabic texts were captured and translated as the Moors were driven out. Gerard of Toledo translated hundreds of works by Aristotle, Avicenna, al-Razi, and Albucasis' *De Chirurgia* ("On Surgery"). The *Qanun* of Avicenna became the cornerstone textbook of medicine at the University of Montpelier, the largest non-clerical institution in Europe, until 1650.

THE *ARTICELLA*

Translations continued over the next few centuries, including some directly from surviving Greek texts. Something like the Arabic translation movement occurred in Padua, Montpellier and even in England and France.
The *Articella* was translated into English, French, and even Gaelic and
Welsh. There was some resistance by church officials to dissection and to
medical practice. St. Bernard of Clairvaux declared, "to consult physicians
and take medicines befits not religion and is contrary to purity," but this
was a minority view. There was a popular gibe, "*tres physici, dui athei*" ("three
physicians, two atheists"), but the care of the sick was important to
Christian charity and the Church considered it man's duty to preserve life,
although it was more important to have the dying blessed by the priest
than bled by the doctor. Considering the efficacy of Galenical medicine,
this was sound advice.

Petrus Hispanus was a cleric and physician who became Pope John XXI in
1276. His book *Thesaurus pauperum* ("Treasury of the Poor") was highly regarded although it recommended "pig shit" for stanching nosebleeds. He died
in the collapse of the roof of a palace he had just constructed; perhaps he
was a better doctor than architect. The Lateran Council of 1215 forbade
clerics in higher orders (priests) from shedding blood, an attempt to separate physicians from surgeons just as Hippocrates did. In 1482, Pope Sixtus
IV informed the University of Tübingen that dissection was permissible if
the body was that of an executed criminal and was given a Christian burial.
Thus the study of anatomy was allowed, contrary to some accounts of the
Church's role in science. Monasteries became medical centers, more
important than universities until 1300.

The association between certain saints and healing, or even specific
organs, developed, as in other cultures, and Damian and Cosmas became
patron saints of healing, replacing Asclepius. They were brothers martyred
by Diocletian (by burning, stoning, crucifixion, and being sawn in half-
they survived all this and were finally decapitated) and became patrons
especially of surgeons. Their first miracle involved transplanting a foot
from a Moor to a white man with gangrene. Paintings of the scene depict
the patient with one white and one black leg. St. Anthony was invoked for
relief of erysipelas (St. Anthony's fire), St. Artemis for genital infections
(herpes is forever), St. Sebastian for pestilence, and St. Vitus for chorea
(St. Vitus' dance). Healing shrines were established, some of which survive
today. Mistletoe was widely believed to cure epilepsy, the belief originat-
ing with an account, in the Old Testament, of young David curing a woman
with a fit, and, in the seventeenth century, Robert Boyle, founder of the

Royal Society, was still convinced of its efficacy. Of course, some other folk remedies, like cinchona bark for malaria, turned out to be effective, so we should not be too critical.

Hospitals began as monastery additions to treat the sick but by the twelfth century major institutions that survive today, St. Bartholomew's and St. Thomas's in London being prime examples, had been founded. Many were combinations of hospital and poor house with some (called lazarettos) set aside for lepers who were shunned and needed shelter. The Crusaders built hospitals and some orders, like the Knights of Malta, spent more effort on such matters than in battling Muslims. The High Middle Ages began around 1100 in northern Europe with the founding of universities in Paris, Bologna, Oxford, and Cambridge. Most of these universities were dominated by clerical faculty although at Montpelier and in Italy secular faculty founded law and medical schools. In the northern universities, like Oxford and Paris, medical instruction was informal at first with organized faculty developing later. Padua was the greatest of the medical schools at the time with sixteen medical professors in 1436 while Oxford had only one that year. The curriculum was based on books like *Articella* and Avicenna's Canon. Thomas Aquinas (1226-74) introduced a new emphasis on Aristotle although his principle interests were science and theology, not medicine. By 1300 Bologna, and thirty years later, Montpelier, required attendance at a dissection of a human body to supplement studies of animal anatomy. Paris required an apprenticeship with a physician as did Montpelier.

The duties of a physician at the court of Henry III of England included counseling the steward about the choice of meat and drink served the king, checking for evidence of pestilence or the presence of lepers, and warning the king if one should appear. Medical practice followed the *Aphorisms* and the teaching of Hippocrates and Galen, with diet and drugs the only remedies available. Examination of the pulse and the study of urine (uroscopy – examination of urine in a flask held to the light) were the principle diagnostic aids. Medications were compounded by the physician and were called "Galenicals." Astrology was part of medicine and "critical days", *dies mali* in Latin, were recorded. The Physician of Chaucer's *Canterbury Tales* was "grounded in astronomye". Pharmacy included exotic substances, many imported from the East, and shops in Venice, which stocked these materials, were called *apothecai*.

Science progressed at a pace far slower than during the Greek, Roman, or even Arabic ages. Technology added such mundane developments as the invention of the wheelbarrow, the horse collar, and the horseshoe. While not of a sophistication equal to the calculation of *pi*, or the hypotenuse of a right triangle, these advances lessened the load on the peasant and improved productivity in an agricultural society. The invention of the stirrup has been credited with the development of the feudal system in Europe. It allowed the rider to finally achieve superiority over the foot soldier. The Greek phalanx and Roman legion defeated the bareback cavalry of antiquity. The stirrup mounted horseman could use armor and was invincible until another technological revolution came with the long bow in 1346 at Crecy. The cost of the knight's armor and horses required a new social system and the changes in argriculture permitted the manorial system to survive into the eighteenth century in some parts of Europe (nineteenth century in Russia).[67] The windmill appeared in Yorkshire in 1185 and the technology quickly spread across Europe. The mill and sail beams were mounted on a pivot to accommodate the variable wind of Europe and the European version differed from those of Asia and the Muslim world, because it had gears and a horizontal axle. Ship construction improved, with carvel planking (side-by-side planking with caulking like modern construction) and, by 1400, ships of 1,000 tons were being built. The compass was first mentioned in 1180 (by Alexander Neckham in *De Utensilibus*) and the translation of Ptolomey's *Geography* into Latin led to new voyages by the Portugese and Columbus. In 1202, Leonardo Fibonacci of Pisa introduced the use of Arabic numerals in his *Liber Abaci*. Double-entry bookkeeping appeared in the next century leading to the Medicis and banking. Italians' interest in mathamatics was to grow and, in the fifteenth century, Venice established a university chair devoted to navigation.

For centuries after the fall of Rome, the peasant population was held in check by poor nutrition as much as by disease. Roman agricultural methods were not suitable for northern European areas, and Roman technology was deficient. The adoption of an improved plow followed the horse collar, but horses consumed grain that was in short supply until crop rotation became established. Ironically, the practice of allowing one third of the land to lie fallow for a season, restoring fertility, was a consequence of Viking and Magyar invasions that killed large numbers of peasants. With reduced population, some fields could not be cultivated and the practice of three-field crop rotation, with one field left unplanted, increased productivity so much that the practice was retained after the population recovered. The Black Death would have a similar effect in altering peasant life. The early Middle Ages saw little consumption of animal protein by the peasants, but legume production, which increased with the agricultural revolution, reduced the dependence on carbohydrates and led to rapid population growth again. The Church's practice of fasting from animal flesh on feast days did not appear until the fourteenth century.

Women had shorter lives than men in the Middle Ages and ninth century records confirm that, while more women survived to age fifteen, men had longer life expectancy. This is attributed to the hazards of childbirth, but also to an iron deficient diet when protein, especially animal protein, was not available. By 1422 (Rheims) and 1499 (Nuremburg), women were outnumbering men in the population records. Menarche was occurring at age twelve to fourteen in medieval times and, once animal protein was plentiful, necessary iron replacement for menstrual loss was available.[68] The improvements in agriculture, and the associated presence of domestic animals, increased availability of meat in the diet and provided the necessary iron.

Higher productivity provides the opportunity for leisure, during which other inventions might be conceived. The invention of the mechanical clock in the thirteenth century was an enormous development with an effect on medicine as well as all other human activities. In 1271, Robert the Englishman described the progress of clockmakers and, in 1300, the verge-and-foliot mechanism solved the problem of pendulum clocks.[69] The precision allowed by such devices advanced the cause of science in a very fundamental way. The first such clocks did not measure minutes and seconds, but the potential was inherent and only awaited the next step. The spring-driven mechanisms necessary for watches did not appear until the fifteenth century. The *fusee* mechanism, which converts the declining pressure of the spring-driven mechanism of watches to a steady force, appeared about 1430. The flywheel appeared and allowed the spinning wheel to progress, until Adam Smith estimated that it had improved productivity by a factor of three to one.[70] The canal lock added to transportation and, by 1500, Europe was well beyond the farthest point of Arab science. The opening of the Languedoc Canal in 1681 connected the Atlantic Ocean with the Mediterranian Sea completing the greatest engineering feat of the era of human and animal energy. The mixture of science and theology proved a barrier to progress, but not an impervious one.

ALBERTUS MAGNUS AND THOMAS AQUINAS

Albertus Magnus was a priest born in Germany around 1200. He was educated at Padua and went on to become the finest teacher of his age in Paris. Thomas Aquinas walked from southern Italy to Paris at the age of twenty to become his pupil. Albertus was the first to isolate the element arsenic and his lab notes survive to show that he was the first European since

Rome to use the scientific method in his thinking and studies. He was comfortable with the Aristotelian system of the day and, yet, he was able to consider the possibility of chemical change, a concept foreign to Aristotle. His brilliance stimulated jealousy in contemporaries, who suspected him of being a wizard, but the Church ultimately canonized him and he is the patron saint of scientists.

Roger Bacon, a contemporary of Albertus, was a Franciscan monk who studied at Oxford and Paris. He was nearly as brilliant as Albertus and attracted the attention of Pope Clement IV, who became a patron. Unfortunately, when Clement died, Bacon's enemies (he had many, as he was a brilliant man who did not suffer fools) were able to induce the head of the Franciscan order to imprison him for fifteen years. His books, those not hidden by like-minded monks, were burned. His *opus majus* was finally published in 1733, 450 years after his death. Bacon anticipated Leonardo da Vinci in predicting steamships, automobiles, submarines, and flying machines. In 1230, he anticipated the circumnavigation of the world, 260 years before Columbus. One of his letters contains the first European reference to gunpowder. His was the first mention of spectacles for vision correction and he may have had something to do with the invention. Like Albertus, but with even more certainty, he emphasized experimentation as the basis of science and knowledge. An abrasive personality, however, helped put him on a very different path than Albertus.

FALSE GERBER

A Spanish monk, who called himself "Gerber" after the Arabic mathematician and chemist Jabir ibn-Hayyan, was known to his contemporaries as "False Gerber." In spite of the derision of his critics, and a strong predilection to alchemy, False Gerber discovered *vitriol* in 1300. This was the greatest chemical advance since the discovery of iron smelting 3,000 years before. Vitriol is sulphuric acid and, until the mid-twentieth century, the index of a country's development was measured by the volume of sulphuric acid its industries used each year. It was the first strong acid (acetic, a weak acid, was discovered by the Greeks) discovered and, soon after that momentous discovery, False Gerber described how to make *aqua fortis*, strong nitric acid. Jabir ibn Hayyan, the "real Gerber," had described how to make weak nitric acid in the eighth century but these were the first strong acids to be prepared and the discoveries launched chemistry toward modern science.

Arnold of Villanova was a physician born in Spain during the fourteenth century. He had read the Arabic texts in the original Arabic, rather than the spotty translation of Constantinus Africanus and studied Jabir ibn-Hayyan's description of the preparation of elixirs. Elixirs had become popular in Europe, but their true nature, a solution of the substance in alcohol, was vague. Arnold learned to isolate alcohol by distilling wine and named it *aqua vitae*, the "water of life." He also observed that burning wood in a poorly ventilated room produced a poisonous gas, carbon monoxide. Arnold was the greatest physician of his day, and was given a castle by the king of Aragon and a professorship by Montpellier University. He treated the royalty and twenty popes during his lifetime. While scientific progress proceeded at a crawl during this era, the role of the Church was not as negative as some accounts would assert.

SURGERY IN THE MIDDLE AGES

Barber-surgeons continued to perform most surgery and military wound care was primitive but a few learned surgeons did attempt to raise the standards. Lanfranc of Milan (1250-1306) settled in Paris where he produced *Chirurgia magna*, a later version of his popular work *Chirurgia parva*. There were sections on anatomy, embryology, ulcers, fistulae, fractures, and dislocations and other subjects. There was also a section on herbs and pharmacy. The works were translated into many languages from English to Hebrew. Successors included Henri de Mondeville (1269-1320) who served as military surgeon to the French royal family and who advocated, in his unfinished book, primary closure of wounds. This contradicted the advice of Hippocrates, who described "laudable pus" and encouraged wound treatment designed to induce it. Conventional wound treatment of the time advocated wound plasters and powders to produce suppuration in the belief that laudable pus (the thick yellow pus of staphylococcus infection) conveyed poisoned blood from the body. The school at Salerno and its followers recommended leaving wounds open to heal by "secondary intention" or from the bottom up. This results in slow healing and prominent scars, but in an age ignorant of the cause of infection, it may have been prudent. Laudable pus was distinguished from the deadly streptococcal infection that produced only small amounts of thin, blood tinged pus and spreading wound sepsis.

A subsequent disciple of de Mondeville was Guy de Chauliac (1298-1368) who wrote a later edition of *Chirurgia magna* and included 3,299 references to other works and 890 quotations from Galen in an effort to produce learned surgeons. Since Galen had little to say about surgery that was helpful, these references contributed little, but may have served the purpose.

Modern medical authors (and historians) show the same tendencies. The most prominent English surgeon of the time was John of Arderne, who served John of Gaunt in the Hundred Years War. He wrote a text on treatment of anal fistula, which followed Hippocrates's method of passing a thread through the fistula tract, but then advocated immediate incision of the bridge of tissue between the fistula and anal canal. In a deep fistula, this may leave the patient incontinent and is not an improvement on Hippocrates.

After 1200, towns reappeared with a merchant class as the feudal system gave way to a more modern society. The larger towns began to see the formation of medical guilds, the first of which was formed in Florence in 1236. Physicians and pharmacists were admitted but surgeons were not, although surgery was included in the medical curriculum in Sicily by 1231. In northern Europe, surgeons formed their own guilds, one of which, formed in 1210, was the College of St. Côme, in Paris. In German states and in England, the barber-surgeon persisted. In 1368 a Fellowship of Surgeons was formed in London and a Company of Barbers in 1376. A small group of physicians with university training formed a guild in 1423, but not until 1518 was the College of Physicians of London chartered. Public physicians, called *medici condotti*, were employed by the Italian city of Reggio in 1211 to assist at inquests, treat plague, and tend injuries inflicted on prisoners. By 1300, Bruges, in modern Belgium, had established a municipal water supply, returning to the Roman model after 1,000 years of squalor. Streets in Paris were paved and sewers were functioning but the health of city dwellers was poor.

THE BLACK DEATH

The Black Death was a catastrophe for those living in Europe in the fourteenth century but it ushered in (by destroying feudalism, at least in England) the modern age. The Plague of Justinian did not cross the Bosphorus Strait and the black rat was unknown in Europe until the appearance of the Black Death in 1346.[71] Mice are described in manuscripts, few as they are in the Middle Ages, but not rats. The increase in population, the rise of towns with their more concentrated population, and the appearance of the rat brought to Europe a disease known in China for millennia. The organism responsible requires iron for growth and plague victims were disproportionately men. Perhaps iron deficiency, described above, was actually protective for the female population. There have also been theories that population growth had outstripped food production once again and rats fled empty granaries for homes, but the weak were not the principle victims. Whatever the causes, population once again would be devastated by this new scourge.

The black rat, unlike the brown rat, tends to live in houses and ships and is well adapted to living with man. They were known to inhabit the fields of North Africa back to the beginning of history. The disease is caused by the organism *Yersinia pestis*, formerly known as *Pasteurella pestis* (Alexander Yersin was an associate of Pasteur who discovered the organism in 1894), a gram negative bacterium that is transmitted by fleas' saliva. The flea lives on rats, its preferred host, but will parasitize and bite humans if rats are not available. Bubonic plague epidemics are often precipitated by massive die-offs of infected rats sending their fleas on a search for new hosts. Increased trade with the East was probably the immediate source of the pestilence. It began in Tashkent in central Asia and arrived at the Black Sea, where it broke out among Muslim Tatars fighting Italian merchants in Crimea. The Christians took refuge in the citadel at Kaffia where they were besieged. The plague forced the Tatars to raise the siege, much as the Carthaginians had done in Sicily 1,600 years earlier, but before leaving, they invented bio-logical warfare by catapulting the bodies of plague victims into the citadel. The escaping Christians brought the plague (and presumably the infected rats and fleas) back to Messina and Genoa where it spread across Europe.

A contemporary account, by Fra Michele di Piazze, recounts, "In the first days of October, 1347, twelve Genoese galleys fleeing before the wrath of our Lord over their wicked deeds, entered the port of Messina. The sailors brought in their bones a disease so violent that whoever spoke a word to them was infected and could in no way save himself from death."[72] Perhaps this is a description of pneumonic plague, which, unlike the bubonic form, can be passed from person to person. Another account, by Gabriel de Mussis, declared that no cases occurred on the ship but the plague appeared two days after the ship docked, a suggestion of the rat-flea association. It was noted in all outbreaks of bubonic plague that care-givers were no more likely to contract the disease than the general popu-lation; another bit of evidence of the rat-flea route, rather than person-to-person as occurs in pneumonic plague. Both forms may occur in the same epidemic although the pneumonic form is much less common. During the next three years approximately twenty million people, one quarter of the population of Europe, would die of the plague. Thousands of villages were abandoned and by 1427 Florence's population had decreased by sixty per-cent. Poll tax records in England show a population of 4.5 to 6 million in 1347, but only 2.5 to 3 million in 1377, a drop of 2 million or nearly one third in thirty years. This reversed a trend of increasing population dating back to 1066. Children also seemed to be more severely affected leading to the use of the term *Pestis puerorum*, in 1361. In England, crowded walled towns and coastal areas were most severely affected, while some rural areas with poor communications escaped entirely.

England was more severely affected than most countries for several reasons. The appearance of money had already weakened the feudal system. In the thirteenth century, Edward I had expelled the Jews from England as a reaction to land purchase from spendthrift nobles who had mortgaged land held in feud from the king.[73] Agriculture had grown enormously and by the end of the fourteenth century, there was more land under cultivation than ever before. The country was exporting grain and the road system had been restored to the condition that preceded the Roman collapse. Population increase had produced a glut of labor. Prosperity began a decline after 1295, possibly a result of weather changes. By 1347, the previous prosperity had given way to lean times and a series of bad winters made things worse. The plague, killing off one third of the population and a larger proportion near the coasts, resulted in economic deflation and relative prosperity for the survivors. By 1350, only three years after the plague arrived, there was a shortage of labor and an excess of land with no one to work it. The irregular distribution of the plague resulted in labor shortages in some areas and glut in others.

Peasant mobility developed, for the first time since the Romans left, because of these changes. Landowners were obliged to hire laborers and pay cash wages, although the government, for a time, attempted to restrict the mobility of labor. By 1360, the economy had partially recovered as the birth rate began to catch up. The plague returned in 1361 and this was the *Pestis peurorum*, carrying off the children. The adults may have developed some residual immunity or the disease that year might have been diphtheria or some other infection rather than plague. The result was a return of the labor shortage and a desperate attempt to restore the feudal system resulted in the Peasants' Revolt of 1381. By the fifteenth century, England had become a land of tenant farmers. The peasant had ceased to exist. In continental Europe, feudalism persisted for another 300 years, especially in France. Another effect of the depopulation of England was a marked increase in the raising of sheep as the manpower required was much less than for farming. Tudor prosperity in the sixteenth century was based on wool. The Wars of the Roses, in an example of the irony of fate, accelerated the trend, by wiping out large numbers of the land-owning aristocracy. The rich wool merchants who replaced them were Saxons, not Normans, and they came from the small farmers who survived the Black Death.

Until the coming of the Black Death, Europe had been free of major epidemics for 800 years, perhaps due to the collapse of the Roman Empire with its roads reaching out to new diseases in Asia. Now, with the rise of trade and travel from European towns like Venice and Genoa, the contacts with Asia brought more disasters.[74] Boccacio provides a vivid description of the year 1348 in his *Decameron*. "Between March and the following July (1349) it is estimated that more than 100,000 human beings lost their lives within the walls of Florence." That is equal to the entire population prior to the plague. The descriptions of the disease are identical to more recent plague epidemics, but the physicians of the time had no idea of the cause. Some blamed a "pestilential atmosphere," others God's Will. Severe persecution of the Jews, who were accused of poisoning wells, followed in some areas with 12,000 Jews slaughtered in Mainz (Germany). Finally, Pope Clement VI acted to suppress the worst of the persecutors, called "flagellants," and stop the persecution of the Jews. The authority and power of the Church suffered from the Black Death. Large numbers of clergy died and many contemporary writers commented on a loosening of moral standards. John Wyclif was a theologian and Master of Balliol College, Oxford. He questioned the Church's power in the aftermath of the plague, translated the Bible into English, and attacked other abuses such as the sale of offices and pardons. His followers, known as the "Lollards" (celebrated in the music of Carl Orff's composition, *Carmina Burana*, which puts their poems to music), included many disillusioned monks. The Church survived the attacks by Wyclif and persecuted the Lollards. Wyclif died in 1384 and they were finally suppressed but re-emerged with Martin Luther.

Public health measures, which might, and in some instances probably did, help to control the plague, were not the province of physicians except those few in official positions. The magistrates, as in Venice, laid down burial regulations and banned the sick from entering the city. In Milan, the council sealed the occupants of affected houses in and left them to die. This may have helped in controlling the epidemic as the mortality rate in Milan was only fifteen percent. In Florence a committee of eight was given dictatorial powers but one of their measures, the killing of all cats and dogs, made things worse since the rat population could increase unimpeded by natural enemies. Of course, the physicians of the time had no idea of the role of rats. In 1377, the town of Ragus, in Italy, detained travelers for thirty days (*trentini giorni*) and when this proved ineffective the period of isolation was increased to forty days (*quarantini giorni*); they were "quarantined."

The Galen-based medical knowledge of the time was useless in controlling the epidemic. Bubonic plague would reappear from time to time for the next three centuries in Europe. In the early years of the eighteenth century, it disappeared from Europe, but continued to be endemic in Africa and Asia. Yersin, a Swiss working with Pasteur, and Kitasato, a Japanese bacteriologist also trained by Pasteur, finally discovered the causative organism in Hong Kong in 1894. Discovery of the plague organism in dead rats by Paul Louis Simond, a French scientist studying an epidemic in Bombay in 1898, was the first evidence of the route of transmission. In 1901, the new *Journal of Public Health* printed an article (concerning an outbreak in Australia) in which the source of plague was still uncertain although the rat and flea connection was suspected. Development of a vaccine, of doubtful efficacy, followed the discovery but the epidemic had ceased a century earlier. Why did plague stop in Europe after being such a pestilence for centuries?[75] One theory, widely considered to be the best explanation, is that the black rat, comfortable in ships and houses, was killed off or driven out by the ferocious brown Norwegian rat, which first appeared in 1720 in Europe. The brown rat, more at home in sewers, is infested with a different flea that is less likely to transfer to humans. Evidence against this theory is the fact that the two varieties, having different habitats, do not compete for living space. A second point against this theory is that the black rat, absent from Europe for two centuries, has returned since 1910. Another consideration is the introduction of arsenic as a rat poison, which may have reduced the level of contact between human and rats and their fleas. Whatever the explanation, the plague vanished from Europe after three centuries and medical practice can claim no credit.

66   Lynn White, *Dynamo and Virgin Reconsidered*, page 63,, MIT Press (1968).

67   Lynn White, *Medieval Technology and Social Change*, page 28, Oxford Press (1962).

68   Vern Bullough and Cameron Campbell, "Female longevity and diet in the Middle Ages," *Speculum* 55:317-25 (1980).

69   David Landes, *Revolution in Time*, Harvard University Press (1983).

70   Adam Smith, *The Wealth of Nations*, University of Chicago Press (1976).

71   Hans Zinnsser, *Rats, Lice and History*, Little, Brown and Co. (1934). Zinsser discusses the rat and its presence in Europe prior to the Black Death in Chapter IX

72   Roy Porter, *The Greatest Benefit to Mankind*, page 123.

73   Winston Churchill, *A History of the English Speaking Peoples*. Volume I *The Birth of Britain*, pages 288-291, Dorsett Press (1956).

74   This point is controversial but is commented on by Kiple in *The Cambridge World History of Disease*, p 38 and by McNeil, (1976). David E. Stannard, author of the section I.4 in Cambridge, attributes this to a "parasite-host equilibrium." Endemic disease took a toll, but epidemics did not reappear in Europe until the Black Death.

75   Edward A Eckert, "The Retreat of Plague from Central Europe, 1640-1720: A Geomedical Approach," *Bulletin of the History of Medicine* 74:1-28 (2000).

7
The Beginning of Modern Science

THE RENAISSANCE, AND THE REFORMATION WHICH BROKE THE stranglehold of the Church on learning and science, introduced the first glimmerings of European progress in the sciences. Aristotle's four humours of matter (earth, water, air, and fire) and Galen's four humours of biology (bile, blood, phlegm and black bile) were giving way to better explanations of natural science. Mondino de Luzzi conducted the first recorded human dissection in Europe, in Bologna around 1315. His *Anatomia mundini* (1316) was a brief practical guide to human anatomy based on human dissection. Unfortunately, he perpetuated a number of errors from Galen and the Arabs such as a five-lobed liver and a three-chambered heart. The first printed version appeared in 1478 and forty editions followed. This marked a change from the Salerni School and the *Articella*, based on pig dissection. The corpse was an executed criminal and the procedure became a public spectacle as physicians adopted human dissection. Autopsies for forensic purposes were also beginning to occur after 1250. The practice of human dissection spread slowly from Bologna to Spain in 1404 and finally to England and Germany no earlier than 1550. A Galen revival with the early Renaissance brought a few backward steps.

PARACELSUS

Theophrastus Bombastus von Hohenheim was born in Switzerland in 1493, a year after Columbus's momentous discovery. Lorenzo the Magnificent had died in Florence, and gunpowder had revolutionized warfare. Double entry bookkeeping had transformed banking and Gutenberg had introduced the printing press to the West. Theophrastus was born poor; his father was illegitimate and his mother was a bondswoman who died when he was a child. To add to his troubles, he was emasculated in infancy, though the reason is unknown. His father, a physician, taught alchemy, what we would call metallurgy, at a mining college in Austria. The son, who called himself "Paracelsus" in homage to the famous Roman writer Celsus (he planned to surpass his deeds), became an expert chemist and later a wandering scholar. In Paris, he studied under Ambroise Paré, the army surgeon who invented the instruments of modern surgery, the hemostat and the ligature. Paracelsus claimed a medical degree from Ferrara and, like many educated men of science in that era, combined medicine and chemistry. His contribution was to challenge the primacy of Galen and Avicenna, a dangerous doctrine at the time. He rejected academic medicine with its narrow book-bound dogma and declared that the place to learn medicine was to "seek out old wives, gypsies, sorcerers, wandering tribes, old robbers, and such outlaws and take lessons from them." He supported himself as an army surgeon and itinerant doctor. He was no court physician. A contemporary described him: "He lived like a pig and looked like a sheep drover. He found his greatest pleasure amongst the company of the most dissolute rabble and spent most of his time drunk."[76] Others called him the "German Hermes" because he had learned from the "rabble," and his learning, uninhibited by Galen and Avicenna, was vast.

In Constantinople, the capital of Suleiman the Magnificent in 1522, he learned of a peasant remedy to prevent smallpox. The peasant women would "insert in a vein a needle which had been infected with smallpox." He returned to Europe to become the first to recommend inoculation, two centuries before Jenner and Lady Montague. He also had a bit of the charlatan in him and extended the inoculation concept to include other diseases, inventing homeopathy (which advocates the administration of tiny doses of the supposed cause of disease to produce resistance in the recipient). He was a contemporary of Martin Luther and met him, but remained a Catholic. His revolutionary interest was to place chemistry at the center of medicine. He insisted on mixing chemical compounds from pure ingredients with standard formulas, a truism now, but unknown at that time of patent remedies with exotic ingredients. In 1527, he accomplished a spectacular cure of a prominent citizen of Basel-no one seems to know how-and this act brought him into contact with the famous scholar Erasmus. Paracelsus succeeded in curing Erasmus of gout and, through the influence of both his patients, was awarded the position of town medical officer of Basel

Paracelsus characteristically created problems for himself, when he declared that his lectures in Basel would be in German, not Latin, and that barber-surgeons and midwives were welcome to attend. Luther had adopted German for religious writing and now Paracelsus followed the example. He rejected the four humours theory of disease and added that fermentation and putrefaction were at the center of biological functions. He advocated the use of chemistry in treatment of disease although he continued to hold some primitive beliefs similar to those of other cultures. He believed in the theory of "signatures" in which plants that resembled an organ would cure its maladies. An orchid resembles a testicle (and in fact the term is used for testis as in "orchidectomy"-removal of a testis). In Paracelsus' theory, the orchid should be used in treatment of testicular diseases. He burned the works of Galen and Avicenna, sprinkling sulphur and nitre on the flames with spectacular results. His rejection of Galen extended to a rather dramatic statement that, "All the universities and all the ancient writers put together have less talent than my arse." Not surprisingly, his students worshipped him and his lectures became public events. He attacked the local apothecaries, declaring their potions worthless and the physicians fared no better as he rejected their bleeding and purging of patients. He attacked the use of moss and dung on wounds stating, "If you prevent infection, Nature will heal the wound all by herself." He distributed free medicines that he had made himself and introduced the use of arsenic for skin diseases, possibly a preview of the use of arsenicals in syphilis therapy. Finally, his patron, the wealthy printer he had cured, died of a stroke and Paracelsus' enemies succeeded in having him expelled from his position. Not for the last time, the threat of a reformer would unite the quacks and charlatans in a successful rejection of modern medicine.

He returned to the road and turned up in Nuremberg in 1528, where he upset the authorities by again ridiculing Galen and Avicenna, still the foundation of medical education at the time. He was asked to demonstrate his methods by curing a few cases of syphilis, a disease introduced by the returning sailors of Columbus and much more virulent than the modern disease. He cured nine of fourteen cases held in quarantine outside the city. The city records confirm the feat. In 1530, he published the first accurate clinical description of the disease and recommended the use of mercury compounds as treatment. Mercury remained the treatment of choice until 1909, when Paul Erlich discovered Salvarsan, the first arsenical compound. A popular saying up to the last century was "A night with Venus leads to a life with Mercury." In 1536, Paracelsus published *Die Grosse Wundartzney,* "The Great Surgery Book." It quickly made him wealthy for the first time in his life and his services were in great demand, even from princes. He continued to be a difficult figure but his work remained outstanding. He referred to gout and stone diseases as "Diseases of Tartar" and concluded that tartar accumulated from a chemical reaction similar to that in wine barrels and on teeth. He attempted, with some success, to treat the conditions with Rochelle Salt, potassium sodium tartrate. He introduced laudanum to Europe from Constantinople, although characteristically he claimed to have invented it. He kept the composition, an alcohol solution of opium, secret and charged high prices to wealthy patients for the drug. He continued to dazzle audiences with his chemical wizardry and Goethe is supposed to have modeled his character Faust on Paracelsus. His notorious debauchery kept him in bad repute with towns and, when his father died, the town of Vallach refused to permit him to remain in his father's home. He was driven out. In 1540, he landed in Salzberg, given a position by the Prince-Archbishop, but, a year later, he died after a suspicious fall in the street near the inn where he resided. It was rumored that thugs hired by angry physicians had attacked him.

Less than two years later, Copernicus, a contemporary (and more cautious than Paracelsus, since he waited until his deathbed to publish), published his work on the sun-centered planetary system. The scientific revolution had begun. Renaissance science would accelerate over the next century; in 1585, Simon Stevin, a Flemish engineer, suggested the use of what came to be known as the decimal point. A decade later, Scottish mathematician John Napier discovered the logarithm, which was put to use calculating compound interest. William Oughtred, in 1621, invented the slide rule. Blaise Pascal invented a calculating machine that could add and subtract in 1641 although it was too expensive to be practical. Liebnitz constructed a machine that could also multiply and divide. Gallileo, in addition to his astronomical discoveries, described in the next chapter, wrote *Motion and Mechanics,* a theoretical treatise that established the principles of machines.

ANATOMY

New translations of the original Greek texts increased the enthusiasm for Galen, in spite of Paracelsus' fulminations. In 1492, Nicolas Leoniceno published a book on errors in Pliny's classification of plants and contributed to the rediscovery of Hippocrates and Galen in new translations. Leonardo da Vinci produced over 750 anatomical drawings but never understood the circulation, relying on Galen's description of "pores" between the ventricles even though his drawings and dissections did not reveal them. If anatomy disagreed with Galen, Galen must be correct. Perhaps the anatomy of the ancient body was "more perfect" than the modern and any deviation must be the result of degeneration. Andreas Vesalius had no such qualms about Galen and his anatomy drawings, beginning with *Tabulae anatomicae sex,* ("six anatomical drawings"), in 1538 were intended for students and based on dissection. He still included errors from Galen in these first works but he soon realized that Galen's dissections had been of animals, not humans. In 1543, he published his masterpiece *De humanae corporis fabrica*, which rejected Galen's errors in anatomy but continued the belief in the origin of blood in the liver. In spite of accurate anatomy, the hold of Galen on physiology continued. Vesalius did comment on the absence of visible pores between right and left ventricle and this eventually led to the correct interpretation of the circulation by Harvey in 1615.

Vesalius' successor at Padua was Realdo Colombo, an apothecary's son who studied surgery and did experiments on living animals. He discovered the passage of blood through the lungs from right heart to left heart and noted that the pulmonary veins contained bright red blood, not air as Galen had concluded (Lower would repeat this observation in 1667). His discovery of the pulmonary circulation has been attributed to the Spanish scholar and physician Michael Servetus (see Chapter 5). Servetus became aware of the works of an Arabic physician, al-Nafis, who described the presence of arterial blood in pulmonary veins in the thirteenth century. Colombo may have read Servetus writings, which survived his death in 1553.[77] He also described the heartbeat accurately and observed that systole (contrary to tradition) was more forceful than diastole, a conclusion crucial for Harvey and his study of the circulation. Colombo criticized Vesalius' anatomical drawings and corrected some errors.

Gabriele Fallopia was appointed in 1551 to perform the annual anatomy demonstrations at Padua and, four years later, his students supported him when the authorities attempted to bring back the old ways based on Galen's texts. He added better descriptions of the inner ear, the carotid arteries and the muscles of the eye. He described the uterus and the tubes that bear his name and kept up a large clinical practice claiming to have examined 10,000 syphilitics. Progress continued with Bartolomeo Eustachio who described the ossicles of the ear, the tube named for him and the tensor tympani muscle (a tiny muscle that tenses the eardrum in response to loud sound) in humans and dogs. His other discoveries included the correct anatomy of the kidney, the sympathetic nervous system, and the suprarenal glands (adrenals). His book included an accurate depiction of the thoracic duct (which returns lymph to the venous system) that was to be ignored for centuries. One of Eustachio's pupils, Hieronymous Fabricius, succeeded to the Padua chair in 1565 and produced a work that, for the first time, compared human and animal anatomy and stressed the function of the structures, what we now call "comparative anatomy." In 1603, he wrote *De venarum ostiolis*, which described the valves of the veins. Another step to Harvey's discovery of the circulation of the blood was taken. Fabricius missed the true significance of the valves speculating, based on the Galen concept of circulation, that valves prevented excessive flow of (non-circulating) blood to the limbs when the subject stood up.

SURGERY

Surgery was unchanged by the new developments in anatomy because, with the absence of anesthesia, operations were largely limited to the surface of the body and to amputations. Neither of these fields required details of internal anatomy or physiology. John Halle, in 1560, described the properties of a surgeon: "a heart as the heart of a lion, his eyes like the eye of a hawk, and his hands as the hands of a woman." Surgery in Europe was taught as an apprenticeship and the surgeons were organized in guilds. The Guild of Surgeons merged with the Barbers Company to form the Barber-Surgeons Company of London in 1540. One member, William Clowes (1544-1603), worked as a navy surgeon then set up in practice in London with an appointment at St. Bartholomew's Hospital in 1575. He gained considerable further experience during military operations in the Low Countries in 1586 and in 1588, he was appointed surgeon to the fleet. He wrote treatises on wounds, venereal diseases and scrofula. Other English surgeons wrote workmanlike manuals for naval surgeons and the English Civil War provided ample opportunities for learning about wounds.

AMBROISE PARÉ

Ambroise Paré (1510-1590) was the most able surgeon of the era and invented many of the instruments and techniques that were in use until modern times (Some, like the hemostat clamp are still in use with modifications). He began as a surgeon, after having learned his craft as a barber-surgeon's apprentice at the Paris hospital Hotel Dieu in 1533. From 1537 until nearly 1587, he alternated in serving the poor (and, after his reputation grew, the rich) of Paris and the army on campaign. In 1544, during an interval in the wars of the sixteenth century, he described his ideas about the treatment of wounds to Jacques Dubois, a teacher of Vesalius, who encouraged him to publish his experiences. The next year he published his *Treatise on Wounds*, a classic that was in print for many decades. When Dubois died, Paré openly acknowledged his acceptance of Vesalius' new anatomical descriptions. In 1559, he attempted to save the life of King Henri II, wounded in a joust during the tourney to celebrate the marriage of his sister to the Duke of Savoy, a recent enemy, and his daughter to King Philip of Spain. The marriages to the two former enemies were to cement the peace after years of war. The king suffered the wound during the last joust of the day. Vesalius also attended the unfortunate king who had suffered a head wound from the splintered end of a lance that penetrated his helmet. Henri was paralyzed on his left side and, in spite of bleeding and purging (or more probably finished off by them), he died after ten days. Vesalius attended the autopsy, which revealed a subdural hematoma on the right side of the brain. No conclusion was drawn regarding the location of the injury, on the right side, and the paralysis on the left; neuroanatomy would wait another century. A modern medical student would recognize the association between the side paralyzed and the brain injury on the opposite side.

Paré's greatest innovation was the rejection of the use of cautery, the hot iron or hot oil, on wounds. In his treatise on gunshot wounds, he described how, during a furious battle, he ran out of boiling oil. He was forced to use an alternative: egg white, rose-oil, and turpentine. He could not sleep that night worrying about the men who had been deprived of the standard treatment and who, therefore, would probably die. Gunshot wounds were believed to be poisoned, hence the boiling oil. The next day he rose early, fearing the worst, but found that the patients treated after the boiling oil ran out were in less pain with wounds showing less inflammation. Cautery was unnecessary. He resolved never again to use such cruel methods. He invented the ligature, although others had advocated mass tying off of amputated limbs, and described the ligation of individual vessels using his hemostat clamp, which he called the "crow's beak."

The "Five Duties" of a surgeon, in Paré's estimation, were to "to remove what is superfluous, to restore what is dislocated, to separate what has grown together, to reunite what has been divided, and to redress the defects of nature." He described techniques in obstetrics such as version (turning) of the fetus to permit breech birth. In a sign of the times, the faculty of the Paris school criticized him in 1575 for publishing on "medical topics." He wrote a treatise attacking the use of powdered mummy as an ointment on wounds. In his treatise, he described the manufacture of fake mummies in Egypt to cater to the trade. Surgeons were not permitted to encroach on the turf of physicians and the *Facultié de Médecine* responded with a rebuttal; similar sentiments, about surgeons, persist to the present. In 1584, Paré responded with another treatise on the uselessness of unicorn horn. Civilian practice by surgeons was more mundane. Anesthesia was centuries away, although opium offered some relief of pain and, until the anesthesia era, speed was the sign of the good surgeon.

A sixteenth century account of a thigh amputation describes all the attendants running away when the patient "began to roare out." The surgeon's eldest son and his pregnant wife ran into the room and succeeded in holding the patient down until the amputation was completed. The most common procedures involved draining abscesses, pulling teeth, and treatment of gonorrhea and syphilis. The other common procedure was blood letting, as the principles of Galen still held sway. The surgeon applied a tourniquet to the arm and a vein was opened. A few major operations were developed such as Tagliacozzi's adoption (in 1597) of the ancient Indian practice of rhinoplasty, repair of the nose. See the chapter on Indian medicine. Until the time of the American Civil War amputation was the most common military operation and wounds of the trunk, the abdomen and thorax, were left to Nature's powers alone.

PHARMACY

Renewed interest in ancient texts and the knowledge of the Greeks and Romans led to re-discoveries of ancient drugs and new discoveries in the New World after Columbus. Single herb preparations were called "simples" and more complicated preparations, which included multiple ingredients of all types, were called "Galenicals." Botany was revived and a systematic nomenclature adopted. The Paris humanist Symphorien Champier poured scorn on the concoctions of the pharmacists with "The Mirror of the Apothecaries and Druggists in Which is Demonstrated How the Apothecaries Commonly Make Mistakes in Several Medicines Contrary to the Intentions of the Greeks…on the Basis of the Wicked and Faulty Teachings of the Arabs." He did not reject Galen's remedies; he just wanted to return to the pure formulas of the ancients. Discovery of Dioscorides' *De Materia Medica* contributed to the revival and the return to the Greeks' remedies. Rediscovery of some of the more questionable preparations of the ancients, like *Theriac*, a concoction of over one hundred components, contributed little to the health of the sick, but provided work for botanists and translators of Greek manuscripts. Rhubarb, a useful laxative, was rediscovered and the seeds were imported from Bulgaria to the West. The "true rhubarb," described by Marco Polo in China, was sought unsuccessfully. New drugs like cocoa, sarsaparilla, and sassafras were brought back from the New World, studied and used. The latter two herbs were thought useful for "cleansing the blood." Potatoes, cultivated in South America for thousands of years, were very useful as food and the "filthy weed" tobacco enjoyed a considerable reputation for efficacy in various ailments. The terrifying import of syphilis stimulated a search for New World cures for this scourge and natives were observed using guaiac wood decoctions. The belief that God provided cures for diseases, and a more modern concept that local tribes had had more time to experiment with local remedies, prompted a huge trade in *Guaiacum officinalis*, the bark of certain trees (also known as "holy wood"). Opium was imported from the East and Thomas Sydenham wrote, "None is so universal and efficacious as opium."

THE EUROPEAN DISCOVERY OF AMERICA AND ITS MEDICAL CONSEQUENCES

Infectious diseases were uncommon in primitive societies because the available pool of susceptible individuals was too small and contact with other groups was not common. The introduction of agriculture with larger populations, who remained in a circumscribed geographic area, allowed transmission between animal hosts and human hosts but, with developing immunity, the endemic incidence of disease (the rate of new cases per year) stabilized at a tolerable level or the community would not have survived. The spread of the Roman Empire introduced a new factor, travel to other communities with exposure to new diseases and return to the susceptible home community. The Greek Empire of Alexander did not involve such round-trip travel; Alexander and most of his men never returned to Greece. Possibly, the few that did return brought leprosy.[78]

The appearance of plague in the Byzantine Empire was a warning of the consequence of trade and round-trip travel. The disease outbreaks of earlier antiquity, like the plague of Athens and the epidemic in the Carthaginian army in Sicily, were mostly the consequences of war with crowded camps and poor nutrition and hygiene. Rome, with her great roads that permitted frequent travel to and from distant lands, was devastated by disease as much as by barbarian invasion. After the fall of Rome, travel in Europe was severely curtailed by the Dark Ages. The Crusaders were gone for years and many died, minimizing the transmission of infectious disease. The resumption of trade by the Italian city-states of Venice and Genoa exposed Europe to new epidemics and the Black Death followed. Ships could return in time for infected crew to carry the disease back home, and rats hitchhiked in the holds.

The continents of North and South America had been isolated from other populations (with the brief exception of the Leif Ericson colony in Newfoundland) for 10,000 years. The appearance of the crew of Columbus and the succeeding expeditions and colonists wrought havoc in both societies. Europe was to be exposed to a new disease, which devastated society, and the "Indies" were exposed to Old World diseases that had evolved since the last contact between the continents during the Ice Age. Both populations suffered immensely.

SYPHILIS

Syphilis suddenly emerged in Europe at the end of the fifteenth century. The disease in modern society is transmitted by sexual contact in almost all cases. It produces a primary lesion, called a chancre, which occurs near the site of infection, usually the genitals. It is painless and disappears spontaneously in a month or so. The secondary stage may occur from a month to a year after infection and usually involves a rash and some mild systemic symptoms like fever and headache. Again, the rash disappears without treatment and the next phase is called the early latent stage. The patient is highly infectious during all this time. The late latent stage begins about two years after infection and there are many manifestations from aortic aneurysms to insanity. The insanity stage, called General Paresis of the Insane or GPI, often includes delusions and a manic sort of behavior. The disease is also passed from mother to fetus and results in a characteristic appearance of the newborn and the older child. Hutchinson's Triad, described by Jonathan Hutchinson in 1861, includes peg shaped teeth, called "Hutchinson's teeth," deafness and impaired vision. Bone defects occur in the tertiary stage (after late latent) in both children and adults. In the fifteenth century, the disease progression was much more aggressive and the skin manifestations were horrendous.

The new disease appeared in 1495 in Europe then spread to India, Asia, and China. The first reports came from the army of Charles VIII of France who was attacking Naples in 1495 as part of his invasion of Italy that began in 1494. The French army developed numerous cases of this new disease and was accused of transmitting it to the population of conquered territory. Thereafter it was known as the "French Disease" or the "French Pox" throughout Europe. The army, about 30,000 men, included many mercenaries from other countries. The disease spread rapidly and forced Charles to abandon the conquest of Italy. The army dispersed when the campaign ended and the mercenaries returned to their homes carrying the disease all over Europe. Columbus first visited the New World on October 12, 1492, a date that used to be celebrated by schoolchildren. He returned to Spain four months later with ten natives of the islands and forty-four crewmen. He arrived in Palos, the port in Spain from which he had sailed, on March 15, 1493. One of the natives died soon after arriving in Spain and, at the end of April, six male natives of the surviving nine were displayed, naked, to the Spanish court. There is no mention in contemporary accounts of any disease affecting these natives. Meanwhile, many of the paid-off crewmen from his expedition joined the army of Charles VIII in Italy.[79] In 1518, a book printed in Venice first mentioned the theory of a "Spanish disease" imported from America. Gonzalo Oviedo, who had been a page in the Spanish court at the time of Columbus' return, made voyages to the Indies and reported evidence of a similar disease among the natives. In 1539, Rodrigo Ruiz Diaz de Isla, a physician, published a description of the "West Indian disease" and claimed to have treated at least one of Columbus' men in Barcelona. Another bit of evidence for the American origin of syphilis is the supposed efficacy of *guaiacum*, the resin mentioned in the last chapter. It is obtained from evergreen trees indigenous to South America and the West Indies and was introduced as a remedy in Europe in 1508, many years prior to the first published mention of the origin in the West Indies.

There is a second theory of the origin of syphilis involving African slaves brought back to Portugal after Prince Henry's expeditions in 1442.[80] In 1502, slaves were shipped to the West Indies until the governor of Haiti became alarmed at the large number of African slaves. There is an African disease called yaws, which is almost indistinguishable from syphilis scientifically, since it is caused by a related (or the same) organism. It is transmitted by skin contact, especially among children who play together naked in hot climates. Its clinical features are mostly limited to the skin and it does not have the severe later stage complications. The African origin theory suggests that yaws, introduced into a cold climate where clothing is worn covering the skin, might become a venereal disease since the only skin-to-skin contact would be sexual. Equatorial Africans, presumably exposed to yaws, have been in contact with Europeans and Middle Easterners for thousands of years before Columbus. Early European explorers in Africa, including the famous Dr. Livingstone, found yaws common, but saw no syphilis. Father Giovanni Cavazzi, a Portuguese missionary, described "mal Frances" spreading rapidly through the population of Congo and Angola in the sixteenth century. This may have been syphilis infecting an African population previously unexposed or it may have been the arrival of leprosy. It is impossible to be certain from his description.

Did syphilis actually exist in Europe before the contact with America and only become more virulent in 1495? Syphilis, especially congenital syphilis, leaves characteristic bone lesions. The bone lesions have been found in European skeletons from the post Columbus era but not before. Evidence from the Americas is more controversial. Lesions thought to be syphilitic have been found in pre-Columbian bones from South America and the West Indies, but there are only small numbers. Pinta, a skin disease transmitted by a spirochete, was clearly present in the Americas. The spirochete is related to syphilis and transmitted like yaws in Africa.

Perhaps pinta was transformed in the susceptible European population. In modern times, pinta is limited to the Americas and is purely a skin disease. In its late stages it causes patchy depigmentation in dark-skinned individuals but has no other manifestations. Serological study of primitive Amazon Indian populations has shown the presence of positive serology but no evidence of disease. Either the population has resistance to the organism or it is non-virulent. This evidence further supports the theory of American origin of syphilis.[81] The organism, although called a species (*T. pallidum careteum* or simply *T. careteum*), is indistinguishable from *T. pallidum* and *T. pallidum ssp. Pertenue,* the cause of yaws.[82]

In 1519, Ulrich von Hutten published a description of the new disease, which he said had first appeared in Germany in 1497. His account includes the initial stage which, at the time, produced "disgusting sores" and lasted for seven years. The skin lesions then tended to disappear and the patient no longer appeared revolting. The mode of transmission reported by von Hutten was sexual. Diaz de Isla, in his description of 1539, listed the stages seen today but added a final stage of fever, emaciation, diarrhea, jaundice, delirium, coma and death. Girollamo Fracastoro gave the new disease its name derived from a shepherd he named Syphilis. His book in 1546 described the chancre lesion and a pustular rash which became ulcerated with some ulcers deep enough to expose bone. The pharynx was ulcerated and in some patients, the lips and even the eyes were entirely eaten away. His description also concluded that the disease had changed its nature during the previous twenty years with a reduction in the skin rash and an increase in the gumma (skin ulcer) lesions still characteristic of tertiary syphilis today. The spread of the disease across Europe was not as rapid as that of plague in the fourteenth century. It appeared in England in 1496, in Poland in 1499, in Russia in 1500, and, finally, in China in 1505. Japan escaped until 1569 and Iceland was free of syphilis until 1753. One puzzle, which has contributed to the alternate theories of origin, is an outbreak in India in 1498. Vasco de Gama led an expedition of four ships around the Cape of Good Hope in 1497 and landed in Calicut on the Malabar River on May 20, 1498. The crew of 160 men may have included some from Columbus' crew who carried syphilis to India.

By the end of the sixteenth century (1599), one-third of the residents of Paris was infected. In 1519, Erasmus the scholar said that any nobleman who had not contracted syphilis was a "country bumpkin." The disease seemed to subside in its prevalence or its severity because Sir Thomas More, in 1529, wrote that there were only one-fifth of the syphilis cases ("French Pocks") in the monastic hospitals that year compared with thirty years before. The observations of Fracastoro and Thomas More suggest that the disease was changing with time. Since preventive immunity does not develop to the organism, only a change in the disease or a reduction of exposure would explain the accounts. The European population (according to the New World theory) had not been exposed to this organism before 1493, but it is possible that either the most susceptible died off or the organism became less virulent with passage through many new hosts. Both phenomena occur in infectious diseases. Kissing was a common form of greeting at the time in some societies, especially the Tudor society of England. Perhaps the different transmission method, as in smallpox inoculation, produced differences in virulence. Oral transmission, by kissing, might have resulted in oral chancres and different manifestations in other ways.

Yaws, which chiefly infects children, does have destructive oral and facial lesions in some cases. "Late yaws," which occurs in about ten percent of cases, can destroy the mouth, pharynx and even the face. "Endemic syphilis" is a disease of African children (which is not congenital and without any of the abnormal teeth or visual impairment), which is transmitted by kissing and food contamination, and is the least virulent of the *Treponema* infections. The virulent version of the infection seems to be the venereal one and the organism, while indistinguishable in all four diseases by either antigenicity or even genetic differences, behaves differently depending on the route of infection. One of the bits of evidence for the African origin of syphilis is the fact that the organism of yaws and syphilis are identical even though they are called by different subspecies. Yaws, however, does leave skeletal lesions similar to those of syphilis and neither has been found in pre-Columbus Europe.

ROYAL SYPHILIS

The social and historical consequences of syphilis have been enormous. Kings, including Francis I of France and, possibly, Henry VIII of England have been affected. Czar Ivan the Terrible was born in 1530 as the Grand Duke of Muscovy and spent his youth, as did many of his peers, drinking and womanizing. He was crowned Czar in 1547 and showed promise as a serious and studious young ruler. He established a legal code, banished many oppressive nobles, founded schools and extended his empire as far as Prussia by 1560. In 1552 his wife Anastasia gave birth to a son, Dimitri, who died at six months of age, perhaps of congenital syphilis. Two more sons were born before Anastasia died in 1560.

After her death, Ivan developed a fantasy that his closest advisors, friends from his days as Grand Duke, had caused the death of his wife by witch-craft. He dismissed and imprisoned them. He proceeded to condemn a number of friends and their children to death, and then, in 1561, he married a Circassian princess. This marriage did not prevent him from offering a proposal of marriage to Elizabeth I, Queen of England in 1563. His younger son was described as unhealthy looking and of weak wits, suggesting congenital syphilis here as well. In 1563, his new Tzaritsa bore another son, but this child died at six weeks of age. Stillbirths, neonatal mortality, and late miscarriages are common in maternal syphilis.

In 1564, Ivan began to demonstrate bizarre behavior strongly suggestive of cerebral syphilis. He loaded a sleigh with treasure and took off from Moscow with his wife and two surviving children, giving no indication of their destination. He left a message saying that he could no longer tolerate "the treachery by which I was surrounded." Russian officials finally found him in a small village and induced him to return to Moscow with a promise that he could "execute any traitors he desired." He returned to Moscow in February 1565 and began the executions two days later. He established a monastery-like residence and clothed his bodyguards in black habits. He alternated fervent praying with visits to the torture chambers. A reign of terror began and continued for nineteen years with thousands flogged to death for imaginary conspiracies and nobles hung while Ivan and his son raped their wives and daughters.

In 1581, he murdered his own son, also named Ivan. He pursued his fantasy of marrying Queen Elizabeth and even offered to marry a kinswoman in spite of his own existing marriage. Finally, fortunately for some young relative of Elizabeth, he died in 1584. His last days were horrible with sleeplessness and terror as the insanity overwhelmed him. During the period of Soviet rule, his remains were exhumed and clear evidence of tertiary syphilis was found. His death, and the murder of his son Ivan, left the throne to an idiot, the other son Feodor, who was dominated by advisors, chiefly Boris Godunov and, on Boris' death in 1605, the result was chaos. Finally, in 1613, the Romanovs began their dynasty, but the consequences of Ivan's syphilis and its effect on his behavior left long-lasting damage to the Russian monarchy.

The case of Henry VIII is less certain and there are controversies over his personality change in his mid-forties. He led an active life as a young man with several serious injuries but, as he aged, he became grossly obese. His problems obtaining a male heir led to the break with Rome, wars with European rulers including his daughter Elizabeth's war with Spain, and the death of thousands of his subjects in the religious wars of the Tudors.

Catharine of Aragon, his first wife, had a stillborn male infant and at least three late miscarriages, a history consistent with syphilis. Ann Boleyn had three miscarriages in addition to the birth of her daughter Elizabeth. Jane Seymour had one son, King Edward IV, born in 1537 and no other known pregnancies. Henry had four children who survived including one illegitimate boy, Henry Fitzroy, Earl of Richmond, who died at seventeen from what may have been tuberculosis. Elizabeth and Mary Tudor were "short-sighted" and Mary died at forty-two. During her life, she was of short stature and was said to have a flat nose with a chronic discharge. Edward IV died at age fifteen and was never healthy, dying of tuberculosis after a long illness. He developed a rash not long before his death, possibly measles.

Henry as a young man was very handsome and showed evidence of high intelligence. In 1514, he developed small pox, but there was no description of pustules. Was this small pox or secondary syphilis? In 1521, he wrote a scholarly rebuttal to Martin Luther and received the title "Defender of the Faith" by Pope Leo X. Thomas More probably wrote the treatise as ghostwriter. In 1527, he began to complain of headaches and the next year developed a chronic ulcer on his thigh, about the time his character began to change. The divorce from Catharine was no doubt a source of worry and frustration but, in 1531, he enacted the new punishment of boiling alive and saw to the execution of three people in this fashion. The first Treason Act came in 1533, and in 1534 he began the persecution of Catholics, Lutherans, and Lollards. In 1535, he beheaded the abbot and monks of Charterhouse monastery and executed Thomas More, his friend and advisor for years. His treatment of Ann Boleyn was savage and the suppression of the abbeys in 1538-40, while lucrative for the crown, supports an impression of imbalance. The rest of his life, while he never deteriorated as Ivan did, continued a trend toward tyranny and absolutism.

After his death, and the death of his weakling son, Edward IV, his daughter Mary ascended the throne. Her behavior was no improvement and even her husband Philip II of Spain was unable to dissuade her from fierce persecution of Protestants, which produced enduring hatred of the Catholic Church among her subjects. Again, the spirochete may well have affected history. Elizabeth, the "virgin queen", never married although that may have been a political decision for the first English queen rather than the consequence of awareness of disease. The causative organism was only identified in 1905 and its treatment will be described in a later chapter.

SMALLPOX

The Old World received syphilis as an unwanted "gift" from the New World, but reciprocated with an equally savage contribution. Ko Hung in China first described smallpox about 300CE. The first certain description in Europe was by Gregory of Tours in 581CE although earlier plagues might have been smallpox with manifestations later lost in the evolution of the virus. Buddhist missionaries carried it to Japan before 580CE and the Japanese "Age of Plagues" from 750 to 1000 was largely a series of smallpox and measles epidemics. Rhazes, the Persian physician, provided an accurate account in 900 and his description of smallpox and measles identified the two as different diseases for the first time. By the tenth century, there were clearly three varieties: *variola major*-virulent smallpox, *variola minor*- the lesser disease that was used in a few examples of immunization prior to Jenner's writings and also known as alastrim, and *variola vaccinia*-cowpox. Each of the three provides immunity to the other two varieties but the mortality and morbidity differ markedly.

In 1518, Hernando Cortez sailed from the colony of Cuba with an army of 800 Spaniards and Indian allies. After landing at Veracruz, and following a threatened mutiny, he burned his ships to encourage his hesitant army to proceed into the interior of Mexico. After a victorious battle with the Tlascalan tribe, he continued toward Montezuma's capital of Tenochtitlan (Mexico City), accompanied by new Tlascalan allies, who knew a winner when they saw one. In 1520, a second army, commanded by Panfilo de Narvaez the governor of Cuba, approached with the intention of replacing Cortez as commander. Cortez left a small force in Tenochtitlan and took the majority of his army back toward the coast to attack de Narvaez. He defeated Narvaez and his forces in a surprise night attack. Montezuma and the Aztecs attacked the remaining garrison during the absence of Cortez and nearly annihilated them. The returning Cortez was able to extract less than half his army from the city insurrection and took refuge with the Tlascalans. He returned to besiege the city in 1521 and, after defeating a furious defense, entered the city on August 13, 1521. He found the houses filled with dead, not from wounds, but from disease.

Narvaez's army had included many African slaves, some of whom became ill and one of whom may have carried smallpox. The Indian population became infected and the disease, called by the Indians the "great leprosy," produced a rash and spread rapidly, unlike true leprosy. It was undoubtedly smallpox and a virulent strain. The Spaniards, many of whom had had smallpox or variola minor-alastrim, were not affected. When Cortez entered Tenochtitlan in August, one half of the population had died.

Almost half the Aztec population perished in this first smallpox epidemic in the New World. A second epidemic in 1531, brought by another ship, continued the devastation and by 1576 the population had fallen to two million from as high as 25 million in 1492. During the same period, the Inca population of Peru fell from seven million to one-half million. Mumps and measles contributed a significant proportion to this toll and the experience was to be repeated in the South Pacific during the next century when measles was the principle killer.[83] It is unknown whether the disease brought by the Spaniards was caused by *variola major* transmitted by an African slave or whether *variola minor*, carried by an asymptomatic Spanish soldier, gained virulence in this susceptible population.

Mexico remained a reservoir of virulent smallpox until modern times. A traveler carried the disease into New York City in 1947 in one of the last outbreaks in the US. The disease had been relatively mild in Europe prior to the contact with America. In the sixteenth century virulence returned, possibly as a consequence of passage through the susceptible Indian population. By 1629, the Bills of Mortality of London reported less than 1,000 smallpox deaths in a population of 300 to 400 thousand. The disease had changed again. It had become a common disease of children with a low mortality, similar to measles in recent times before the measles vaccine was developed. This changed again with the eighteenth century; in the years 1769 to 1784, in one small town of 5,000 in England, 589 children died of smallpox. All but one of these children were under the age of ten and 466 were three and under. In London eighty-five percent of smallpox deaths were children under five. The immunity of the adults, perhaps provided by exposure to alastrim, protected them but the children were as susceptible as the Indians had been.

Smallpox was not the only disease carried to the New World by the Europeans or their slaves. Swine influenza seems to have wiped out most of the indigenous population of the Caribbean islands before the arrival of smallpox. It arrived with Canary Island pigs in 1493 long before smallpox arrived with Cortez. Typhus took a toll and, in 1529, measles arrived with another epidemic in the susceptible population that had survived smallpox. Chickenpox, diphtheria, scarlet fever, typhoid, whooping cough and bubonic plague, all absent from the New World for 10,000 years appeared in the first few decades after contact with Europeans occurred. The Carib Indians, in an area less exposed to European contact, and fierce enough to discourage it, survived the initial onslaught. The islanders, whose smaller population and exposure to successive waves of immigration left them unable to adapt, died off. The islands' climate was also more like home for the next invader, *P. vivax* malaria, which arrived with the Spaniards. As the islanders died off, the Spanish began to import African slaves who brought with them *P. falciparum* malaria. By 1647, yellow fever had arrived, probably with the *Aedes Aegypti* mosquito, which was not native to the Americas as the Anopheles (which carries malaria) was. The African slaves carried resistance to Old World diseases that killed the Indians, hence their value as slaves. Cholera did not appear until the nineteenth century but when it did, it carried off slaves by the thousands. The Indians had been gone for centuries by then.[84]

76   Paul Strathern, *Mendeleyev's Dream*, page 75, Thomas Dunne Books (2000).

77   J. Schact, "Ibn al-Nafis, Servetus and Colombo," *al-Andalus*, volume xxii:317-36 (1937).

78   E.V. Hulse, "Leprosy and Ancient Egypt," *The Lancet*, (September 23, 1972) page 659. The author attributes the spread to Europe to the Roman army of Pompey in 62 BCE.

79   Roy Porter, page 166-167.

80   Frederick F. Cartwright and Michael Biddis, *Disease and History*, Sutton Publishing (2000), pages 45-46 discuss the African origin theory of syphilis.

81   Francis L. Black, "Infectious Diseases in Primitive Societies," *Science* 187:515 (1975) The Amazon tribes had positive VDRL tests but no disease. Malaria was also present.

82   Charlotte Roberts, pages 150-159 for a lengthy discussion of the origin of the *Treponema* diseases.

83   Francis L. Black, "Measles Epidemicity in Insular Populations: Critical Community Size and Its Evolutionary Implication," *Journal of Theoretical Biology,* 11:207 (1966). This is a study of nineteen island communities and the dynamics of measles virus epidemics.

84   Kenneth F Kiple, "The Geography of Human Disease," in the "Cambridge World History of Human Disease," Cambridge University Press (1993).

8
The Enlightenment and Medicine

RENAISSANCE PHYSICIANS HAD ACQUIRED NEW STATUS AND LEARNING but their patients derived small benefit from this professional progress. Remedies were still mostly Galenicals and bleeding and purging killed more then they cured. Pompous and wealthy physicians were the butt of playwrights although the role of the public physician (it is too early to call them public health physicians) increased. Charles V, in the new Carolina Code in 1532, required judges to consult surgeons in criminal cases and midwives in infanticide. Paré described methods of determining virginity in women, important, as non-consummation was grounds for annulment. He also taught how to determine whether wounds were produced before or after death. In 1518, Henry VIII chartered the College of Physicians but the closure and asset stripping of monasteries by Henry and his son Edward IV closed all the medieval hospitals. St Bartholomew's and St Thomas' hospitals passed to the city of London as secular institutions as did Bethlehem, the lunatic asylum. These three hospitals survived to treat a population of 200,000 by 1600. The treatment was of doubtful efficacy but they did provide shelter to the sick.

The English Civil War brought upheaval in medical as well as social circles. Royal charters meant little when the King had been beheaded. Nicholas Culpepper (1616-1654) had no medical degree but, after an apprenticeship to an apothecary, he set up as a physician to the poor. Having supported the Roundheads and Cromwell in the war, he defied the College of Physicians by publishing an unauthorized translation of their pharmacopoeia, *A Physicall Directory,* in 1649. He declared that the poor could not afford the fees of College physicians and, after they reacted with outrage, he published *The English Physician Enlarged* in 1653, an even more controversial version. It went through scores of editions and became known as "Culpepper's Herbal"; a revised edition is still in print. After the Restoration in 1660, the College never regained its prior status and English medical books continued to be published in the vernacular. The College eventually, after scientific medicine became established, regained its reputation but Galen was discredited forever.

In 1628 William Harvey published *de Motu Cordis et Sanguinus in Animalibus*, the culmination of his studies based on Vesalius' anatomy. Harvey was born in Folkestone in 1578 and attended Caius College, Cambridge. From 1600, he studied under Fabricius at Padua absorbing comparative anatomy and embryology. In 1602, he returned to England and was elected to the College of Physicians in 1607. Two years later he was appointed as physician at St Bartholomew's and in 1615 became Lumleian Lecturer of the College, the lecturer in anatomy and charged with performing public dissections. By 1618, he was a royal physician and, during the Civil War, he was present at the battle of Edgehill as personal physician to Charles I where he is reported to have spent the day reading a book while the battle raged around him.

He confirmed Colombo's observations on the pulmonary circulation and his experiments showed that the volume of blood passing through the heart every minute was so great that Galen's theory, that it was absorbed by the body and regenerated in the liver, must be incorrect. He was the first to measure the volume of blood expelled by the heart in an hour and noted that it far exceeded the total blood volume of the body. He could not see the connection between the arteries and veins (the microscope was invented about 1600 but not applied to anatomy until much later) but he could see the fact that blood did pass through the lungs and the tissues. He tied a ligature around the arm so tightly that arterial circulation was interrupted. Then he loosened it to allow arterial input but kept the veins obstructed. He demonstrated that the veins became distended when the arteries were opened. Finally, he demonstrated that the valves allowed flow in the veins only toward the heart and corrected Fabricius' theory that the valves' function was to prevent a static column of blood from falling into the legs when the individual stood erect.

His explanation of the circulation did not include an understanding of the role of the lungs and oxygen exchange. He wrote, "All things do depend on the motional pulsation of the heart" and attributed the regeneration of the blood, after passage through the body, to the pulse and heartbeat. He noted the constriction of the ductus arteriosus (see the chapter on cardiac surgery) that occurs after birth but drew no conclusions about the role of the lungs from this astute observation.[85]

Harvey was attacked for his presumption in rejecting Galen's concept of the pulse and the role of the heart. One of his attackers was Riolan, the leading advocate of Galen in the faculty of Paris, who reaffirmed his confidence in the role of the liver as the source of new blood and of bleeding in therapeutics. If blood circulates, the sites for bleeding (a subject of treatises) have no significance, as all blood is the same. One of Harvey's most prominent defenders was Rene Descartes, the greatest thinker of the Scientific Revolution (author of the phrase *Cogito Ergo Sum*), the inventor of analytical geometry and, while not a physician, author of three treatises on anatomy and physiology. Descartes erred in having too mechanical a concept of the body and rejected Harvey's description of systole and diastole. To Descartes the diastole was the engine of the circulation in which innate heat rarified drops of blood, caused them to expand and forced them into the arteries. Another supporter was Thomas Hobbes, author of *Leviathan*, and even more controversial as a supposed atheist who believed, like Newton, that the universe was a gigantic clockwork.

Anatomical research continued with the discovery of chyle, the fat filled lymph draining from the intestine, and lacteal vessels (which carry the lymph) in a recently fed dog by Gaspare Aselli (1581-1625), an anatomy professor in Padua. He studied these structures and demonstrated that they became distended after eating. Modern surgeons often observe this phenomenon. Elective abdominal surgery is performed on fasting patients and the mesenteric lymphatics are invisible, the lymph is clear. In trauma, or other emergency cases, the patient may have eaten recently and the lacteals are clearly visible, filled with chyle. Jean Pecquet (1622-1674) rediscovered the thoracic duct, which carries lymph up along the spinal column and empties into the subclavian vein, and demonstrated the return of lymph from the lacteals to the venous circulation via the duct, another blow to Galenism. Thomas Bartholin published a book in 1653, *Vasa Lymphatica et hepaticus exsequiae*, the first book to include color plates, describing the lymphatic system.

The physiology of respiration was next to be delineated beginning with the Italians Viviani and Torricelli who demonstrated air pressure with vacuum experiments. Torricelli demonstrated the pressure of air (the units of which – torr, are named for him) by filling a glass tube, sealed at one end, with mercury. He inverted the tube over a bowl filled with mercury and placed the open end of the tube beneath the surface. The top of the column of mercury in the tube dropped to a point 76 centimeters above the surface of the mercury in the bowl. Something was pressing down on the surface of the mercury in the bowl and pushing the column up into the glass tube. Torricelli concluded that the force pressing down on the mercury was the pressure of air. Over the next few days, he noted that the top of the mercury column moved up and down in height above the bowl of mercury. He had discovered the barometer. Blaise Pascal, the French mathematician, immediately recognized the significance of Torricelli's observation and arranged to duplicate the experiment at the top of a 1,500-foot mountain. The pressure (and the height of the column of mercury) was lower and Pascal discovered the concept of atmosphere and the vacuum of space.

The German inventor von Guericke demonstrated air pressure in spectacular fashion in 1650 by building two carefully constructed hemispheres and pumping the air from the sphere created by fitting them together. (The pumps he constructed to do this were at least as great a scientific advance as the hemispheres.) He then attempted to pull the sphere apart with two teams of horses, each attached to one hemisphere. They could not pull them apart but, when the air was allowed to refill the sphere, the two halves fell apart without any effort to separate them. He repeated the experiment all over Europe and demonstrated that a bell rung within the evacuated sphere could not be heard and a candle would not burn. A garbled version of the experiment gave us the nursery rhyme "Humpty Dumpty."[86] He experimented with Torricelli's device and made a special barometer in which the column of mercury moved the arm of a man, which thus pointed out rising and falling pressure. This was the *Wettermännchen*.

Robert Boyle, working with his assistant Robert Hooke, continued the study of air and gases. They proved that animals and birds could not survive without air and that it caused rust on iron and a green discoloration of copper. When compressed it seemed to have elasticity. Van Helmont, a Flemish physician born in 1577, had preceded Boyle in these studies by growing a tree in a large earthenware vessel. He carefully weighed the soil and protected it from dust and other impurities. After watering the plant with distilled water for five years he measured it and found that it had increased from five pounds to 169 pounds but the soil in the pot had decreased by only two ounces. He concluded that the tree was composed only of water after what must have been the first modern scientific experiment. He then investigated the role of air since the plant and its leaves and branches seemed to consist of more than water alone. His next major experiment consisted of burning sixty-two pounds of charcoal. He was left with a quantity of gas and one pound of ash. The gas given off had characteristics very different from air and he named it *spiritus Sylvester* ("spirit of wood"); we call it carbon dioxide. Von Helmont discovered that fermentation produced the same gas. In the absence of adequate laboratory apparatus to collect the gas, his experiments were limited and he called the air-like substances he collected "chaos," a sort of pre-matter described by the Greeks as the origin of the universe. The Flemish pronunciation of the word "chaos" resulted in the term being translated as "gas" and the word has been used for that form of matter since Von Helmont's time. These experiments provided a fertile field for later scientists as progress in physical science and physiology accelerated.

Boyle continued Torricelli's experiments with gases, this time using a J-shaped tube, and learned that, as he added mercury to the open end of the tube, the gas was compressed in the sealed end. Torricelli's experiment, by filling the tube with mercury and then inverting it, had produced a vacuum above the mercury in the tube. Boyle did not invert his tube and adding mercury produced compression of the gas in the closed end. The weight of the mercury and the volume of the air could be measured and compared; from this experiment we have Boyle's Laws of the properties of gas. Heating the gas added the third component of Boyle's Law. In one of History's ironies Boyle's experiments were anticipated by Heron of Alexandria (also called Hero although this seems to be incorrect) in about 62CE. Heron studied air and concluded that it was composed of compressible particles. He demonstrated a vacuum in an upturned water glass and determined that steam expanded. He used this property of steam to construct a working steam engine (which he called an *aeolipile*) which turned a wheel by expelling steam from two jet-like arm tubes. The steam jets turned the wheel using the principle currently employed by rotating lawn sprinklers. No application of the invention was apparent in 62CE (although it was used to open temple doors) and knowledge of the entire matter was lost for centuries after the Library at Alexandria was destroyed. Heron's works were rediscovered in the last century, long after Boyle's time. Boyle also invented a method to distinguish between acids and alkalis using syrup of violets which turns red in acid and green in alkali. Boyle's assistant Robert Hooke continued his work with gases after Boyle's death in 1661.

Richard Lower (1631-1691) studied blood to learn why arterial blood was bright red and venous blood was darker. In October 1667, while working with Hooke, he noted that pulmonary artery blood was still dark and pulmonary venous blood, returning to the heart from the lungs, was bright red. The change occurred not in the heart, as Galen and everyone since, including Harvey, believed, but in the lungs. He concluded that a "nitrous spirit of the air" mixed with the blood in the lungs and produced the bright color. John Mayow (1641-1679) assisted Boyle in his air pump experiments and learned that the same "nitrous spirit" was necessary for combustion and was consumed by respiration and combustion leaving "vitiated air". It would take another century and the discovery of oxygen to explain the observations of Lower and Mayow.

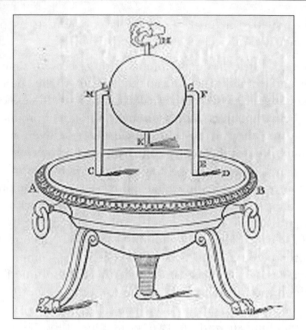

*Figure 5 – Heron's steam engine, the movable part
suspended (at G and L) to allow rotation as jet arms
produce the force rotating the sphere. The steam
was generated in the vessel AB.*

The Microscope

Three Dutch spectacle makers constructed the first microscopes about
1600. The spectacle, unknown to the ancients, was mentioned, in his *opus
majus* (sometime before 1294), by Roger Bacon in the thirteenth century,
the earliest reference to be found. Initially, only convex lenses were made
but eventually concave lenses, to correct nearsightedness, were discovered. The process of manufacturing was by trial and error since optics was
poorly understood. Roger Bacon's description gave the best explanation
of the principle for centuries. A Dutch spectacle maker, named Jansen, is
credited with the compound microscope, in 1590. Robert Lippershey is
given credit for the binocular microscope, although the power of these
devices was poor until the nineteenth century. The telescope, which
preceded the microscope, was actually discovered by an anonymous
apprentice who was polishing lenses and put one in front of the other. He
found that the image of a church was magnified by this maneuver and the
master immediately recognized the significance of the observation.
Reducing the focal length produced the microscope.

In 1621, Jacob Kuffler presented a microscope to a Roman cardinal but Kuffler died before he could explain what it was. The device remained a mystery until Galileo arrived in Rome two years later. He explained its use and mentioned that he had constructed many such instruments in the previous years.[87] Initially it was a curiosity allowing the observation of gnats and grubs. Robert Hooke, while working as Robert Boyle's assistant, adopted the microscope as a tool and in 1665 published *Micrographia* in which he coined the term "cell" (describing the structure of cork, which looks like a honeycomb in the microscope). Malpighi, a professor of Medicine in Pisa, continued this work discovering the fine structure of the lungs and, in 1661, published *De pulmonibus* describing the alveoli, the missing link in Harvey's theory of the circulation. He studied the lungs of living frogs and saw blood flowing through the capillaries in the walls of the alveoli. His studies included the microscopic anatomy of the tongue and the organs of sensation in the skin, both of which contain structures bearing his name. He showed that the liver, not the gallbladder, secretes bile and that the kidney functions as a filter. He also first described red blood cells.

Von Leeuwenhoek, using extremely well made simple (one lens only) microscopes, of which he built 247, extended the study of anatomy including that of insects. Beginning in 1671 he saw the crystals of uric acid in gout and, in his most famous discovery; saw "animalcules" in various fluids setting off a furious debate on spontaneous generation of life that raged for another 200 years until Pasteur. His animalcules include human spermatozoa, protozoa and other microscopic creatures. The discovery of female ova by Graaf and Stenson, both Dutch anatomists, fueled the controversy. Stenson first used the term "ovary" to describe the female gonad. A feud between "ovists" and "animalculists" ensued with the animalculists asserting that the spermatozoa contained a tiny complete human called a "homunculus." Harvey had conducted experiments on deer embryos and demonstrated the differentiation of limbs in the fetus, a fact that contradicted the theories of a fully formed homunculus, but the controversy continued for a long time.

Actual medical practice was not affected by these scientific advances and the typical physician, often still in the thrall of Galen, was parodied by Moliere in his play *Le medicine malgre lui* ("The Doctor Despite Himself"-1666-67) and a number of other comedies with physicians as fools and scoundrels. Malpighi's assistant Giorgio Baglivi (1668-1707) pictured the body as a machine with the teeth functioning as scissors, the heart and vessels as waterworks, etc. His work with the microscope delineated the difference between striated and smooth muscle but, in his treatment of patients, he reiterated Hippocratic ideals. Thomas Sydenham (1624-1689) was called the "English Hippocrates" but he rejected anatomy and dissection saying "I know an old woman in Covent Garden (the flower market) who understands botany better, and, as for anatomy, my butcher can dissect a joint full and well. Now young man, all that is stuff, you must go to the bedside, it is there alone you can learn disease." He was observant and, while rejecting the theoretical basis of scientific medicine, which was developing at the time, he drew appropriate conclusions and used Peruvian bark in the treatment of malaria, endemic in England at the time. This, the first disease-specific effective drug (and source of quinine), seemed to strike at the basis of the disease, in contrast to the Hippocratic regimen, which was directed at a general sense of health. The bark was brought to Europe by the Jesuits around 1630 causing it to be called "Jesuits' Bark," a fact that prompted Oliver Cromwell to refuse it and suffer from malaria rather than accept a remedy discovered by the hated Jesuits. It appeared in the *London Pharmacopoeia* in 1677. Sydenham wrote, "All diseases should be reduced to definite and certain species with the same care which we see exhibited by Botanick Writers in their Phytologies." Diseases were specific entities possessing unique natural histories. He did not reject the humours of Hippocrates, believing that malaria occurred in the spring and summer because the sun warmed humours accumulated in the blood during winter.

Midwives continued to attend childbirth and a few were educated in anatomy and enjoyed large practices. William Chamberlen, a French Huguenot who fled to England to escape persecution, invented the obstetrical forceps and kept it a family secret through many generations. Chamberlen brought the instrument into the patient's room in a box and assembled it beneath the sheets covering the patient, out of the view of bystanders. The Chamberlen family kept the secret from about 1570 until nearly 1720, when the last of the family, Hugh Chamberlen, died.

With the exception of quinine, remedies continued in the Hippocratic and ineffective tradition. The death of Charles II was a particularly grim example as he was treated for his stroke with sixteen ounces of bleeding, cupping, and another eight ounces of bleeding (which might possibly benefit a hypertensive crisis). He was then given an emetic, which he could not be induced to swallow and finally a cautery iron was applied to his scalp in numerous places. Samuel Pepys (1633-1703), in his famous diary, recounts witnessing Richard Lower transfuse a "crack-brained" student with sheep's blood in an attempt to treat his mental illness. This procedure prompted a satirist of the time to speculate on possible consequences such as growing magnificent fleeces on such patients. Pepys speculated on the effect of transfusing an archbishop with the blood of a Quaker. Cutting for stone existed in seventeenth century England and Pepys was himself subjected to the procedure in 1657 by surgeon Thomas Hollyer at St. Thomas's Hospital. The stone was the size of a tennis ball and the fee was twenty-four shillings. Pepys kept the stone in a case and celebrated the anniversary each year. He observed the great plague epidemic of 1665 and, unlike many London physicians, declined to leave the city. He was acquainted with many physicians but sought treatment with few. He wore a rabbit's foot around his neck to ward off sickness.

Physics with Newton's *Principia*, chemistry with the Gas Laws, mathematics with the Calculus (whose origin was disputed by Newton and Leibnitz), and astronomy progressed rapidly while medicine was still tied to the Greeks. Newton was a thoroughly nasty fellow and conducted a feud with two men, John Flamsteed, the Royal Astronomer, and Stephen Gray, an amateur scientist. Flamsteed produced an astronomical catalogue and was responsible for much of Newton's *Principia*. Newton feuded with Hooke, as well, and the story is told in a recent book.[88] Gross and microscopic anatomy progressed but, with the exception of cinchona (Jesuits') bark and opium, medicine remained ineffective. In 1662 haberdasher, John Graunt published the *Natural and Political Observations…Upon the Bills of Mortality* based on the weekly burial lists of parish clerks. This began the study of demographics and, while the causes of death listed were often inaccurate, important information was preserved. Edmund Halley, discoverer of the comet, calculated life-tables and annual mortality rates in 1693. This benefited the new life insurance business but also contained important information for medicine that was put to use in the next century. In 1750, infant mortality in France was over 200 per 1000 live births and in Geneva, it was 296 per 1000. John Locke, philosopher as well as physician, wrote *Essay Concerning Human Understanding* in 1690, an important introduction to the period of the Enlightenment. In 1668, combining surgery with medicine, he drained an infected liver hydatid cyst in Anthony Ashley Cooper, later Earl of Shaftesbury, using a silver tube. As the eighteenth century began, little progress in therapeutics had occurred in spite of great advances in anatomy and, in Harvey's case, the beginnings of physiology.

PHLOGISTON

Gas chemistry progressed rapidly and Lavoisier discovered that the atmosphere was composed of a number of gases. Combustion continued to pose problems in understanding and the science took a wrong turn in 1703 when Stahl, a professor of medicine at the University of Halle, published the concept of *phlogiston*, a new word based on the Greek word *phlogios* which means "fiery." Phlogiston was the substance given off during burning and corresponded to the loss of weight. His theory got into trouble when it tried to explain the rusting of metals since the rust and remaining metal weigh more than the metal did to begin with. Rust and combustion had already been connected (both required the "nitrous spirit" of air discovered by Lower and Hooke) and it was pretty well accepted that they were related. If phlogiston is given off by rusting why should the combination of rust and metal weigh more? His defenders tried to explain the discrepancy by proposing two types of phlogiston, one in wood or paper that had weight and another type in metals that had negative weight. Von Helmont's experiment with the tree was now explained with the conclusion that a growing tree absorbs phlogiston.

This all seems silly now but the phlogiston idea took science on a blind alley for many years and, only with modern chemistry, was it finally dispelled. Henry Cavendish, one of the greatest and most eccentric scientists England has ever produced (and the richest) studied gases in the eighteenth century and his discoveries supported the phlogiston theory although some findings were hard to explain. Among his other interests were electricity and James Maxwell, the discoverer of the laws of electromagnetism and first director of the Cavendish Laboratory at Cambridge, read his unpublished papers a century later and found that Cavendish had anticipated many of the findings of Faraday and Maxwell himself.

Joseph Priestley, a contemporary of Cavendish who corresponded with him, experimented with air and, following a suggestion of Cavendish's, used mercury instead of water to compress the air. This revealed several water-soluble gases previously undiscovered. By creating a calx of mercury, the equivalent of rust, by heating it in air, then heating it again in the absence of air, he returned the mercury to its metallic state and collected a gas. The gas he collected from this experiment caused a candle to burn brightly and supported life. He called this "de-phlogisticated air," for he was also a believer. In 1774, at a scientific exposition, he passed this observation on to Lavoisier, the greatest chemist of the age. Among Priestley's other discoveries was the sap of a Brazilian tree which, when hardened, would rub out pencil marks. For this reason, he called it "rubber."

Lavoisier had already conducted experiments to disprove the phlogiston theory and the gas, which Priestley provided, allowed further work on this subject, that of combustion and its products. Lavoisier named the new element "oxygen" (Lower's "nitrous spirit," as well) and proved that, rather than phlogiston being given off by burning or rusting, the material burned or rusted combined with oxygen from the air. Lavoisier now conducted a number of studies of respiration and concluded that oxygen was the element in air necessary for life. In his book of 1787, *Method of Chemical Nomenclature*, he established a systematic method of naming compounds and elements. Two years later, he published his *Elementary Treatise on Chemistry* and placed the science on a modern footing. Unfortunately, the French Revolution began in 1789 and Lavoisier was a stalwart of the *Ancien Regime*. Jean-Paul Marat, whose scientific paper Lavoisier had once rejected, denounced him and in 1793, he was guillotined after the revolutionary judge remarked, "The Republic has no need of scientists." In spite of Lavoisier's work, the phlogiston theory continued to be debated until the mid-nineteenth century when modern chemistry finally laid it to rest.

EIGHTEENTH CENTURY MEDICINE

During the eighteenth century, fever was the subject of many books, but, with the exception of malaria, little was accomplished in treatment. Giovanni Battista Morgagni, chair of the anatomy department at Padua, published *De sedibus et causis morborum* ("On the Sites and Causes of Disease") in 1761. He reported the findings from 700 autopsies, with extensive drawings, and discussed the pathology of disease. This was a major work and was translated into English in 1769 and into German in 1774. He included case histories and correlated the autopsy findings with ante-mortem symptoms. He described the pathology of myocardial infarction, mitral stenosis, and pulmonary stenosis. He pointed out that stroke was a disease of cerebral blood vessels, not the brain itself. Diseases were located in specific organs and, like Sydenham, he emphasized the specificity of disease.

Matthew Baillie (1761-1823), a student of the Hunter brothers, the anatomist William and the surgeon John, followed up Morgagni's book with further description of pathology. In Baillie's book, he described emphysema and cirrhosis of the liver, which he linked to alcohol. Ovarian cysts and gastric ulcers were illustrated with fine copper plate engravings. A later edition of the book described rheumatic fever of the heart. Baillie remarked, "I know better perhaps than another man, from my knowledge of anatomy, how to discover disease but, when I have done so, I don't know better how to cure it." Some innovations made things worse. The new lying-in hospitals had horrendous mortality rates due to puerperal fever, often a consequence of physicians coming from the autopsy room to examine women without washing their hands. Bloodletting continued with Benjamin Rush, a signer of the Declaration of Independence and "the American Hippocrates," an enthusiastic advocate. Rush was also an advocate of calomel purges and "blue pills," both mixtures of mercury chloride, which had a high risk of toxicity. Reverend Edmund Stone advocated willow bark, which contains *salicin*, a compound similar to aspirin, to the Royal Society for fever but was ignored.

WITHERING AND DIGITALIS

In 1785, William Withering produced *An Account of the Foxglove and Some of its Medical Uses etc; With Practical Remarks on Dropsy and Other Diseases*. Withering was a physician, and England's greatest medical botanist, when he heard, in 1775, from a Shropshire woman about an herbal tea, a family secret, useful in treating swollen legs. He had actually produced a student paper on dropsy during his time at Edinburgh, interesting in light of later developments. The tea had twenty ingredients but Withering concluded that the effective component must be the leaf of the foxglove, a common ornamental flower. He experimented with different preparations to ascertain the best dosage. On December 8, 1775 he gave foxglove tea to a fifty-year-old man with asthma and abdominal fluid, ascites. The patient "made a large quantity of water. His breath gradually drew easier, his belly subsided and in about ten days he began to eat with a keen appetite." The first effective medicine since opium and Jesuits' bark had been discovered. Withering moved to Birmingham that year, at the invitation of Erasmus Darwin, physician and grandfather of the biologist Charles.

Withering quickly became successful in Birmingham, exceeding the expectations of Dr. Darwin and stimulating his jealousy. Withering's fourth case of dropsy treated with foxglove was later published as his own by Darwin, in 1785, just before Withering's report appeared. Darwin claimed credit for the discovery, perhaps stimulated by professional jealousy, but no one accepts his claim of priority. Darwin's first case is obviously the same person as Withering's fourth patient. Withering contracted tuberculosis in Birmingham and was chronically ill for the rest of his life. In spite of this handicap he was active almost to the end, which came in December of 1799. His voluminous writings were later collected and edited by Sir William Osler. Among his patients was Benjamin Franklin who was treated successfully for bladder stone while living in Paris. Richard Bright later learned that *digitalis*, the scientific name of foxglove, was effective against cardiac dropsy-we would call it heart failure-but not against renal dropsy, the disease (renal failure) that for two centuries carried Bright's name.

JENNER AND SMALLPOX

In 1717 Lady Mary Wortley Montague, the wife of the British Consul in Constantinople, reported how Turkish peasant women held smallpox parties at which inoculations of children were carried out. Lady Mary had her five-year-old daughter inoculated by surgeon Charles Maitland after their return to England in 1721. After a series of experiments on prisoners, who were promised clemency in return for their cooperation, King George II had his two daughters inoculated. The procedure was not without complications and about two percent of patients inoculated died. After 1728, because of such deaths, the procedure fell into disfavor. In America, an epidemic occurred in 1721, and Cotton Mather, the well-known minister, learned of the practice of inoculation. Zabdiel Bolyston, a Boston physician, was willing to participate and began by inoculating his six-year-old son and two negro slaves. After initial success, he inoculated 244 people during the summer of 1721 but six patients died of smallpox. He was accused of spreading the infection and narrowly escaped lynching when it was learned that he had used actual smallpox pus.

A severe epidemic in South Carolina in 1738 prompted another physician, James Kilpatrick, to inoculate a large number of people with good success in preventing a high mortality. Benjamin Franklin had lost his only legitimate son to smallpox in 1736, and he became a prominent supporter of Dr. Kilpatrick. Under Franklin's influence, George Washington arranged to have his troops inoculated. Kilpatrick, who used a variation of the usual technique by choosing pus from mild cases and inoculating with a shallow scratch, traveled to London in 1743 and his reports of success prompted a revival of "variolation," as inoculation with the smallpox virus is called, in Europe. Some inoculators made improvements in the method, as had Kilpatrick by choosing pus from a mild case. Robert Sutton and his son Daniel devised the important advance of "passaging" or "removes", in which they selected a mild case and used pus from that patient to inoculate others as Kilpatrick had done. Then they took the mildest of those cases for the next batch of pus.

IngenHousz inoculated The Royal Court of Vienna in 1768. He used two hundred subjects and ten removes to obtain the material for the innoculation. Thomas Dimsdale, another inoculator who, like the Suttons, was not a physician, inoculated Catherine the Great using material passed through two hundred of her servants. The royal sized fee he received established an estate still held by the Baron Dimsdale. The inoculators used "airing houses" to isolate the inoculation subjects, essential to avoid accusations of spreading smallpox to the rest of the population. The procedure became quite common in England in the eighteenth century and parish records record mass inoculations in 1769 and later. Employers began to require that apprentices be inoculated prior to acceptance.

COWPOX

For many years, in rural areas, it was observed that dairy maids and cowhands never contracted smallpox. The cowpox disease in cattle usually affects the udder and is quite infectious. Anyone milking the cow will be infected but human-to-human infection is rare. In 1774, a farmer named Benjamin Jesty took matter from a cowpox lesion and inoculated his wife and two children by scratching their arms with a darning needle and rubbing the matter into the scratches. A smallpox epidemic came through the district, but the Jesty family was spared. The sons were said to have been inoculated with smallpox fifteen years later with no effect. In 1791, a German performed a similar experiment.

Edward Jenner was born in 1749 and studied medicine at St. George's Hospital, London, under John Hunter who stirred his enthusiasm for the experimental approach. The cowpox story came to Jenner's attention in the 1770's when he was serving an apprenticeship with a surgeon at Sodbury. Completing his apprenticeship, Jenner returned to Berkeley, his birthplace, to practice and spent the next twenty years investigating the cowpox phenomenon before attempting any experiment. In May of 1796, he took lymph from a dairymaid named Sarah Nelmes and used it to inoculate a boy named James Phipps. Jenner's report of the boy's course described some discomfort on the seventh day, a chilly feeling on the nineth with some vague general discomfort and a return to normal thereafter. The lesion's appearance was similar to that of variolation. On July first he was inoculated with matter from a smallpox lesion and no disease occurred. Jenner decided to attempt several more cases before publishing his results but cowpox disappeared from the district for the next two years. With the reappearance of cowpox, he took material and "vaccinated" another twenty-three subjects, then followed this in a month with inoculation using smallpox material. Again, no reaction occurred to the second inoculation. He reported his results in his classic publication, *An Inquiry into the Causes and Effects of the Variolae Vaccinae,* a seventy-five-page pamphlet, in 1798.

Within five years, his pamphlet had been translated into all the European languages. There was not universal approval. The "inoculators," driven by self-interest, attacked his method. Clergy denounced the transference of an animal disease to man. Some, who objected that other cattle diseases might be transferred to man, were prescient. It became a popular practice to use a chain of subjects taking matter from a cow for the first vaccination, and then transferring the inoculation from person to person. This solved the problem of cow diseases but added the considerable potential for other human diseases, such as syphilis, to be transferred. By the end of 1800, about 100,000 vaccinations had been performed in England and the method was becoming common worldwide. Jenner had spent a great deal of time and effort on vaccination, which produced no income to him. Parliament took notice of this in 1802 after a committee chaired by Doctor Mathew Baillie reported, "If Doctor Jenner had not chosen openly and honourably to explain to the public all he knew upon the subject he might have acquired a considerable fortune. In my opinion it is the most important discovery ever made in medicine." Jenner was granted £10,000, a sum later doubled. A "Jennerian Institute" was set up in London to "eradicate" smallpox by vaccination and, in 1808, it was replaced by the National Vaccine Establishment.

In 1803, the King of Spain decided to transfer vaccination to the New World and arranged for twenty-two children, who had not had smallpox, to be transported by ship. Two children were vaccinated and, in a human chain, two more children were vaccinated from the preceding pair every ten days. The chain worked until the ship arrived in Caracas, Venezuela following which half of the party went on to Peru where another 50,000 people were vaccinated. Another ship took a second party, using the same human chain procedure, to the Philippines where vaccination was carried on to China. From there American missionaries took vaccination into the interior. In 1802, after several unsuccessful attempts, virus-bearing lymph from Jenner was carried from England to India. Only one vaccination was successful but that case provided material for local vaccination and transport to Ceylon and Madras. The original "Jenner strain" had reached India.

WOODVILLE AND VACCINIA

Another English physician, William Woodville, took material from two cows and inoculated seven subjects in the Smallpox and Inoculation Hospital of London. He then inoculated them with matter from a smallpox case, three of them after only five days. From the original seven he inoculated another 200, then another group of 300 from them. There were three or four deaths among the 500 subjects and Jenner was furious since he considered that not enough time had elapsed to develop immunity, little as that was understood at the time. He believed that Woodville's strain was contaminated with smallpox. The demand for vaccination was so strong that

Woodville's strain, produced in a much greater volume in London than in Jenner's rural area, became the most widely used source for vaccination.

By 1836, Woodville's strain had been passed through at least 2,000 removes and was safe. He provided the material used in America by Dr. Benjamin Woodhouse of Boston in 1800. All vaccinations were performed by the arm-to-arm method until 1881 and excessive passages attenuated the virus so that immunity was decreased. In addition, human infections like erysipelas, tuberculosis and syphilis were passed along as a complication. In England, the Animal Vaccination Establishment inoculated healthy calves with cowpox to provide a source of lymph for vaccination of subjects. The lymph material was variable in potency until it was discovered that the addition of glycerin preserved the cowpox and by 1895 "glycerinated calves lymph" was the preferred source of cowpox for vaccination. Human lymph was available for those who objected to the use of animal matter.

Opposition to vaccination continued into the twentieth century even after it became compulsory. Uneducated poor and working- class people were the most likely to object but, for some reason, they favored variation which continued to be practiced. In 1837-40, a severe epidemic of small-pox caused 35,000 deaths in England, mostly in urban working-class and poor children. The Parliament responded to this event by passing an act making variation a felony and increasing penalties for failure to vaccinate children. Mandatory vaccination became the law in Germany and other countries followed slowly, especially with army recruits. Napoleon had his army vaccinated in the early 1800's and, when Jenner wrote to him asking for the release of a captured English officer, Napoleon complied saying "Anything Jenner wants shall be granted. He has been my most faithful servant in the European campaigns." The officer was released.

A pandemic in 1869 in Europe was followed the next year by the Franco-Prussian War. The German army, with good compliance in vaccination, had 4,835 cases with 278 deaths. Among French prisoners (not the entire French army), with a lower level of immunity (Napoleon's lesson about vaccination of soldiers had been forgotten), there were 14,178 cases with 1,963 deaths. The number of French prisoners has been lost but must have been much smaller than the total numbers of the entire German army. An epidemic in England in 1870 was blamed on French refugees and produced 44,079 deaths. The level of compliance with vaccination, especially among the urban poor had been no better than 50 percent. A quarter of the deaths were in London slums. The mortality rate, however, had declined to 148 deaths per 100,000, much less than the pre-vaccination level of 500 per 100,000 people. Vaccination was working. In 1873, as a consequence of the recent epidemic, ninety-three percent of children born in England and Wales were vaccinated. Over the next seventy years, compliance fell to about seventy percent but the smallpox virus was less virulent as demonstrated by mandatory reporting introduced in 1899. In 1927, 14,767 cases occurred but only forty-seven patients died. In 1928, an experiment of nature occurred when a ship from India brought a new virulent strain of the virus. There were thirty-five cases of smallpox, of which eleven died.[89] The epidemic was easily contained because of the high level of immunity in the population. All contacts were vaccinated and quarantine was enforced. No new cases occurred after the first month.

Who actually defeated smallpox, Jenner or Woodville? Cowpox inoculation did not confer lifetime immunity and the German government eventually instituted seven-year revaccination, no doubt due to failure of immunity in some cases. A distinguished epidemiologist, Arthur Gale, considered the matter in 1956. "One can only make a guess at what happened in London in 1799. The most plausible guess seems to me to be that the bringing together of cowpox and smallpox virus did in some way produce a modified smallpox virus which by an empirical process of selection on the part of the vaccinators gradually became safer and safer." He added that modern work in the laboratory has shown that the modern *vaccinia* virus resembles the smallpox virus more than cowpox although they have the same antigenic structure. Since Gale's writing, virology has progressed enormously along with molecular biology. Vaccinia virus, a large double stranded DNA virus, is only distantly related to the smallpox virus (if at all) and is not cowpox either. It is thought to be related to buffalopox, yet another animal poxvirus, and how it came to be used for immunization against smallpox will most likely never be known.[90] Jenner, of course, knew nothing of viruses but his work was the beginning of attempts to combat infection by immunization. His discovery also introduced profound changes in social relationships as governments adopted compulsory rules of behavior to protect public health.

THE AGE OF QUACKS

Before vaccination, little that was new appeared in eighteenth century medicine and it was called the "Golden Age of Quacks". The term quackery may have come from quicksilver (Dutch- quacksilver), referring to mercury, the common remedy for syphilis. Medicines continued to contain items such as powdered skull of condemned criminal and preparations from the rope that hanged him. Increasing literacy caused a decline in the belief in magic among the more prosperous members of society, but folk healers abounded and many had better results than educated physicians did. If Pepys had lived a hundred years later his rabbit foot would still have been as effective as the physicians' medicines. Some quacks grew rich. Johanna Stephens promoted a remedy to dissolve bladder stones without surgery in mid-century. Parliament raised a £5000 subscription to buy the formula from her. The medical authorities attempted to clamp down on quacks with little success.

Franz Anton Mesmer (1734-1815) obtained a doctorate in Vienna on "the medical effects of the influence of the planets." He developed unorthodox healing methods, as might be expected with such a background, but he obtained some startling results. Franzisca Oesterlin suffered crippling seizures, which included vomiting, fainting fits, convulsions, temporary blindness and episodes of paralysis. Mesmer placed three magnets over places on her body producing seizures and remission of her symptoms. This technique produced the same result on several occasions (she was not permanently cured) and Mesmer concluded that he had discovered a basic principle of life, which he called "animal magnetism." Though he was a qualified physician (by the standards of the day), Mesmer was drummed out of Vienna by faculty opposition to his "quackery." He moved to Paris and became famous for "séances", at which he cured nervously afflicted women. Patients sat in a circle around a tub of "magnetized water" and grasped iron rods protruding from the tub. Many were cured after a convulsive fit while others were "mesmerized" into a trance. Louis XVI appointed a commission to investigate Dr. Mesmer, which decided his practices were charlatanry, and he was forced to leave Paris, as well. "Mesmerists" practiced freely in London and we now know that hypnosis was the basis of his successes.

MEDICAL SCHOOLS

In England, the Royal College of Physicians lost much influence again as it devolved into a gentleman's club with little power. It restricted membership to graduates of Oxford and Cambridge who were members of the Church of England in spite of the fact that most physicians were Dissenters and many were graduates of Leiden and Edinburgh. The London Company of Surgeons separated from the Barbers in 1745, but did not evolve into a teaching body. No uniform system of medical education prevailed and the volume of medical graduates from Oxford and Cambridge declined to a trickle. A similar situation existed in America. John Morgan (1735-1789), a Philadelphian who learned medicine as an apprentice wrote *A Discourse upon the Institution of Medical Schools in America* in 1765. Returning from Edinburgh and further study, he established the University of Pennsylvania Medical Department and held the chair of Practice of Medicine. William Shippen (1736-1808) also studied at Edinburgh and returned to Philadelphia to become professor of anatomy and surgery. In 1769 Benjamin Rush was elected professor of chemistry and became physician to Pennsylvania Hospital from 1783 to 1813. Harvard Medical School opened in 1783 and by 1803, a Harvard diploma was equivalent to an examination for a Massachusetts license. In Europe, the city of Leiden became prominent because of professor Boerhaave who was called the "medical instructor of Europe." As Oxford and Cambridge declined in the number of medical graduates, Edinburgh became the principle source of educated physicians for England. Paris persisted in adhering to Galen and was passed by as a source of learning in medicine. Hospitals opened to English students in the eighteenth century for the first time and lectures and dissections were conducted at St. Thomas' Hospital.

THE HUNTER BROTHERS

In London, in 1768, William Hunter opened the most famous anatomy and obstetrics school in England. In 1743, Hunter had published his first anatomical study, *The Structure and Diseases of Articulating Cartilages.* Instructors included his brother John Hunter, who became the most famous surgeon in England. John Hunter was apprenticed to a cabinet-maker as a boy and his skills with his hands made him the premier anatomical dissector when he joined his brother in his anatomy school. The Hunter brothers worked together for ten years and provided a major source for the new knowledge of anatomy and physiology being discovered in Europe. In spite of a shortage of cadavers, students learned anatomy from dissections often performed on "privately acquired bodies," usually dug up by grave robbers. William Hewson, another instructor, prepared microscopic mounts, many of which may still be examined at the Hunter Museum in London.

In 1760 the brothers separated, John becoming a surgeon and his brother continuing his anatomical teaching. John Hunter became interested in comparative anatomy and acquired a menagerie, preserving the remains of dead animals in a museum. He accepted apprentices the first of which was Edward Jenner, discoverer of vaccination. In 1780, the brothers had a serious dispute concerning which of them had discovered the placental circulation. William claimed the credit while John asserted that he had performed the dissections and the real credit should be his. They never spoke again. William died in 1783 leaving his museum to be donated to the

University of Glasgow. John continued his work although his health began to fail. He did manage to acquire the corpse of Charles Byrne, the Irish Giant, who, knowing that Hunter coveted his body, arranged to be buried at sea from the Irish Sea ferry. Hunter bribed the attendants and the skeleton of Byrne may be seen today in the Hunter Museum in London. See Figure 5.

In 1785, Hunter performed physiology experiments far ahead of their time, ligating the artery to one antler of fallow deer in Richmond Park. He demonstrated that collateral circulation developed and the antler, at first cold after the ligation of its artery, warmed up in a few days. In December 1785, long before anesthesia or antisepsis, Hunter ligated the femoral artery in a man suffering from an aneurysm of the popliteal artery, below the point of ligation. These aneurysms were dangerous and frequently ruptured resulting in death or amputation. The man tolerated the procedure and, after a six-week convalescence, resumed a normal life. Drawing on his military experience Hunter published a great work on gunshot wounds in 1792. His heart disease worsened and, given his irascible nature, he was famously quoted, "My life is in the hands of any rascal who chooses to annoy me." Sure enough, during a dispute with other surgeons at St. George's Hospital over the appointment of an assistant, he flew into a rage and collapsed. An autopsy confirmed Jenner's diagnosis of heart valve disease. His museum was preserved but was badly damaged in the Blitz in 1941. The remaining specimens may be seen today. He had truly been the harbinger of the great progress to be made in the next century.

PUBLIC HEALTH AND SCURVY

Interest in public health increased as European nations began to collect census and vital statistics similar to the records in England. Germany established "medical police" as some countries became increasingly concerned about hygiene and the role of sickness in the conduct of military operations. John Pringle (1707-1782), while physician-general of the British army, studied the relationship between dirt and illness in armies. His book, *Account of Several Persons Seized with the Gaol Fever Working at Newgate*, studied the cause of typhus, which would devastate Napoleon's army in 1812 and end his ambition for European rule. Pringle also proposed to the French commanding officer, at the battle of Dettingen in 1743, that hospital tents on both sides be protected from attack. This began the practice of protecting medical staff and wounded soldiers in war.

Lord Anson's voyage around the world in 1740-44 lost 320 men to fever and 997 from scurvy out of a total of 1,955 men and boys. James Lind (1716-91), a Scottish naval surgeon studied the survivors who were suffering from scurvy. In 1753, he published *Treatise on the Scurvy*, which recommended citrus fruits as prevention.

In 1754, he performed the world's first clinical trial on board the HMS Salisbury and proved that citrus fruit was effective. Lind selected twelve patients suffering from scurvy and gave pairs of them different preparations to be studied. Cider, oil of vitriol (ether), vinegar, seawater, lemons and oranges were tested. Only the citrus fruits restored the men to health. Lind did not understand that scurvy was a deficiency disease and thought that citrus acted like the Jesuits' bark that cured malaria. He thought the cause of scurvy was moist air. The belief in the harmful effects of air, especially night air, seems ridiculous to us in modern times but it is useful to remember that the population who feared night air had no concept of the role of the mosquito, active at night and prevented from biting sleepers by bed curtains, in spreading malaria (which is Latin for "bad air").

The Navy did not act on Lind's recommendations and scurvy plagued Captain Cook's voyages in spite of his enlightened concern with cleanliness. Finally, in 1795, lemon juice was issued to the Navy as a regular practice and a few years later scurvy was virtually absent from the British fleet. These studies influenced the civilian world and concern with cleanliness was such that by 1790 free admission of air and bathing was common in treatment of the sick. Percival Pott (1714-88) linked scrotal cancer in chimney sweeps to soot accumulation in the groin of men who did not wash themselves. He also associated the spine lesion of tuberculosis with the pulmonary form of the disease (he was the first to realize they were the same disease although Hippocrates mentioned the association, as well) although he did not know about the organism that caused both lesions.

Hospitals, unfortunately, continued to be centers of contamination and the new Vienna Allgemeines Krankenhaus, rebuilt with 1600 beds in 1784, would drive Semmelweis to insanity in the mid 1800s with its resistance to hand washing. On December 14, 1799, George Washington died from a combination of pneumonia, contracted after a chill, and vigorous bleeding by his physicians. In 1806, Thomas Jefferson, a lover of enlightened learning but a skeptic toward the profession wrote, "Harvey's discovery of the circulation of the blood was a beautiful addition to our knowledge of the animal economy, but on a review of the practice of medicine before and since that epoch, I do not see any great amelioration which has been derived from that discovery." True enough although Jenner, Withering and Lind had made giant steps in therapeutics.

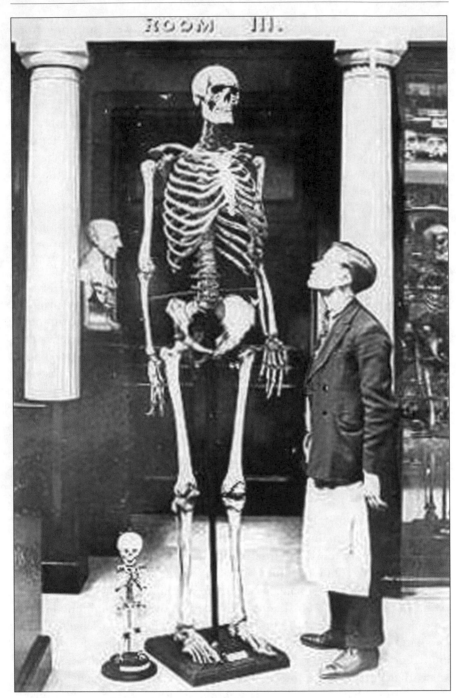

Figure 6 – Byrne's skeleton in the Hunter Museum

85   William Harvey, *The movement of the heart and blood in animals*, Facsimile edition printed at Frankfurt-on-the-Maine (1628).

86   There are other sources attributed for this nursery rhymn including a cannon defending the city of Colchester in 1648 that fell from the city wall and was broken. Kings Richard III and Charles I are also possible figures referred to. Both were toppled in revolutions and could not be restored by their supporters.

87   Elizabeth Genung, "The development of the compound microscope," *Bulletin of the History of Medicine* 12:575-594 (1942).

88   David H. Clark and Stephen P.H. Clark, *Newton's Tyranny*, W.H. Freeman & Co. (2001).

89   There was a strain of smallpox in India that was much more virulent and produced a hemorrhagic form of the disease. The Soviet Union used samples of the virus recovered from Indian hemorrhagic cases to produce a "weaponized" virus. A store of that virus has recently been described on an island in the Aral Sea. In the 1970s a small outbreak resulted from a lab accident. People who were immunized to smallpox developed the disease but survived. Those who had not been immunized all died.

90   Edward K. Wagner and Martinez J. Hewlett, "Basic Virology," page 104, Blackwell Science (1999).

9

The Century of the Surgeon

THE NINETEENTH CENTURY OPENED WITH A RECURRENCE OF THE plagues that had beleaguered armies since Carthage and Athens. The French Revolution, in addition to ordering the execution of Lavoisier, the greatest chemist of the century if not all of history, brought reforms in the Paris faculty of medicine, previously a holdout of Galenical orthodoxy. Dr. Guillotine, of course, offered a humane form of execution with his new machine, and it was put to great use.

René Theophile Hyacinthe Laennec (1781-1826) became chief physician at Salpetriere Hospital in 1814 and at Hôpital Necker two years later, both vast infirmaries for the poor. Two years later, he devised the stethoscope giving access at last to the internal organs. It was the most important advance for objective medicine and diagnosis until the invention of the x-ray. His account of the discovery in 1816 is interesting. A young woman with symptoms of heart disease consulted him. His prior technique of examination was to place his ear against the patient's chest but the rules of polite society inhibited his exam until he recalled a phenomenon he had previously observed. Placing an ear to one end of a wooden beam allows an observer to hear very soft scratches on the other end of the beam. He rolled a sheet of paper into a tight roll and, using this as an aid, was able to hear her heartbeat clearly. In 1819, he published a treatise and described a wooden instrument, which was applied to one ear with the other end placed on the chest. In 1852 an American, George Cammann, invented the familiar instrument with rubber tubing and two earpieces.

Laennec became an expert diagnostician with his instrument and was able to diagnose pulmonary diseases with great accuracy. In addition to his stethoscope, he coined the terms "egophony" (the alteration of a spoken letter "e" to an "a" heard by the examiner when lung consolidation alters transmission of the sound) and "pectoriloquy" (augmentation of whispered speech by lung consolidation) to describe some of his findings with the new instrument. The terms, and the examinations they represent, remain important parts of the physical examination of the chest.

Tuberculosis, one of the diseases he diagnosed quite frequently and was consequently exposed to daily, took his life in 1826.

Leopold Auenbrugger invented percussion examination of the chest, the other essential technique, but it was neglected until Jean Nicholas Corvisart translated his description for his book, *An Essay on the Organic Diseases and Lesions of the Heart and Great Vessels*, in 1806. Auenbrugger was born in 1722 to a father who operated an inn in Graz, Austria. As a boy, he observed his father tapping wine barrels to measure the level of the wine in the barrel. When he was appointed physician to the Military Hospital of Vienna, he recalled the wine barrel tapping. He tried this technique to examine the chest and found that the method was useful. Auenbrugger's book, *Inventum Novum*, was in Latin and was ignored until Corvisart's translation. Another problem in the adoption of this new examination was the fact that the French Revolution produced panic in the Austrian royal family and the Vienna Medical School was placed in the hands of the extremely conservative Joseph von Stifft, the Emperor's personal physician. A number of the more progressive Austrian medical faculty members migrated to Paris, after being purged around 1804, carrying with them Auenbrugger's technique where it was discovered by Corvisart. Physical examination had begun to replace the sole reliance on history as an instrument of diagnosis and French medical science leaped ahead of other countries'.

Pierre Louis (1787-1872), another of the new wave of diagnosticians in Paris, began to use numerical methods to analyze therapy. Mathematics was making continued progress and statistics offered a way to test traditional treatment for efficacy. Galen was truly gone. Louis studied a series of patients with pneumonia and demonstrated that phlebotomy made no difference in the outcome. In fact, every conventional therapy he tested, using his *methodé numerique*, proved ineffective and he was accused of being a therapeutic nihilist (of course, he was correct and none of it was effective). Opponents continued to use phlebotomy and Broussais, a prominent Galenist, recommended using fifty leeches at a time. Broussais did contribute one idea, that of a continuum from health to disease which proved useful in dealing with chronic diseases in the future. Broussais's influence was so powerful that France, an exporter of leeches in 1825, was importing thirty-three million a year by 1837. A student of Broussais, Jean Bouillaud, performed such copious bleeding that he removed up to three liters of blood from patients with pneumonia. Lest the leech be prematurely consigned to the dustbin of history, I would point out that their use has recently been advocated in plastic surgery to improve the microcirculation in ischemic pedicle grafts.[91]

NAPOLEON AND TYPHUS

Before the new Parisian medicine could influence other countries, the Napoleonic Wars had to end. Another plague contributed a major share in this development. In the spring of 1812, Napoleon's empire extended from Russia and Austria in the East to the North Sea in the West. After a childless marriage to Josephine, he divorced her and married Marie Louise, an Archduchess and grandniece of Marie Antoinette, who provided him with a son in 1811. His empire ended at the sea, however, as Britain and the Royal Navy maintained a blockade. Napoleon had attempted to break through the ring and cut Britain's lifeline to India in 1798 by invading Egypt, but Nelson defeated his fleet at Aboukir Bay, trapping the French army and ending the threat. Napoleon proposed a joint invasion of India to the Tsar, at their meeting at Tilsit in 1807, but the two autocrats had a falling out and the plan was stillborn.

In June 1812, Napoleon concentrated his army in Prussia, a huge force consisting of 368,000 infantry, 80,000 cavalry, and a reserve of 100,000 men. Reinforcements during the campaign brought the total to 600,000 men engaged on the French side. The Russian armies totaled about 250,000 men so they were badly outnumbered. The summer was unusually hot and dry so marching was easy and food was abundant in Germany and Prussia. Napoleon had an excellent medical corps and was quite sophisticated about medical and health matters. He had his army (and his son) vaccinated against smallpox, for example. Once the army entered Poland, things began to change. Typhus was endemic in Poland and Napoleon had had no experience with this disease.

Typhus is caused by a Rickettsia organism, an intracellular organism halfway between a virus and bacteria. It infects the human body louse and is excreted by the louse in its feces. Typhus is transmitted to the human host, not by the bite of the louse, but from the droppings, or by crushing the louse, and then scratching the skin, which produces small openings that admit the organism. Lice are common in settings where people are dirty, and do not wash or change clothing. The lice infest the seams of the clothing or bedding and were common in eighteenth century prisons where they caused gaol fever. In the hot dry weather of Poland that summer, water was scarce and washing was impossible. Twenty thousand horses died crossing Poland from lack of water and forage. Hunger and dysentery affected the army but real trouble began when men developed a high fever, a blotchy pink rash and then their faces became bluish. Many died quickly. The great sanitary facilities of the army, established by Napoleon's surgeon Baron D.J. Larrey, were not equal to the task. The cause of the infection was unknown. Good sanitation did not help because the disease was not water-borne. Lack of water and insufficient changes of clothing were the sources and soldiers had been foraging and sleeping in Polish cottages, which were full of lice. The undisciplined foraging had alienated the Polish peasants, so the men slept in large groups for protection. Lice are easily transmitted from person to person, a fact well known to mothers whose children acquire head lice in school.

By the third week of July, after 150 miles, 80,000 men had died or were too ill for duty. The Russians fought rear-guard actions and retreated, so battle casualties were not heavy, although the threat of Cossack cavalry sweeps contributed to the crowded sleeping conditions and transmission of the louse. By the end of July, several of Napoleon's more cautious generals were worried. The failure of the Russians to make a stand was leading the French army into hazardous territory. Half the army was now too ill for duty or had died of illness, mostly typhus. Undecided at first whether to press on, Napoleon finally declared, "Victory will justify and save us." When they reached Smolensk, about halfway to Moscow, they could have halted and spent the winter with good supplies from Germany and adequate shelter. The army surgeons recommended this course, but Napoleon decided to continue marching to Moscow using Smolensk as an advanced base. He was convinced that Alexander would surrender if Moscow were in French hands. His army was now reduced to 160,000 men and 30,000 more contracted typhus by September 5. On September 7, the French and Russians fought the battle of Borodino, in front of Moscow, with both sides sustaining heavy casualties. The Russians retired having fought to a draw in what was really a demonstration defense of the city. Alexander did not believe he could abandon Moscow (not then the capital) without a battle, but was not willing to risk his army in an all-out defense.

The French entered Moscow on September 14 and found it burned and abandoned. Napoleon had 90,000 troops left, having lost another 10,000 to typhus in the previous week. He was convinced that Alexander would surrender and wasted a month sitting in Moscow as winter approached. The Russians hinted at conciliation, but they meant only to lull the French and wait for winter. A warm autumn after the hot summer deceived Napoleon about the coming Russian winter while his army bivouacked in the ruined city with little shelter and no winter clothing. The typhus continued unchecked.

On the eighteenth of October, the Russians, now between Napoleon and his base camp at Smolensk, attacked and he finally realized that they were not going to make peace. The army began the slow retreat from Moscow.

15,000 reinforcements had reached them but another 10,000 had died of typhus leaving 95,000 to begin the retreat. The snow began to fall on November 5 and an attempt to retreat south, toward warmer weather and better forage, was foiled by the Russians. The army turned north, into the winter and the country they had devastated on the way into Russia. Smolensk was reached on November 8, but the troops there were wasted by typhus and the garrison had consumed the supplies. The army continued the retreat on November 13 leaving 20,000 sick behind. When the Grand Army finally reached the German border, fewer than 40,000 of the 600,000 survived and it was later written that only about 1,000 were ever again to return to duty. General Typhus, with the help of the outnumbered Russians, had defeated General Napoleon.

The retreating French Army brought typhus with it and an epidemic devastated central and Eastern Europe in 1813-14. Napoleon recruited a new army of 470,000 after his return from Russia, but by late autumn 1813 only half were fit for service. During the next year Napoleon, himself, succumbed to illness on two critical occasions and lost opportunities to defeat his encircling enemies. His health deteriorated during this period as he was beset with migraine headaches, abdominal pain, and, before Waterloo, with severe hemorrhoids that made it impossible to ride. The morning of Waterloo, he lost six hours, crucial hours while the Prussians joined Wellington after their defeat the day before at Quatre-Bras, because he slept late following a heavy dose of opium to relieve his pain.[92] Six years later he died, of massive upper GI bleeding from cancer of the stomach, an exile in the island of St. Helena. Considerable excitement was generated in 1960 by a report that a hair sample taken from Napoleon at his death showed a high concentration of arsenic, but the autopsy report, and the history of "tarry stools, coffee ground vomiting and persistent hiccups," make the cause of death clear.

POSTWAR PROGRESS

When the wars finally ended in 1815, students from all over the world converged on Paris to learn new methods. Laennec alone taught 300 foreign students. The huge public hospitals allowed medical students free rein and the opportunity for bedside experience and dissections was unmatched in the world. Thomas Hodgkin (1798-1866) was one such student, a Quaker like many of his fellow English physicians, who returned home with a stethoscope and knowledge of morbid anatomy. He became lecturer on what we now call pathology at Guy's Hospital in 1825 and, in 1832, published *On Some Morbid Appearances of the Absorbent Glands and*

Spleen, describing the disease which bears his name. Carl von Rokitansky (1804-78) trained in Paris for a time, after graduation from Vienna Medical School, and then spent his career reviving medical science in Vienna and performing 1,500 necropsies per year to a grand total of 60,000. His *Handbuch der pathologischen Anatomie* ("Handbook of Pathological Anatomy") described peptic ulcer, heart valve abnormalities and pneumonia and his technique of performing an autopsy is still used.

The French example stimulated reforms in medical education in London, but students were still limited in clinical experience in English hospitals. James Paget described teaching in St Bartholomew's Hospital in 1834: "There was very little, or no, personal guidance...for the most part the students guided themselves or one another to evil or to good, to various degrees of work or of idleness. No one was, in any sense, responsible for them." He added, "I am not sure that, being well-disposed for work, I was the worse for this."[93] Things began to improve after the Apothecaries Act of 1815 required that general practitioners, licensed under the Act, must study anatomy, chemistry, botany, *materia medica* (mostly useless at that date), and theory and practice of physic, including six months of bedside experience. By the 1830s, 400 students per year were taking the license and the demand for clinical training forced hospitals to expand teaching. The teaching was, of course, of variable quality as Paget relates. The demand for anatomy teaching produced a shortage of cadavers, a deficiency addressed by a new group of Scottish entrepreneurs. In 1827, two men, William Hare and William Burke, began selling bodies to anatomists. They began with a lodger in Hare's boarding house who died of natural causes, but quickly passed on to abduction and murder. They were caught two years later and Hare turned King's Evidence, confessing to sixteen murders. Burke was hung and the last cadaver procured by the men was found in the dissecting room of a prominent anatomist, Robert Knox, who taught classes of 500 in Edinburgh. An angry crowd burned down Knox's house and drove him from the city. The scandal helped to pass the Anatomy Act of 1832, which awarded the "unclaimed bodies" of paupers without family to anatomy schools. The Act assisted teaching and aided the work of Henry Gray (1827-1861), an anatomy lecturer at St. George's Hospital who published *Gray's Anatomy: Descriptive and Applied* in 1858, three years before he died prematurely of smallpox.

THE MICROSCOPE AND LABORATORY MEDICINE

Germany contributed laboratory medicine as the French developed gross pathology. The microscope had advanced far enough in 1819 to produce the term "histology" for the microscopic examination of tissue. "Learn to see microscopically" was Rudolph Virchow's advice to his students. Joseph Jackson Lister, father of the surgeon, produced a far superior microscope in 1826 and the next year published, with Thomas Hodgkin, the paper that founded histology as a real science by demonstrating that tissue was composed of fibers, not globules. The French were slow to adopt the new science; Rokitansky's first handbook is all gross pathology with no microscopic examination. In 1846, Carl Zeiss opened his workshop in Jena and German lenses quickly became the best in the world. Jacob Henle (1809-85) produced the first textbook of combined gross and microscopic anatomy in 1866 and encouraged the use of microscopes by students. The Royal College of Surgeons in England instituted courses in gross and microscopic anatomy in 1848. German universities invested in academic science, with the support of rulers concerned about national prestige, and Germany quickly adopted research-based medical science, which would pay great dividends by the end of the century. Chemistry at last was to play the role once emphasized by Paracelsus four centuries earlier. The Germans began to study what we now call organic chemistry and the accidental observations of an American surgeon added new understanding of digestion.

William Beaumont (1785-1853) was a US Army surgeon, stationed at Fort Mackinac on Mackinac Island (at the straits between Lake Huron and Lake Michigan), in 1822 when he was summoned to a small trading post to treat Alexis St. Martin. St. Martin was a trapper who had suffered a shotgun wound to the abdomen. He recovered, unusual at the time, but was left with a persistent fistula from the stomach to the outside. He could plug the fistula at mealtime but, when left open, it drained gastric contents. Beaumont was without academic training, but immediately recognized the significance of the situation for research on digestion. In 1833, he published his first work, *Observations on the Gastric Juice and the Physiology of Digestion*, which confirmed the presence of hydrochloric acid and showed that the process consisted of dissolving the food, not putrefaction as had been believed since ancient times. Claude Bernard later based his own studies on Beaumont's pioneering work and Theodore Schwann discovered pepsin, the first digestive enzyme identified. Beaumont spent much of his life following St. Martin around Canada to continue experiments while the trapper tried to elude this annoying intruder into his simple life. After the doctor's death in 1853, St. Martin continued to correspond with Beaumont's son, Israel, until his own death at the age of eighty-one.

Virchow continued his work with the microscope fending off several premature theories of the cell's role in disease. Rokitansky, making up for his hesitancy in adopting histology, promoted a theory of "blastema," a sort of spontaneous generation of cells from a nurturing fluid or matrix called the blastema. The study of cells began with botany and Matthias Schleiden (1804-81), in Jena, declared that plants are made up of cells, which are self-reproducing living units. The problem was, where did cells come from? Schwann believed that cells could be formed from blastema in inflammation and Rokitansky extended this to conclude that abnormal cells, producing disease, could also arise by spontaneous generation from the primitive blastema. Virchow distrusted all this, maintaining that cells always arose from other cells (and attacked Rokitansky in 1846 on this point, prompting Rokitansky eventually to change his mind). In inflammation, he said, pus cells were identical to white blood cells circulating in the blood. He coined the term "leukocytosis" and in 1847, simultaneously with Edinburgh professor John Hughes Bennett, described leukemia. He attacked the concept of blastema writing, *"omnis cellula a cellula*, "each cell from a cell," In 1858, he wrote *Cell Pathology*, which explained that all diseases were due to disturbances in cell structures.

Rokitansky attacked Virchow's assertions warning that all diseases should not be attributed to "solid pathology" and bacteriologists like Klebs opposed him, because he did not explain how external factors (like bacteria) produced disease. Still, Virchow's work was enormously important in the development of modern medicine. He studied thrombosis and embolism (identifying the first cases of pulmonary embolism), cardiovascular disease, cancer, bilirubin and hemoglobin. He was active in German politics and was forced to leave Berlin in 1848 during the political unrest all over Europe. He returned in triumph from internal exile in Wurtzburg to become, in 1856, Director of the Pathological Institute of Berlin. He served in the Prussian House of Representatives as leader of the Progressive Party, wrote articles attacking the new racial theories of Teutonic supremacists and nearly fought a duel with Bismarck over political differences. He traveled to Troy with Heinrich Schliemann in 1879 to participate in the excavations. In 1902, he was given a state funeral, although his politics were at odds with the new German state.

Pharmacology had progressed considerably since Withering identified the usefulness of digitalis. Poisons were identified and the new science of toxicology emerged in Paris. Francois Magendie (1783-1855), professor of anatomy at the College de France, studied nerve function and experimented with a Javanese arrow poison whose active ingredient proved to be strychnine. The active ingredients of a number of herbal remedies and natural substances were identified between 1818 and 1821 including strychnine, brucine, veratrine, cinchonine, quinine, and caffeine. Nicotine was discovered in 1828 and atropine in 1833. Opium was analyzed and an opium ingredient of crystalline purity was named Morphium (for Morpheus,the god of sleep). Codeine was isolated in 1832, then colchicine (whose effect had been reported by Paul of Aegina in 640CE) and hyoscyamine and, finally, in 1860, cocaine. With all this progress, few new, effective medicines were introduced. The science of medicine and the understanding of mechanisms of disease improved rapidly, but it was surgery that first broke free with major advances in treatment.

SURGERY BEFORE ANESTHESIA

In 1800, surgery was conducted exactly as Paré had practiced in 1537. Operations were limited to amputations and drainage of abscesses with anal fistula surgery the most sophisticated and closest to modern physiological concepts. Fractures were set, but open fractures were fraught with danger from infection and amputation was often the safest course. A few famous surgeons performed operations with masses of spectators like theatrical productions. Astley Cooper (1768-1841) at Guy's Hospital earned the stupendous income of £15,000 per year in the pre-anesthesia days. His largest fee was £1,000 from a wealthy West Indian planter named Hyatt. Cooper's servant, a man named Charles, earned several hundred pounds per year himself in bribes from eager prospective patients. Cooper began at St. Thomas' Hospital but, after a dispute about the appointment of his successor as Lecturer in Anatomy, he left and established a surgery lecture series at the Guy's Hospital medical school. The two schools were across from each other on St. Thomas Street and Guy's had conducted lectures in medicine while surgery was taught at St. Thomas. That changed with Cooper's move in 1800.[94]

In 1824, he amputated a limb by hip disarticulation (amputation through the joint) in twenty minutes. Ten years later, James Syme (1799-1870) performed a hip disarticulation in ninety seconds. Speed was essential when pain could not be relieved. Baron Larrey, Napoleon's chief surgeon, reported performing 200 amputations at the battle of Borodino in twenty-four hours[95]: one amputation every seven minutes. No mention was made of how many survived, but in good conditions, the mortality rate was about forty percent. Great advances were being made in spite of the limits early in the century.

THE FIRST INTERNAL OPERATIONS

Ephraim McDowell (1771-1830) practiced surgery near the frontier in Danville, Kentucky. He had trained in Edinburgh with John Bell, one of the famous Edinburgh physicians, and, when he visited his patient Jane Todd in 1809, he was ready. She had requested his services for delivery of a pregnancy but, when he examined her in her home, he realized that, although she appeared to be nine months pregnant, she had a huge ovarian mass, not a pregnant uterus. Ovariotomy (surgery of the abdomen, specifically on the ovary) had never before been successfully performed but "she appeared willing to undergo an experiment."[96] She rode a mule over the mountains to Danville after McDowell agreed to remove the mass in her abdomen. Working at home, McDowell took twenty-five minutes to remove the twenty-two-pound tumor from the conscious patient. The mass, a tumor involving the left ovary and Fallopian tube, contained fifteen pounds of gelatinous material and the tumor itself weighed another seven pounds making the total. Mrs. Todd sang hymns to dull the pain, survived the operation, and lived another thirty-two years. McDowell, perhaps because he believed that his success would be doubted by big city surgeons, waited until he had two more successful cases before reporting his results to his teacher John Bell.

He did publish a report in the *Eclectic Repertory and Analytical Review*, in Philadelphia in 1817 but relied on his teacher to inform the European surgical profession. Unfortunately, Bell was ill and died shortly after receiving McDowell's letter. Bell's assistant, John Lizars, did not disseminate McDowell's report and only quoted the letter in his own publication of successful ovariotomy (one of two cases survived) in 1825. Even then, the priority of McDowell's achievement was disputed until he published another report in 1826 with additional successful cases, up to a total of twelve operations. He is now acknowledged as the father of abdominal surgery. The operation was performed on many occasions over the coming years but the mortality rate exceeded twenty-five percent, in the best hands, until antisepsis came.

James Marion Sims (1813-1883) achieved another milestone with the first successful correction of vesico-vaginal fistula (an abnormal connection between bladder and vagina, usually the result of complicated childbirth). This distressing condition resulted in continuous, uncontrollable urine drainage from the vagina and could condemn a woman to a life of misery. Sims had studied medicine in Philadelphia and practiced in Alabama. One day, Sims examined a woman who had been injured in a riding accident. Using a new position (now called Sims' position, but one he had been taught to help return a prolapsed uterus to normal position) and a new pattern speculum (made from bending a spoon), he examined her vagina and found that he could see the fistula clearly. He had previously refused to operate on women who sought treatment for fistula, since no one had ever been successful with repair. Now, with his new position and speculum, he decided to try. It took thirty-three operations (without anesthesia) on his first successful candidate before the fistula did not recur. In 1853, he moved to New York and opened a Women's Hospital where he performed many such procedures.

ANESTHESIA

English novelist Fanny Burney, in a letter to her sister from Paris described surgery without anesthesia, after Baron Larrey performed a mastectomy on her in 1810. She wrote, "I refused to be held; but when, bright through the cambric (a cloth over her eyes) I saw the glitter of polished steel – I closed my eyes... Yet – when the dreadful steel was plunged into the breast– cutting through veins– arteries– flesh– nerves– I needed no injunctions not to restrain my cries. I began a scream that lasted unintermittantly during the whole time of the incision- & I almost marvel that it rings not in my ears still!!! So excruciating was the agony. When the wound was made & the instrument was withdrawn, the pain seemed undiminished, for the air that rushed suddenly into those delicate parts felt like a mass of minute but sharp & forked poniards that were tearing the edges of the wound..." The operation continued for twenty-five minutes. It was however, a success and she lived to the age of eighty-eight, dying in 1840. Of course, without the microscope, it is impossible to determine whether the breast lesion was cancer.

NITROUS OXIDE

Previous attempts at pain relief had used opium, mandrake root (which produced Juliet's death-like coma in Shakespeare's play), hyoscyamine (called henbane or poor man's opium) and atropine; all with inadequate effect. In 1795 the young Humphrey Davy (1778-1829), while working as a laboratory assistant to Thomas Beddoes, tried inhaling nitrous oxide. Joseph Priestley had discovered nitrous oxide in 1793, but its anesthetic properties were undiscovered until Davy. Priestley's discovery of multiple gases in the atmosphere led to a faddish enthusiasm for "pneumatic medicine," the inhalation of the various gases. Davy, the son of a wealthy family, had an interest in science stimulated by a local saddler who conducted experiments in electricity, building Voltaic piles and Leyden jars. After the death of his father, Davy was apprenticed to a surgeon, John Tonkin, who allowed him to continue his chemical experiments in the attic. Through the acquaintance of several notable scholars, his knowledge increased. He befriended the son of James Watt, inventor of the steam engine.

During the 1790s, Beddoes, a physician from Berkeley (and neighbor of Jenner's), who had been experimenting with pneumatic medicine, left his position as lecturer in chemistry at Oxford and moved to Bristol where he established the "Pneumatic Medicine Institute." Watt and Josiah Wedgwood, wealthy heir of the pottery family, supported this new concept and suggested Davy as Beddoes' assistant. The association of Watt, Wedgewood, Erasmus Darwin (grandfather of Charles and partner of Jenner in Birmingham), Matthew Boulton and Joseph Priestley has been commemorated in two books: *The Lunar Society of Birmingham*, by Robert E. Schofield, in 1963[97] and a recent book, *The Lunar Men*, by Jenny Uglow.[98] The only person who seems to have taken the medical implications of Davy's work seriously was a Dr. Henry Hickman of Shropshire. He conducted animal experiments with carbon *dioxide* and reported that the subjects became unconscious and insensitive to pain. His suggestion that this might prove useful in surgery was not taken seriously and he was considered a crank. Nothing came of it.

In the United States, laughing gas became popular at parties and fairs, but no medical application was considered until December 1844 when Horace Wells, a graduate of Baltimore Dental School, attended a fair in Hartford, Connecticut and watched a demonstration. The idea of using it for tooth extraction occurred to him and he offered himself as a candidate. While under its effect, his molar was extracted by dentist John Riggs. Gardner Colton, the man giving the exhibition at the fair, administered the gas. Wells constructed an apparatus for the administration of nitrous oxide and, after some experience, offered to demonstrate anesthesia at the Massachusetts General Hospital. The demonstration was arranged by a Harvard medical student named William T. Morton, a strange character (also a dentist and a former partner of Wells) soon to play another major role. Surgeon John Collins Warren accepted his offer but the patient chosen, a large man with a mass to be removed from his bull neck (there are several versions of his attempt-this is the classic one), was not a good candidate for nitrous oxide. Wells' apparatus was not capable of producing enough depth of anesthesia for a surgical operation, however well it may have functioned for dental anesthesia. The demonstration was a failure and Wells was disgraced. He eventually became addicted to chloroform and committed suicide.

ETHER

In 1842, two years before Well's attempt, William Clarke, a physician and dentist in Rochester, New York, suggested the use of ether for extracting teeth to his own dentist, Dr. Elija Pope. Raymundus Lullius, a Spanish alchemist, first produced ether in 1275. He found that, if vitriol (sulphuric acid) was mixed with alcohol and distilled, a sweet white fluid resulted. Valerius Cordus rediscovered ether in 1540 and named it "sweet oil of vitriol." Paracelsus used the same chemical to relieve pain about the same time, but the concept of surgical anesthesia did not occur to him. It was renamed ether (or sulphuric ether) in 1730 and was used as an expectorant to bring up phlegm in respiratory illnesses. In 1815, Michael Faraday, Davy's assistant, noted that ether could produce an effect similar to laughing gas and "ether frolics" soon became popular. Pope's use of ether in dentistry, in January 1842, was successful.

Crawford Long, a doctor in Jefferson, Georgia, had also attended ether parties and, noting that pain was absent under its effect, used ether to open a cyst in the neck of a boy named James Venable. Long had attended the University of Pennsylvania medical school and then trained in surgery in New York City for eighteen months. He returned to Georgia in 1841 and, before long, his practice had become very successful in spite of his rural location. Some of the young men in town asked Long to make ether for them and he complied. After one of the ether frolics, Long noted that he had suffered several bruises, although he could not recall any pain associated with the injury. James Venable had cancelled the removal of the cyst in his neck several times because of fear of pain. Finally, Long invited Venable to an ether frolic to see the effect for himself. On March 30, 1842 the surgeon poured ether onto a towel held over Venable's face, saw that he was unconscious and removed two cysts without any pain being suffered by his patient. Long continued to use ether for anesthesia and in 1846 performed six surgeries under its effects. In December 1845, he used ether during childbirth. He moved to Atlanta and continued to practice surgery with the use of anesthesia until his death in 1878. He did not publish his experience until 1849 and is usually ignored in the history of anesthesia.

WILLIAM T MORTON AND THE ETHER CONTROVERSY

William T. Morton, who had arranged Wells' attempt, used ether for anesthesia on dogs and for dental procedures, or so he claimed. A visit to Georgia in 1842, at the time that Dr. Long performed his first anesthesia, may have stimulated his interest[99] It is difficult to imagine that he was unaware of the event since it was a sensation in the state. During a later dispute about who had actually discovered ether anesthesia, other Harvard students denied that Morton had performed any experiments. Morton was acquainted with another unusual character, Charles Jackson, who had graduated from Harvard Medical School in 1829 and became a member of the faculty. Jackson had a distinguished career and his chair is still exhibited in the Ether Dome at the Massachusetts General Hospital.

Unfortunately, Jackson also had a history of claiming credit for other people's discoveries. In 1834, Jackson attempted to claim credit for the discovery of the function of gastric juice. He was acquainted with William Beaumont and, when Beaumont sent a sample of gastric secretion from his patient Alexis St. Martin, Jackson attempted to have Congress assign St. Martin to his care. The US Surgeon general became aware of Jackson's intrigue and stopped it. In 1832, during an ocean passage, Jackson met Samuel Morse who mentioned the possibility of transmitting messages on an electric wire. In 1837, Morse patented the telegraph, but Jackson attempted to dispute his invention claiming that he, Jackson, had come up with the idea. The matter went to the US Supreme Court, which ruled in Morse's favor.

In October 1846, Morton convinced Warren to allow a second demonstration, this time using ether. The procedure was a success and Warren declared, "Gentlemen, this is no humbug."[100] Unfortunately for Morton, a bit of a charlatan, ether was a common chemical and he saw no way to profit from his discovery. He attempted to disguise the drug he was using by adding a coloring agent and another gas to mask the smell. Anyone who has smelled ether realizes that this was a forlorn hope. He named his new gas "Letheon," and he and Jackson sought a patent, but other doctors immediately dismissed him as a fake and he lost any chance for success in the new field of anesthesia. Jackson, who had assisted Morton in purifying the ether and teaching him science, distanced himself from the Letheon fiasco, but obtained a written agreement to share any profits with Morton. Eventually they cancelled the patent application.

Ether, stronger and more effective than nitrous oxide, was tried in Europe with equal success and a new age dawned. Robert Liston, an English surgeon known for speed, who held his knife in his teeth when not using it for cutting, performed an amputation of the thigh under ether anesthesia in December 1846, only two months after Morton's demonstration. Present in the audience was medical student Joseph Lister who would conquer the next hurdle in surgery. After completing the pain-free operation Liston declared, "This Yankee dodge, gentlemen, beats mesmerism (hypnotism) hollow." World acceptance was rapid and ether was used in the Crimean War on battle casualties.

Morton, Jackson, and even Wells attempted to claim credit for the new discovery. Then, Morton and Jackson signed an agreement claiming credit and excluding Wells. Not long after this became public, Wells took his life. Jackson, ever the intriguer, then wrote to the French Academy of Sciences claiming credit for himself. When Morton heard of Jackson's claim, he revoked the agreement and claimed sole credit, as well. In 1847, the US Congress became involved in what came to be known as the "Ether Controversy." Morton was supported by Daniel Webster, a powerful Senator (and Massachusetts neighbor), and Oliver Wendell Holmes, professor of anatomy at Harvard. In spite of this support and the facts of the first demonstration, Congress decided that Morton was not the discoverer of ether anesthesia! Long had refused to become involved in the controversy but the senator from Georgia stated his claim to priority and Congress decided that Jackson and Long should settle the issue between themselves! Jackson visited Long, but nothing was decided. Jackson soon became deranged and Long remained the sole discoverer who carried on his normal life. During the Civil War he asked his daughter to hide the documents relating to his discovery in a glass jar buried in the yard until Union soldiers left the area.

In 1864, the American Dental Association passed a resolution crediting Wells with discovering anesthesia. In 1870 and 1872, the American Medical Association passed similar resolutions. Long's Confederate associations may have influenced these deliberations. In 1913, the New York University Hall of Fame decided to credit Morton with the discovery reasoning, at the suggestion of William Osler, that Long was not responsible for the worldwide dissemination of the information. Osler was unaware of Morton's visit to Georgia in 1842. A recent book, *Ether Day* by Julie Fenster, does not mention a visit to Georgia by Morton in 1842, but does suggest that Morton was in Rochester, New York in 1842 when ether was successfully used by dentist and physician William E. Clarke (mentioned above) to extract a patient's tooth.[101] In 1921, the American College of Surgeons named Crawford Long the discoverer of ether anesthesia and created the Crawford Long Association. A statue of Long was erected in Statuary Hall in Washington, DC.

CHLOROFORM

Chloroform, discovered in 1831, caused less vomiting and lung irritation, was equally powerful for pain relief, and soon displaced ether. A New York chemist named Guthrie discovered a new chemical he called the "spirituous solution of chloric ether" and reported his findings in 1831. The same year, M. Soubeirian, in France, reported the same results, independently discovered. Von Liebig reported his own studies of the drug in 1832. In 1835, M. Jean-Baptiste Dumas named the drug "chloroform," but none of the chemists imagined that it had any medical usefulness. The story of how chloroform came to be used as an anesthetic may be apocryphal but it was said that James Simpson, a professor of midwifery at Edinburgh, had been testing chemicals with his assistants when someone overturned a bottle of chloroform. David Waldie, a chemist in Edinburgh, had suggested the chloroform and it was one of several chemicals being studied by Simpson. His wife came into the lab with his dinner to find them asleep.

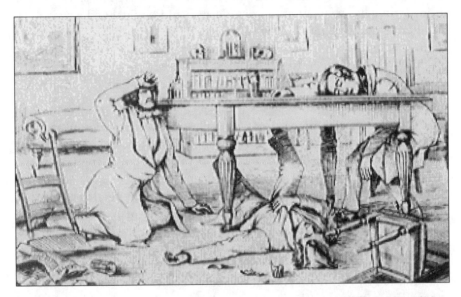

Figure 7 – A contemporary depiction of the discovery of chloroform anesthesia

Simpson tested it on a woman in labor and was so pleased with the effect that he used it on thirty patients during the next week. On April 7, 1853, Queen Victoria took chloroform during the birth of Prince Leopold. John Snow, who will be discussed more completely later, administered the chloroform. Snow published a book on chloroform in 1853 describing its use in anesthesia. There were protests, some on religious grounds (the biblical admonition to bring forth children in pain), but most (and mostly from men, no doubt) were on medical grounds. There were risks of general anesthesia, and ether would eventually prove to be safer in the end, partly because of the lung irritation, which stimulated breathing. Chloroform also has a risk of liver damage and the mortality rate of surgery under chloroform was eventually shown to higher than that using ether.[102]

General anesthesia would prove to have another serious consequence as it caused a great many more operations to be performed before the problems of infection were solved.

THE ETHER CHART

At the Massachusetts General Hospital, ether was administered by medical students (still true in 1965), but, in 1893, there was no good method of determining the dose. The irritable surgeon, on being inhibited by movement of the patient during an operation, would often demand that the student administer more ether. Fortunately, ether is quite safe because it does stimulate respiration but overdoses could be fatal and a system of monitoring depth of anesthesia was needed. The first real progress in controlling administration of anesthesia resulted from a tragedy. Harvey Cushing, destined to be the great founder of neurosurgery and professor of surgery at Harvard, administered ether to one of his first cases as a medical student on January 10, 1893.

The patient suffered from a strangulated hernia and had been ill for over forty-eight hours. The surgeon, Arthur Cabot, found black, dead bowel and the patient died during the operation, probably of a combination of sepsis, poorly treated at the time and, possibly, an overdose of ether in a sick patient. Cushing was very upset and talked of quitting medicine. He had substituted for another student and friend, Frank Lyman, and a few days later, while substituting again, another patient died during surgery. The surgeon, Arthur Cabot again, was anxious for an autopsy and Lyman went in to ask the patient's wife for permission. He found a wake in progress and was attacked by the mourners and chased when his errand became clear to them. These two cases had a profound impression on Cushing. Lyman called him a damned fool for thinking of quitting and he persevered, but was determined to do something to improve care.

In 1895, after some experimentation, Cushing and his classmate, Amory Codman, devised an anesthesia record. They made up a chart divided into fifteen-minute intervals and recorded pulse, temperature and respiration rate in a graphic fashion. Codman and Cushing wagered a dinner on who gave the best anesthesia on their assigned days. They used as their criterion of quality the status of the patient at the end of the surgery. There was no recovery room and patients were taken straight to the ward at the end of the case. A second criterion was the absence of vomiting. Some of these old records have been preserved and contain other notes such as intraoperative hemorrhage and estimates of blood loss. In 1901, during a European trip, Cushing learned of a device invented by Italian Professor

Riva-Rocci that measured blood pressure by inflating an arm cuff and watching a mercury-filled tube to determine the pressure by the height of the column of mercury. He promptly adopted it and brought it back to Johns Hopkins Hospital where it joined the ether chart as another measurement tool. The modern anesthesia record was then essentially complete.

LOCAL ANESTHESIA

As the risks of general anesthesia became clear, a search for agents which would prevent pain without producing unconsciousness began. Cocoa leaves had been used in South America before the arrival of Columbus to relieve pain and as a stimulant. Many of the trephined skulls found in Peru may be examples of anesthesia practice in pre-Columbian America. There are reports of the surgeon performing the trephination chewing cocoa leaves during the procedure and dripping saliva into the wound to produce local anesthesia. It is difficult to imagine how wound infections would have been avoided with this practice and there is no evidence to support the theory. The active chemical, cocaine, was isolated in 1859 by Albert Nieman, who also named the new drug, and it was soon to be included as an ingredient of Coca-Cola and other non-alcoholic drinks.

Sigmund Freud experimented with cocaine in 1884 and wrote to his future wife that it had relieved his depression: "In my last severe depression, I took coca again and a small dose lifted me to the heights in a wonderful fashion. I am now busy collecting the literature for a song of praise for this magical substance."[103] He experimented with it as a cure for morphine addiction, already recognized as a problem. He mentioned its effect of numbing the tongue to Karl Koller, an ophthalmologist friend who was seeking a topical anesthetic. It became the first local anesthetic and was marketed by the Merck drug company in 1885.

Surgeons began experimenting with cocaine as a local anesthetic and many, including William Halsted who reported on 1,000 cases of local anesthesia,[104] became addicted. In 1888, Leonard Corning of New York injected cocaine into the epidural space, the space between the dura mater surrounding the spinal cord and the vertebral bony arch. The method is called epidural anesthesia and is today widely used. In 1899, August Bier, a German, injected cocaine into the spinal fluid, itself, and obtained anesthesia of the entire body below the site of injection. This is now called spinal anesthesia. Epidural anesthesia anesthetizes only the area supplied by the spinal nerves, which pass through the epidural space at the location of the injection (producing a band of anesthesia without affecting the legs below). The two techniques are in wide use and have different applications. Epidural anesthesia has replaced general anesthesia in obstetrical practice, as it does not affect the baby

In 1899, the problem of cocaine addiction was partly solved (at least in medical terms) with the invention of procaine, an artificial compound synthesized by Alfred Einhorn and called "Novocain." In 1905, Braun used it for local anesthesia and cocaine was no longer necessary.[105] Cocaine is still used in ear, nose and throat surgery because the drug causes vasoconstriction, as well as local anesthesia, reducing bleeding and shrinking swollen mucus membranes in the nose. The same effect is responsible for perforation of the nasal septum in chronic cocaine users who sniff, or snort, the powder. The prolonged vasoconstriction causes death of the mucus membrane and cartilage and nasal septum perforation is a classic finding in cocaine addicts.

ANTISEPSIS

Surgeons in the early nineteenth century had no notion that the old, dirty, pus-encrusted frock coats they wore to operate were killing their patients. Simpson candidly admitted that those entering the hospital were "exposed to more chances of death than was the English soldier on the field of Waterloo." The question was why. Especially tragic was puerperal fever which, as more women chose to deliver their babies in hospitals, took a progressively greater toll. At mid-century, there were more survivors from farm accidents in which pregnant women had their abdomen and uterus ripped open by a bull, than from caesarian section operations. The development of anesthesia increased the toll as more operations were performed. Alexander Gordon, in 1795, wrote that the fever was caused by "putrid matter" introduced into the uterus by the midwife or doctor. He recommended washing of the operator's hands and person. In 1843, Boston physician and Harvard anatomy professor Oliver Wendell Holmes regarded childbed fever as an infection whose "germs" were transmitted by birth attendants. He recommended washing with chlorinated water and changing clothes. Two prominent obstetricians in Philadelphia disputed this theory and scoffed that puerperal fever was neither contagious nor caused by the doctors' examinations. Patients continued to die of infection and surgeons resisted hand washing while medical students followed their example.

In the 1840s, Ignaz Semmelweiss, at the Vienna General Hospital, noted that the two maternity wards had very different rates of infection. Ward One, staffed by medical students, had an epidemic of childbed fever and a twenty-nine percent mortality rate. Ward Two, staffed by midwifery pupils who did not attend autopsies, had a three percent mortality rate. Semmelweiss had the wards switched with medical students attending Ward Two and the midwives, Ward One. The mortality rate followed the medical students. His suspicion was confirmed when a friend and professor, Jacob Kolletschka, cut his finger during an autopsy and died of sepsis. At Kolletschka's autopsy, the findings in the professor's body were identical to those in victims of puerperal sepsis. Semmelweiss wrote, "Day and night, the image of Kolletschka's illness pursued me." In May 1847, he ordered hand washing with chlorinated water and sepsis rates plummeted. His colleagues resisted his changes and in 1851, he finally resigned and moved to Budapest where he became head of St. Rochus Hospital. He introduced chlorine disinfection and puerperal fever mortality rates fell below one percent. In 1861, he published *The Cause, Concept, and Prophylaxis of Childbed Fever,* but still he could not convince his colleagues of the hazard of microscopic organisms they could not see. Bacteriology was in its infancy and spontaneous generation of life would not be disproved until Pasteur. In 1865, Semmelweiss' mind failed, possibly from thinking of the thousands of women who had died unnecessarily. He spent time in a mental institution and finally, in a last irony, he is reported to have died of streptococcal sepsis contracted while performing an autopsy.

FLORENCE NIGHTINGALE

The advocates of antisepsis (or at least hand washing) could show better results, but could not explain why they occurred. Florence Nightingale was born in 1820 (in Florence, Italy during her parents' two-year European wedding trip) to a wealthy, cultured family and developed at age seventeen, possibly as a reaction to her hothouse sheltered existence, a "call from God." At first, the "call" was only a vague mission to serve mankind in some fashion. For young ladies of her station this was decidedly abnormal and she kept this secret for many years. In 1844, she decided upon a mission to serve mankind by nursing the sick, hitherto an occupation carried out by those thought worthless for anything else. She confided her thoughts to the visiting American doctor and philanthropist Samuel Gridley Howe, whose wife Julia Ward Howe would later write "The Battle Hymn of the Republic." He encouraged her interest. The next year she gained confidence by nursing two elderly family members and finally confided her ambitions to her family, but they recoiled in disgust, even her devoted father who had encouraged her studies. Her mother accused her of forming some attachment to "a low and disgusting surgeon."

For families like the Nightingales, surgeons were beyond the Pale, let alone nurses. In 1851, a surgeon remarked that every nurse he knew was a drunkard and even Florence related being told in 1854 that all nurses were drunkards and immoral practices were common on wards of a hospital. Even though she believed that she had found her calling in 1845, she had to endure eight more years of resistance from her family until she was free. She risked madness, but the experience made her a woman of steel. At the suggestion of Lord Ashley, a friend, she began to study the Blue Books, reports of the new public health authorities. She read hospital reports and kept voluminous notebooks during early morning hours before her family was awake. She wrote to friends in France and Germany and acquired copies of similar public health reports. She refused an offer of marriage from a family friend, an event that caused a rupture in the family's social circle as Florence was very beautiful and the young man had courted her for several years.

In 1847, she became friends with another exceptional woman, Lady Ada Lovelace, the daughter of Lord Byron and the first computer programmer, for whom the programming language ADA is named. Ada Lovelace suggested the programming for Babbage's "Analytical Engine" and believed that graphics could eventually be generated by a similar, but more advanced device.

In Rome, in 1848, Florence met Sidney Herbert, an extremely wealthy philanthropist interested in hospital reform. Little by little, Florence was, because of her secret study, becoming known to her circle of friends as an expert on health-care matters. An opportunity to visit a nursing school in Germany was cancelled due to the political unrest in Europe in 1848. Florence refused another offer of marriage and a battle of wills between her and her mother resulted. The mother was determined to thwart her willful daughter's unsuitable ambitions. Finally, in 1851, in spite of furious scenes with her mother and sister, she was able to spend three months at Kaiserwerth, a nursing home and orphanage in Germany. Her mother and sister remained unreconciled to her ambition, but she eventually converted her father to an ally. An experience with the Anglican Church, which refused to aid an orphan girl that Florence was trying to rescue from prostitution because she was Irish, led her to contemplate conversion to the Roman Catholic Church. The priest who aided in the rescue of the orphan, arranged for Florence to enter nurses' training with the Sisters of Charity. Her mother and sister had hysterics. Others in the family began to side with Florence, recognizing that her mother was obsessed. Finally, in February 1853, Florence was able to wrench herself away from her family and arrived in Paris on February 4, 1853, able at last to seek her mission from God. Just as she was about to enter the convent to train as a nurse, the family reached out again and she was obliged to return to England to care for an elderly relative.

Later in 1853, she acquired an appointment as superintendent of the Establishment for Gentlewomen During Illness, a private clinic. This followed lengthy negotiations with the committee supervising the Establishment and she was obliged, because of her youth and beauty, to bring with her a matron who would act as a sort of chaperone. She never was able to spend any time with the Sisters of Charity. The committee was soon dazed by the furious energy of their new superintendent who quickly arranged for hot water on all floors and a dumb waiter to bring food from the kitchen, so that nurses might never be obliged to leave their patients. The committee wanted to exclude Catholic patients, but Florence threatened to leave unless all, including "Jews and their Rabbis," were also welcome. Her devotion to good works was evident through organization, not romantic frivolities, a trend that would last her lifetime. She reorganized the purchasing of food and obtained wholesale prices, a detail previously neglected by the committee. Within six months, opposition to her innovations had collapsed and support for her efforts grew among her social circle in London. By 1854, she had the Establishment organized and began to study other hospitals and collect information on the working conditions of nurses. A cholera epidemic in the summer of 1854 brought new responsibilities and she worked with Dr. Bowman, a senior surgeon at King's College Hospital, to found a nursing school where she might train the kind of nurses she needed in her reformed hospitals. By the end of the year, she was also Superintendent of Nurses at King's College Hospital. New acquaintances were taken with her delicate beauty, although a few were later disturbed when they discovered the steel beneath. Her mother wailed that, "We are ducks that have hatched a wild swan."

The Crimean War began in early 1854 and, by September, a disaster was in the making. Supplies were inadequate, the quartermaster corps was incompetent (the Purveyor's Department for the entire British Army had a staff of four) and a cholera epidemic had produced 1,000 cases at Scutari where a hospital was established in a Turkish barracks. An attack at Varna saw 30,000 troops landed with only thirty-one wagons to carry supplies. Newspaper reporters, the first war correspondents in history, at the scene of the battles reported the utter incompetence of the army medical establishment. William Russell, a *Times* correspondent, reported "Not only are there not sufficient surgeons... Not only are there no dressers and nurses… There is not even linen to make bandages."[106] Soldiers died in droves, of illness as well as wounds. All of this news arrived in England in October as a thunderclap. The French army had the Sisters of Charity, with whom Florence had wished to train. The Times wrote, "Why have we no Sisters of Charity?" Sidney Herbert, Florence's old friend and now Secretary of War, stated, "There is but one person in England that I know of who would be capable of organizing and superintending such a scheme." He asked for her services and his letter crossed in the mail her offer to go with a private party. She traveled to the Middle East with thirty-eight nurses: ten Catholic sisters (through the intervention of Father Manning, her friend with the orphanage), eight Anglican sisters, six St. John's Hospital nurses, and fourteen others (who were described as "stout and elderly" and who were allowed a pint of ale each evening). The military protested, but the newspaper accounts of horrors gave her enormous power.

She had a formal appointment as "Superintendent of the Female Nursing Establishment of the English General Hospitals in Turkey," but her power was greater than the appointment would seem to provide. On November 4, 1854, she arrived at Scutari where two thousand sick and wounded lay in foul, rat-infested wards. Three hundred scrubbing brushes were quickly applied to the scene. The Battle of Inkerman occurred soon after her arrival and the hospitals were flooded with wounded. She obtained eighty more nurses as reinforcements and took over the management of the entire facility ordering supplies, meals, bedding, and organizing a system for tracking infection. She had the entire sewer system rebuilt and discovered that the fresh water pipeline was obstructed by a dead horse. Within six months, in spite of constant resistance by the military command, she had cut the mortality rate from forty percent to two percent and, in doing so, invented the science of epidemiology and biostatistics, as well the profession of nursing. Among her other innovations were the first graphical charts ever produced, summarizing the statistics she collected on disease and mortality. The reports prior to her arrival stated, "The orderlies are drawn from the ranks, without any regard to their aptitude or their inclination for the employment."

She returned to Britain in 1856 a national hero. Her contributions to scientific medicine have not been given sufficient credit. She has been called the founder of the nursing profession but she also founded biostatistics and hospital infection control, even though bacteria had yet to be demonstrated to cause disease. Her statistical records of hospital cases are still studied in epidemiology training. After her return to England, she continued for twenty years to try to improve military health care and the lot of the common soldier against incredible resistance by the bureaucracy. The Duke of Wellington, fifty years before, had illustrated the officer corps contempt for the ranks saying that the soldiers enlisted "for the drink." She collected massive amounts of data and wrote, without a secretary, enormous reports in longhand. She established a cost accounting system for the Army Medical Services that was still in use eighty years later. In 1947, the Select Committee on Estimates was evaluating government accounting systems. Several systems had been adopted within the past twenty years but proved less than successful. When the committee investigated the Army Medical Services system, it found the source to be Florence Nightingale in the 1860s. She continued her work on reform of sanitary systems, hospitals and nursing. She was slow to accept the new science of bacteriology, although her own work in statistical analysis of disease had set the stage.

LISTER AND PASTEUR

Joseph Lister was born to a well-off Yorkshire Quaker family. His father Joseph Jackson Lister had developed improved microscopes by discovering a means of avoiding chromatic aberration. After the elder Lister's discovery, microscope development progressed rapidly and would soon make major contributions to the new science of microbiology. The son studied medicine at University College and became an assistant surgeon, under Syme, at Edinburgh in 1854. He married Syme's daughter and was obliged to leave the Quaker Society of Friends because they would not accept "marrying out." By 1860, he had advanced to the Regius Chair in Surgery at Glasgow. He was presented with the problem of sepsis, which was still considered to be caused by "miasma," bad air. His interest was principally in orthopedics and he developed a new operation for tuberculosis of the wrist. When the wound healed cleanly, the results were good but six of sixteen patients developed wound sepsis and died. Lister studied gangrene in frogs and found that rotting and sepsis were related; both involved the decomposition of organic material.

Louis Pasteur had been appointed to a chair in chemistry in Lille, a French manufacturing center, in the same year that Lister joined Syme as assistant surgeon. Pasteur studied tartaric acid, a byproduct of winemaking, and its chemical twin racemic acid. They have identical chemical composition and differ only in crystal formation. Solutions of each rotate polarized light in opposite directions. His studies led him to biology and the composition of life, organic chemistry. Liebig, Director of the Institute of Chemistry at

Giessen, had concluded that fermentation was a chemical process and regarded ferments as unstable chemical products. Pasteur, working ten years later, believed that ferments were living microorganisms and studied the souring of milk and the fermentation of wine and beer. He returned to Paris as the new chairman of chemistry and centered his work on these two phenomena.

By 1860, he had established that fermentation was biological, not chemical, and called this characteristic "vitalism." He showed that fermentation did not occur without yeast and discovered anaerobic organisms. Felix Pouchet proposed spontaneous generation of life in 1854 and the competition between his adherents and those of Pasteur was intense for years. These experiments will be discussed in more detail in the next chapter. Lister was aware of Pasteur's work and became convinced that the cause of wound infection was not air but microorganisms carried by the air. Lister was also familiar with sewage treatment and the studies of early public health advocates who realized that cholera epidemics were related to water and sewage treatment.

John Snow and the Broad Street Pump

John Snow, who administered the chloroform to Queen Victoria in 1853, became convinced, during a London cholera epidemic in 1849, that the disease was not caused by miasma but was carried on the hands from person to person contaminating food. In addition he, much like Florence Nightingale a few years later, did a statistical analysis of the epidemic using the weekly death lists compiled by town clerks. He plotted cases of cholera on a map of London (using the victims' addresses) and realized that they were clustered around water wells. One cluster, in the houses of the wealthy around Golden Square, centered on the Broad Street pump. This pump provided a good flow of water and was used by most residents of the area. In August of 1849, there were 600 cases of cholera in the vicinity of the pump. There were 344 deaths in four days in the Golden Square neighborhood. Eighty-nine deaths occurred on Broad Street itself and all had used that well.[107] The local vestryman, aware of Snow's interest, asked his advice and was told: "Remove the handle on the pump." The legend is that the official declined and Snow stole the pump handle during the night. The epidemic in the neighborhood stopped. He did not stop there, but mapped the water companies supplying homes with piped water.[108] He showed that one company had many cholera cases among its subscribers, while the other had few or none.

Four years later, during another epidemic, Snow repeated his studies and showed that one water company had a death rate of 315 per 10,000 customers and another had only fifty-seven deaths per 10,000 subscribers. He was by now convinced that a living organism caused cholera. Snow, and William Budd, another English physician, came very close to anticipating the Pasteur germ theory. The public health reformers finally established a system of carrying sewage to "sewage farms" where the solid waste was spread on the ground. London at the time had about 200,000 cesspools and the contents had been used for years as fertilizer. The cesspools would be emptied and the contents removed to farms. About the time of the epidemic, chicken manure had become popular as fertilizer, population growth had reduced the value of human feces as fertilizer (the growth of the city had moved the farms farther away) and cesspool maintenance had been neglected. Resuming the practice of cleaning the cesspools and removing the contents to farms reduced contamination of the water supplies, especially town wells, but caused a bad odor and disease among cattle that grazed in the sewage farm fields.

Carbolic acid, phenol, had been discovered in the 1830s by a German industrial chemist, Friedlieb Runge, who isolated it from coal tar. It was found to have antiseptic properties and was widely applied to sewage farms to reduce odor. It was then discovered that the diseases of the cattle grazing in the fields of the sewage farms were much reduced by the application.

THE COMING OF "LISTERISM"

Lister, in his search for a substance that would protect wounds from infection, became aware of this experience and believed that carbolic acid would be effective. His first trial of the antiseptic was in the case of James Greenlees, an eleven-year-old boy with a compound fracture, in August 1865. Lister used lint, soaked in carbolic acid and linseed oil, as a dressing and left it in place for four days. The boy recovered and walked out of the infirmary in six weeks. Nine months later, Lister tried the regimen on another case with the same result. Compound fractures had been a lethal injury without amputation. All this now changed in Glasgow. Lister developed a rigid protocol, including bathing the wound in carbolic acid, lint soaked in carbolic was then applied and covered with foil to prevent evaporation. Dressings were changed periodically using carbolic-soaked lint and, in 1870, he began spraying carbolic acid into the air while the wound was exposed. In May 1867, he published eleven cases of compound fracture with no infections in *Lancet*, the medical journal.[109] Acceptance was not immediate as the presence of bacteria and their role in infection was still unproven. Skeptics abounded among other surgeons. Some of this, as had occurred with Semmelweis twenty years before, may have been a natural reluctance to admit that they had been carrying infection to their patients with unclean hands and clothing. Other surgeons had adopted hand washing and clean operating rooms because of Florence Nightingale's work but refused to accept the "germ theory," as it was termed. Lister's work was accepted in Germany by Karl Thiersch, in 1867, and the technique spread, although not in time for the Franco-Prussian War. During the war the French performed 13,200 amputations with a mortality rate of seventy-six percent.

In the 1870s, Johann Ritter von Nussbaum, who conducted a surgical clinic in Munich, had an eighty percent mortality rate in his surgical cases until his assistant, Lindpainter, returned from Glasgow a convert to Listerism. The mortality rate plummeted and von Nussbaum said, "Behold now my wards, which so recently were ravaged by death. I can only say that I and my assistants and nurses are overwhelmed with joy and gladly submit to all the trouble this treatment involves." In England, the response was less positive. John Bennett, professor of surgery in Edinburgh, said, "Where are these little beasts? Show them to us and we shall believe in them. Has anyone seen them yet?" Lister began to treat the source of infection before anyone could prove the existence of bacteria or their role in infection. He was mistaken in some details: He believed that abscesses were germ free, and that streptococcus and staphylococcus were ubiquitous and often non-pathogenic. He was wrong on both of these details, but he had the right answer for the main issue. Florence Nightingale and John Snow had recognized that disease was related to filth and contamination of water supplies. Lister was able to focus the principle of cleanliness on the individual patient with the use of carbolic acid to sterilize wounds. The bacteriologists would eventually explain why they were correct.

91   BA Kraemer, KE Korber, TI Aquino, A Engleman, "The Use of Leeches in Plastic and Reconstructive Surgery," *Journal of Reconstructive Microsurgery*, 4:381-6 (1988).

92   J. Henry Dible, *Napoleon's Surgeon*, page 237, William Heinemann (1970).

93   Roy Porter, *The Greatest Benefit to Mankind*, page 316.

94   Harold Ellis, *A History of Surgery*, Greenwich Medical Media (2001).

95   J. Henry Dible, *Napoleon's Surgeon*, p 166.

96   Quoted in: Ira M. Rutkow, *American Surgery. An Illustrated History*, p 68, Lippincott-Raven (1998).

97   Robert E. Schofield, *The Lunar Society of Birmingham*, Oxford University Press (1963).

98   Jenny Uglow, *The Lunar Men*, Farrar, Straus and Giroux (2002).

99   F.K. Boland, *The First Anesthetic: The Story of Crawford Long*, University of Georgia Press (1950).

100   Bigelow HJ. "Insensibility during surgical operations produced by inhalation." *Boston Medical and Surgical Journal* 35:309-317 (1846).

101   Julie M. Fenster, *Ether Day* p 194, Harper Collins (2002).

102   William W Keen, *Papers and Addresses*, Chapter "Dangers of Ether" where he discusses the complications of both ether and chloroform and refers to a JAMA study by the Committee on Anesthesia of the American Medical Association. He also quotes a study in Britain in which, of 700 deaths from anesthetics, chloroform was responsible for 478 and ether only twenty-eight., George W Jacobs and Co. (1923).

103   Ernest Jones, *Freud*, Basic Books (1963).

104   W.S. Halsted, "Practical Comments on the Use and Abuse of Cocaine: Suggested by its Invariably Successful Employment in More Than a Thousand Minor Surgical Operations," *New York Medical Journal* v 42: 294-295 (1885).

105   H.F.W. Braun, "Ueber einige neue orthohe Anesthetica (Stovain, Alypin, Novocaine)," *Deutsche Medizinische Wochenschrift* 32: 1667-71 (1904).

106   William Russell, *The Times* , October 9, 1854, quoted in *Florence Nightingale*, by Cecil Woodham Smith, McGraw-Hill (1951) page 85.

107   Nigel Paneth, Peter Vinten-Johansen, Howard Brody and Michael Rip, "A Rivalry of Foulness: Official and Unofficial Investigations of the London Cholera Epidemic of 1854," *American Journal of Public Health* 88:1545-1553 (1998). This study includes considerable detail on the epidemic and the analysis of the cause carried out by authorities at the time.

108   A map of the London water companies is reproduced by the UCLA School of Public Health web site and may be viewed at http://www.ph.ucla.edu/epi/snow/watermap1856/watermap_1856.html.

109   Joseph Lister, "On a new method of treating compound fracture, abscess, etc. with observations on the conditions of suppuration," *Lancet* i:326, 357, 387, 507; vol ii p 95 (1867).

10
The Germans

BILLROTH

THE GERMANS CONTINUED TO BE THE STRONGEST LISTERIANS AND MOST of the rapid progress in surgery for the rest of the century was made by them and by German trained surgeons. Theodore Billroth was born on the island of Rügen in the Baltic Sea. His family was poor and only the assistance of an aunt allowed him to scrape by financially during his education and training. He obtained his medical degree in 1852, after passing examinations and submitting his thesis. He obtained an assistantship in the Berlin clinic of Bernard von Langenbeck, the greatest academic and practical surgeon of the 1850s. Surgery had only been freed of its dominance by medical practitioners for thirty years when Langenbeck took over in 1847. Chloroform anesthesia was in use at the clinic but surgical cases were still mostly limited to amputations, although a predecessor of Langenbeck's, von Gräfe, had corrected cleft palate in 1816 and performed blepharoplasty (correction of eyelid droop or paralysis) in 1818.

In his early career, Billroth spent most of his time on pathology and even considered a career as a pathologist. In 1856, he and Virchow were the finalists for the position of Professor of Pathology in Berlin. Virchow's radical political views had been a barrier to his appointment until the King intervened and told the faculty that his politics were to be disregarded. Billroth was flattered to even be considered as the alternate candidate and believed that the decision was "a voice of destiny calling me to serve surgery faithfully." He continued with pathology investigation, however, and tried to understand the relationship between primary tumors and metastases. In addition to his medical interests, Billroth was an accomplished musician and friend of the composer Brahms and the Swedish soprano Jenny Lind.

On April 1, 1860, Billroth was appointed Professor of Surgery at Zurich. There he continued his study of lymphatic tissue and took an interest in bone and joint surgery. His hospital department had ninety beds for patients and he adopted the practices of Florence Nightingale in terms of hygienic measures and also in his treatment of nurses. He initially required that male patients be cared for by male nurses, but he treated his nurses well and even sent one to a health spa after he contracted an infection. His views evolved and, years later, he would write a book on nursing and establish a nursing school in Vienna. He introduced the practice of taking a patient's medical history, a detail previously neglected for preoperative surgical candidates. Shortly after his arrival in Zurich, he introduced the use of the thermometer for surgical cases after observing Ludwig Traube, professor of medicine at Charité Hospital in Berlin, use body temperature to follow infectious diseases. Prior to Traube's work, the measurement of body temperature was unknown and he established the normal value as well as demonstrating its role in disease, particularly syphilis. In spite of a negative reception from Virchow, still unconvinced of the role of contagion in wound sepsis, Billroth studied septic emboli and endocarditis. By 1862, he was trying to connect wound infection, fever and other types of infection like erysipelas (spreading streptococcal sepsis). He was the first to apply the statistical methods of John Snow and Florence Nightingale to surgery. He discussed the effect of surgery and trauma on body temperature and used postoperative fever to identify developing wound infection, the first surgeon to do so.

Prior to his adoption of Listerism, he used chlorine or lead solutions to treat clean wounds but was disappointed with the results. Many wounds he left open anticipating suppuration. His methods resulted in thirteen percent mortality from infection, far superior to most other clinics and it was 1875 before he adopted Lister's methods. He studied sepsis and wound infection but remained ignorant of the role of bacteria although he recognized the significance of contact with contaminated material. None of his writings refer to Semmelweis and it appears that Billroth never learned of him or his work. Miasma was still the source of infection to most physicians and surgeons but Billroth introduced statistical analysis of the results of surgery and recognized that something was happening that he could not understand. In 1864, he was able to install water tanks and running water in the operating room and used the same techniques that Semmelweis had adopted to keep his infection rate down. He continued his histological studies and attempted to determine the difference between benign and malignant tumors. He was the first to mention a connection between colon polyps and colon cancer. In 1862, he succeeded in having a chair in pathology established and Edward von Rindfleisch, a qualified pathologist, was hired. In 1866, he was offered the chair in surgery at Heidelberg but he remained in Zurich. He was becoming disillusioned with Prussian nationalism and he used the offer to negotiate better terms with the Zurich faculty, including a facility for research. In 1867, he produced his *Handbuch der allgemeinen und speciellen Chirurgie* ("Handbook of General and Special Surgery"), including descriptions of burn treatment and gunshot wounds. This huge book, with a number of other authors contributing chapters, included 8,225 pages. He became fluent in French and taught students from both French and German speaking cantons.

In 1866, Billroth received an offer of the chair in surgery in Vienna. A brief war between Prussia and Austria complicated the situation, and he feared that the defeated Austrians would resent his Prussian origins. As he waited for a decision by the faculty, he continued his work on fever. The experimental lab had shown that wound pus, injected into animals, produces fever, but the "cold pus" from tuberculosis nodules did not. He studied circadian rhythm and discussed conservation of energy with the physicist Clausius (who invented a double lumen tube later used to purify U-235 for the atomic bomb). He had now progressed to the concept of "infectious bodies" in his analysis of infection and recognized the similarity to fermentation but he lacked the chemistry knowledge that finally led Pasteur to the answer. In 1867, he also produced the third edition of his *Die allgemeine chirurgische Pathologie und Therapie* ("General Surgical Pathology and Therapeutics"). Soon after, he decided to accept the Austrian offer although he worried about political influence and a sense of impermanence in the Habsburg monarchy. On May 12, 1867, the Emperor signed his appointment and he assumed his new position.

Vienna

The huge new hospital in Vienna, the Allgemeine Krankenhaus, built in 1784, had a weak surgical department from its establishment. Vincenz Kern, "Magister" of Surgery from 1784 to 1826 was known chiefly as a lithotomist ("cutting for stone"). By 1825, Civiale and others had introduced lithotripsy, via the newly-invented instruments that broke up the stone in the bladder, but Kern resisted the innovation. I have already referred to the influence of the monarchy on the politics of medicine in Vienna, but Napoleon had been dead twenty years when Rokitansky returned to Vienna in 1844 after two years in Paris to absorb the new developments in French clinical medicine. He was appointed full professor of pathology having served as a junior pathologist after accepting an unpaid position in 1827 on his graduation from the medical school. The conservative establishment had permitted this deviation from orthodoxy, but in 1848 the students and faculty rebelled against the stultifying regime and a new constitution for the medical school was drafted. Reform had developed gradually with new professors, like Jacob Kolletschka (Semmelweis' friend) who took over forensic medicine only to die of sepsis contracted at an autopsy. Ludwig von Türkheim was responsible for most of this improvement, but he died in 1846 before his task was accomplished. Had he lived until 1850 he might have approved Semmelweis' application for a lectureship in obstetrics. Instead, with his loss, and with the political revolution of 1848, which sent Prince Metternich into exile, others finally instituted the reforms and von Türkheim has not received credit. The reformed curriculum has been called the "Second Vienna Medical School" so revolutionary were the changes. For the next twenty years, Rokitansky, with his 60,000 autopsy reports, would dominate the curriculum. A second surgical clinic was established and its head raised to full professor. It was this position that Billroth assumed in 1867.

Virchow had emphasized the role of the cell in pathology in 1858, but Rokitansky resisted this innovation, clinging to the "blastema" concept. The arrival of Billroth brought a surgeon who was also an experienced microscopic pathologist, and who was well versed in Virchow's approach. Billroth brought with him the measurement of temperature, a routine postoperative examination since 1860, and considerable sophistication in statistical analysis. In 1870, he recognized the role of cocco-bacteria in wound sepsis although he was uncertain of their nature; thinking perhaps these microscopic organisms were plant forms. He studied botany in an attempt to understand what he was seeing. At the same time, Pasteur was studying fungi so they were on parallel paths. In 1874, he published his work and named one organism *Streptococcus*. He also identified the *Staphylococcus*, but named it *"Gliacoccus,"* later changed by Ogston to the current name. Ten years later, Hans Christian Gram, while he was working with Karl Friedländer (1847-1887) in Berlin, began to use gentian violet (also called crystal violet) to stain organisms which he found, at autopsy, in pneumonia victim's lungs. Gram's method was published in Friedländer's journal *Fortschritte der Medizin* in 1884. A few years later, German pathologist Carl Weigert (1845-1904), director of the Senckenberg Foundation in Frankfurt, added a final step of staining with safranine, which turns gramnegative bacteria red. Gram himself never used counterstaining for gramnegative microbes. Billroth had made his discoveries without the aid of vital stains like that of Gram.

In his studies, Billroth anticipated Koch and Pasteur and introduced the entire field of bacteriology to the Vienna School. In a striking section of his publication, called *Coccobacteria Septica*, he mentions the antibacterial properties of *Penicillium* mold fifty-four years before Fleming![110] In 1884, he sent one of his outstanding students, Anton von Eisenberg, to Koch's lab for advanced study. In 1874, Volkmann convinced Billroth to adopt Lister's antisepsis protocol, a step he had resisted because of his own good results (compared to others at the time) and the laborious wound dressings needed. He began to perform abdominal surgery beginning with six ovariotomies between 1865 and 1870. In the first few years, some of the older physicians, whose practices predated the reforms and who resisted them, frustrated him. Visits from, and musical collaboration with, Brahms relaxed him. He was criticized for his informality with students and it was noted with disdain by old-timers that he even attended student parties. This was not the traditional German and Austrian way of doing things. He experimented with attempts to transplant human tumors to laboratory animals, a shocking concept to the Viennese physicians. A series of cardiac arrests with chloroform anesthesia prompted him to turn to ether or a combination of ether and chloroform.

In 1870, the Franco-Prussian War diverted Billroth's attention and he became involved with military surgery. He had written a historical review of military surgery but had no direct experience himself. He had studied the writing of George A. Otis MD, an American military surgeon who had written about the Civil War.[111] Now, he would have the chance to apply all the recent advances, including antisepsis, to war casualties, but Billroth was still not convinced of Lister's principles and that opportunity was lost. He and Pasteur agreed that France had fallen behind scientifically and the war was a consequence of a change in the balance of power in science as well as in politics. Billroth and his assistant Czerny volunteered to be consultant surgeons in German military hospitals and were accepted. Technically, being residents of Austria, they were neutral. The Prussian Army Medical Corps was poorly organized and Billroth enjoyed his chance to follow in the footsteps of Paré and Larrey as he set up field hospitals. His German nationalism is apparent as he complains that the Alsatians, who speak German and whose territory is coveted by the Prussians, do not want to be separated from France. He writes to his wife, "in five or ten years they will all be good Germans."[112] He does, however, understand that Prussian rule is not good for Germany and complains of Prussian "Caesarism." He cannot understand why the Austrians do not support Bismarck and the war, showing that he was still a Northern German, not an Austrian, in his heart. Soon, he and Czerny were overwhelmed with patients. By October 1870, they had treated thousands of gunshot wounds and he was becoming bored with trauma. His experience was extremely valuable for his subsequent career and he and Czerny reported their experience in medical journals. His views about infection, wound infection in particular, were strongly influenced by the experience. Vascular injuries were invariably treated by ligation, but delayed hemorrhage resulted in a high mortality rate. Billroth still had not accepted Lister's work completely, but he did prohibit his assistants from probing such wounds with fingers. In October, he returned to Vienna.

In late 1870, he began his work on surgery of the esophagus, first constructing lateral esophagotomies in dogs. This procedure opens the esophagus in the neck, attaching it to the skin, and is still useful in patients with esophageal obstruction by cancer. The saliva drains from the fistula instead of filling the mouth requiring frequent expectoration. He performed excision of half the tongue for cancer and even some more radical procedures involving excision of the posterior tongue through the neck were successful. On December 31, 1873, he performed the first total laryngectomy for cancer. The patient was a young theology teacher with a three-year history of hoarseness. In November, his larynx was split and the tumor removed locally. It immediately recurred. The second operation was a success, and Billroth immediately applied his musical talents to an attempt to restore the patient's speech. The folly of local excision will be discussed again in recounting the story of Freidrich, the German Crown Prince.

On January 29, 1881, Billroth successfully resected a cancer of the stomach, restoring the anatomy by connecting the stomach to the duodenum, a technique since called the Billroth I operation and studied by every surgical resident. By 1892, Billroth and his assistant Czerny had performed thirty-seven of these operations with a forty-six percent mortality rate. Part of the high mortality was due to the advanced stage of the patients' disease and part to the primitive state of postoperative care in which blood transfusion and even intravenous fluid infusion were still far in the future. Billroth established a formal surgery training program in Vienna; much like the one William Halsted was to develop at Johns Hopkins a few years later. His residents included Winiwarter, who first performed cholecyst-enterostomy (bypass of biliary obstruction), Mikulicz-Radecki who devised pyloroplasty (to relieve gastric outlet obstruction) in 1887, and many others whose intestinal suture techniques were in use twenty-five years before they became common in North America. Walter von Heineke described the pyloroplasty in 1886, and he and Mickulicz share the credit. Czerny adopted carbolic acid sterilized silk for suture material after disappointing failures with improperly prepared catgut.

RUBBER GLOVES, AND ASEPSIS

In America, William Halsted adopted antisepsis at Bellevue Hospital, New York, but the operating rooms were so filthy he erected a tent on the lawn and used it for his operating room. In 1889, after his move to the newly opened Johns Hopkins Hospital, his instrument nurse, Miss Caroline Hampton, developed a skin irritation from the carbolic acid. Hasted had the Goodyear Rubber Company manufacture thin rubber gloves to protect her hands. Miss Hampton eventually retired from the operating room, when she and Halsted were married, and his residents began to use the remaining rubber gloves. Old, dirty frock coats were still used until late in the century and the realization slowly dawned that carbolic acid spray was not enough. Lister did not, at first, scrub his hands or wear surgical gowns. Halsted was responsible for advancing the cause taken up by the Germans. His innovations were soon adopted in Europe.

Ernst von Bergmann, a Prussian who would figure in the tragedy of Freidrich III, pioneered steam sterilization and asepsis in 1881, and this technique would gradually replace antisepsis by 1900. The first doubts about carbolic acid appeared in 1874 when Ranke published a study of wound secretions in which fourteen of fifteen cases showed bacteria present in spite of antisepsis.[113] He could not see the rod-shaped bacteria, that we now call gram-negative organisms, but cocci (round gram-positive organisms) were present. In 1881 Ogston, who named *Staphylococcus*, drew attention to German studies of the limitations of Listerism. He concluded that carbolic acid was ineffective in preventing airborne contamination. Robert Koch, the same year, published a study concluding that mercuric chloride, called "corrosive sublimate," was the only effective antiseptic. In 1884, Lister accepted Koch's conclusions and adopted corrosive sublimate in place of carbolic acid. Carbolic acid had served its purpose and was now superseded by better methods. It is important to remember that carbolic acid brought about the revolution and Lister, although he apologized for his delay in accepting Koch's conclusion, was the pioneer. One problem was the skin irritation produced by the chemical, worse than that caused by carbolic spray. The mercuric compounds persisted until modern times as "Mercurochrome," used as a topical wound preparation by mothers on their children's scrapes until antibiotic ointment replaced it in the 1970s. Mercuric chloride was too toxic to use as a spray and it reacted with metal instruments so it could not be used for sterilization of equipment.

In his 1881 presentation, Koch reported on the effectiveness of steam sterilization of instruments. The method required a new technology, steam boilers that left textile materials dry and avoided rusting of instruments.

Lister objected that dressings must be treated with antiseptics to avoid subsequent contamination. Schimmelbusch described further investigations at von Bergmann's clinic, the Ziegelgasse Klinik, in his book, which was to become the bible of modern surgical technique when it was published in 1892 and translated into English two years later.[114] When Osler visited Berlin in 1884 he observed surgeons working inside the abdomen, using "Edison electric lamps" and asepsis was the standard protocol in the operating room. The methods used in von Bergmann's clinic were described at the 1890 Tenth International Medical Congress. That same Congress saw Koch's announcement of tuberculin and the apology by Lister for his resistance to the new concept of asepsis. The new method was adopted in the United States after an address to the Obstetrical Society of Philadelphia by Howard Kelly in 1886. England was slow to change even though a steam sterilizer had been purchased for the Aberdeen Infirmary in 1890. Finally, the Schimmelbusch book brought adoption of asepsis by 1896 in Aberdeen, although it was 1900 before antisepsis had been fully eclipsed. St. Thomas Hospital in London installed an autoclave in the operating rooms in 1894, but it was 1901 before antiseptic dressings were gone.

By 1890, Halsted had abandoned the carbolic spray for aseptic technique, including steam sterilization of instruments, hand washing, surgical gowns, and careful wound handling. He also adopted Czerny's silk suture material, using suture ligatures for bleeding vessels. Billroth's assistant Johannes von Mikulicz-Radecki began wearing a mask during operations to avoid contamination by mouth and nose, although few were covering noses before 1920. Berkley Moynihan described his student days in Leeds in the 1880s: "He (the surgeon) rolled up his sleeves and, in the corridor to the operation room, took an ancient frock from a cupboard; it bore signs of a chequered past, and was utterly stiff with old blood. One of these coats was worn with special pride, indeed joy, as it had belonged to a retired member of the staff." Moynihan, himself, would become a distinguished surgeon, adopt the aseptic procedure and was the first in Britain to wear rubber gloves. The times were changing. In 1873, Sir John Erichsen, surgeon to University College Hospital London, declared, "The abdomen, the chest and the brain [will] be forever shut from the intrusion of the wise and human surgeon."[115]

In 1882, Carl Langenbuch, surgeon at Lazarus Hospital in Berlin, first removed a gallbladder for stones causing pain and inflammation. Langenbuch had noted the absence of the gallbladder in some animals and concluded that it was not necessary for life. Even before this date, Marion

Sims, who had first corrected vesico-vaginal fistula in the pre-anesthetic days, and Lawson Tait, of Birmingham, England, had performed cholecystotomy, opening the gallbladder and removing the stones without removing it. Sims had adopted antisepsis, as well as anesthesia, but Tait did not and still obtained good results; probably because he did take care with cleanliness. Tait, with the stubbornness and backwardness typical of many British surgeons in this era, refused to adopt the principles of prevention of infection and opposed complete removal of the gallbladder, successfully in England, until he died of uremia in 1899. He was not the only one as many feared to remove the organ in spite of Langenbuch's studies.

A Royal Cancer

The limitations of English surgeons would have serious consequences, not only for their patients, but also for world history. Queen Victoria's children married into the royal families of Europe and, by 1900, most European monarchs were related to the Queen Empress directly or by marriage. In 1887, Crown Prince Freidrich III developed hoarseness. Freidrich was fifty-six years old and healthy, but had been hoarse since a cold several months before. His father was ninety years old and the Prince had been waiting to play his own part in German history for a long time. The Crown Princess, Victoria, was the eldest daughter of the English queen. Examination of the larynx and vocal cords was a recent development; a Doctor Mende, in the early nineteenth century, had first glimpsed the function of the vocal cords in a living person when he examined a man who had cut his own throat in a suicide attempt. The man lived a day and the larynx was exposed by the laceration. The study of diseases of the larynx had begun in Vienna after it was finally learned how to visualize it with mirrors and reflected sunlight. Turck and Czermack, in Vienna, had invented the laryngoscope and were able to use artificial light. Karl Gerhardt, the professor of medicine at Berlin University who had become well known for pediatrics (including tonsillitis), examined the Prince with a mirror and saw a nodule on a vocal cord. The treatment of laryngeal diseases had progressed to the point that he proposed to remove it using the mirror for visualization. This had become a common procedure. He did so using a heated platinum wire and cocaine anesthesia. It grew back within a few weeks. Another removal was followed by another recurrence.

Gerhardt, at this point, suggested that the Prince be examined by a German surgeon, Ernst von Bergmann (inventor of asepsis), who had successfully removed a laryngeal cancer by removing half of the larynx, hemi-laryngectomy. This left the patient permanently hoarse, but cured the malignancy. The Prince was examined by von Bergmann who agreed with the diagnosis and recommended surgery. The operation would be complicated by the need to provide anesthetic and an adequate airway during the procedure. This required a tracheotomy, a procedure performed for 200 years and perfected by Fabricius' invention of the tracheotomy cannula. Laryngectomy, total laryngectomy with removal of both vocal cords and the larynx, had been performed by Billroth in 1873, but the new operation of hemi-laryngectomy had been successful in a few early cases like that of the Prince and would allow the voice to be retained. The physicians, however, were intimidated by the responsibility of treating the Crown Prince of Germany for cancer in the presence of an ailing ninety-year-old monarch who might die at any time. When the Crown Princess, who had never been comfortable with her German subjects, suggested another opinion with an English physician they agreed.

Morell Mackenzie had an interest in throat diseases, but was not up to date on the surgical aspects. Mackenzie had studied in Vienna and afterward took a laryngoscope back to England with him where it had previously been unknown. Since he was the only specialist in diseases of the throat in London, he developed a large practice. He performed tonsillectomies in his office but had not adopted the newer and more complex procedures being developed in Germany. He had a reputation for greediness and the Queen's letter to her daughter, which accompanied Mackenzie to Berlin, mentioned this fact as a warning to her. Further examination of the Prince in Berlin had confirmed the diagnosis and surgery was planned to follow the second opinion consultation. Fatefully, Mackenzie disagreed with the plan for surgery and recommended another attempt at local excision, this time to be performed by him. He was not convinced that the mass was cancer in spite of the history of previous attempts to remove it.

It is characteristic of second opinion physicians, especially surgeons, that they feel confident the preceding care was less skillful than their own would be. After all, seeking a second opinion is evidence of uncertainty. The second surgeon is usually an "expert" and therefore tempted to "take over the case." This is one of the reasons that second opinion programs sponsored by insurance companies in modern times prohibited the second surgeon from doing the surgery, a rule that might affect the recommendation for or against surgery. Mackenzie, by all accounts, was susceptible to the temptation and took over in spite of his limited experience with laryngeal cancer. Mackenzie performed another local excision of the lesion and Virchow examined the biopsy in the microscope. He declared that the lesion did not show cancer! Mackenzie was vindicated. Virchow asked for more tissue but Mackenzie now took control, conversing with the Crown Princess in English and dismissing the German doctors' advice. The royal couple chose the optimistic advice of Mackenzie and no more biopsies were taken although another attempt at excision was made and failed. Mackenzie recommended a trip to England and, at this point, the first accounts of the illness reached the newspapers.

Mackenzie, with a well-known penchant for publicity, wrote to the *Deutche Revue* on July 1, 1887 and declared that there was no cancer. Furthermore, there was speculation in English newspapers that the German surgeons had been about to make a terrible mistake and only the intervention of the expert, Dr. Mackenzie, had saved the Prince from an unnecessary operation and possible death. Henry Butlin, the foremost English laryngologist, published a warning in the *British Medical Journal* that biopsy of laryngeal carcinoma was fraught with false negative results because of the tiny amount of tissue available for examination. He described cases from his own experience in which this had occurred. It was to no avail. The trip to England, for the Queen's Jubilee, was on.

In London, Mackenzie made another attempt to remove the tumor through the mouth with the laryngoscope. A young German laryngologist, who accompanied the party to England, over Mackenzie's protests about a "spy," was kept away from the Prince. He was allowed one examination in June and expressed concern about possible involvement of the other vocal cord and increased inflammation of the larynx. These concerns were dismissed. In August, another excision, with cautery this time, was attempted. A few days later, the German laryngologist was again allowed an examination. He "quivered with horror" as he saw that involvement of the entire larynx had taken place. Confident of Mackenzie's prognosis, the Prince refused the pleas of the German to allow another examination by von Bergmann and the other German surgeons. On Mackenzie's advice, the royal party left for Scotland. A month later, the German laryngologist was allowed another examination and saw that the cancer was now incurable even with total laryngectomy. He documented his findings for the inevitable inquiry. The Princess clung to the optimistic prognosis long after it was obvious that the Prince was failing. At this point Mackenzie, perhaps sensing failure and fearing the consequences, began to qualify his optimism and even suggested a return to Germany. The Princess, by now in a rage at the German doctors who persisted in pessimistic appraisals that frustrated her hopes, refused.

An optimistic report from Mackenzie was published in Berlin, in the *Berliner Tageblatt*, and other German newspapers, in September and resulted in abuse being hurled at the "inept" German surgeons who had wanted to risk the Prince's life with an operation when there was no cancer. Mackenzie was given all the credit and there was talk of a knighthood. By October, Mackenzie began to voice doubts about the negative biopsy report five months before in a letter to another physician. He denied disregarding the German surgeons' advice and invited their assistance if problems arose. None of this was mentioned to the newspaper reporters.

On November 6, another examination showed evidence which could no longer be denied and he admitted to the Prince that the condition was indeed cancer. On November 13, the *Deutche Reichs-Anzieger* reported the true state of affairs and the repercussions were immediate. The Kaiser asked how had the operation been delayed until it was too late? Soon, a newspaper war, between the Princess and Mackenzie on one side and the German doctors on the other, developed. She refused to have anything to do with Professor von Bergmann and even convinced the Crown Prince that it was not cancer after all. On January 7, 1888, the *British Medical Journal* reported that Mackenzie now believed that the Prince was improving and maybe it was not really cancer. By early February, the Prince was having trouble breathing. The young German doctor present attempted to send for von Bergmann to perform a tracheostomy, but the telegram was blocked by the Princess, and by Mackenzie, who did not want to see his hated rival at the Prince's bedside. The young assistant, Bramann, in a scene of incredible chaos and interference by others, performed the tracheostomy successfully. At the order of the Kaiser, von Bergmann came to the Prince's side, but the hostility from the Princess and Mackenzie, who incredibly still retained her confidence, continued and the newspaper war persisted, now with nationalistic overtones.

English newspapers attributed relapses in the dying Prince to the tracheostomy technique or the use of a German design cannula versus an English one. By the end of February, the Princess was insisting that von Bergmann return to Berlin, but, just as he was about to leave, he was ordered by the Kaiser to remain. She rejected the diagnosis of cancer and Mackenzie constantly intrigued with her, turning her against all the other doctors including Professor Kussmaul who had been asked to consult on suspected pneumonia but who immediately recognized the cancer. Prince Wilhelm (the future Kaiser) was now dispatched by his grandfather, the Kaiser, to ensure that his father, the Crown Prince, returned to Berlin so that the Kaiser could see him once more. The monarch had no illusions. In spite of all this, the Princess refused to move her husband and the young

Prince and von Bergmann returned to Berlin.

A week later, the Kaiser died, leaving the dying Freidrich on the throne. The new Emperor must now return to Berlin although the Empress made certain that Mackenzie was still in complete control of his care. He continued to give optimistic bulletins to the newspapers but the Germans, by now, were suspicious. On April 12, the developing cancer extruded the cannula and it could not be replaced. Von Bergmann succeeded in inserting a longer cannula only to learn that the deterioration in the Emperor's condition was now being attributed to the cannula insertion. The *British Medical Journal* participated in this nationalist war of press releases assuring its readers that "the Emperor's English medical attendants" were not responsible for the setback. Still, there was no mention of cancer in the press. At the end of April, in view of the newspaper calumnies, von Bergmann asked to be relieved of his role in the case. The Empress obliged. Years later, after the death of von Bergmann, Mackenzie's young assistant, Mark Hovell, wrote that von Bergmann was apparently intoxicated when he changed the tracheostomy cannula on April 12 and produced a false passage, inserting the cannula into the neck in front of the trachea. He then described the development of an abscess in the neck, which finally drained on April 19. A note written by the Emperor at the time which says, "Bergmann ill treated me" was printed in the *British Medical Journal* in October 1888 and was produced as evidence of the charge.

In June, the Emperor began to cough up food he had swallowed. Incredibly, the *British Medical Journal* printed another optimistic report from Mackenzie. On June 15, the Emperor died, a consequence of the tracheal-esophageal fistula that had developed. The next battle began immediately over a possible autopsy. The Empress-mother was adamant against it, but the German doctors insisted, in view of the long denial of the truth and the allegations of misadventures with the tracheostomy and reinsertion of the cannula. The new Kaiser Wilhelm, never comfortable with his mother or with the English, and convinced that the German doctors had been right all along, gave his consent. Mackenzie witnessed the autopsy and, on his way back to England, gave a newspaper interview stating that he had always known about the cancer, but had denied it to protect the Crown Prince's succession. There were allegations, untrue but widely believed, that a law would have blocked Freidrich's accession to the throne if he were incurably ill. The official report of the autopsy and the German doctors' findings was marred by personal attacks on Mackenzie but his reply *The Fatal Illness of Frederick the Noble* was filled with falsehoods and ruined his reputation as they became clear. He was asked to resign from the medical societies to which he had been elected and finally, after four years of criticism, died in 1892 from complications of asthma. Kaiser Wilhelm indulged his hostility to all things English and began to build battleships after dismissing his chancellor, von Bismarck. His father, had he lived, was a much more liberal and patient man and had no such prejudices against the English, as evidenced by his marrying an English princess. The son was volatile and impulsive and Europe would pay dearly for these characteristics.

110   Karel B. Absolon, *The Surgeon's Surgeon, Theodor Billroth*, Volume III, figure 62 is a photograph of Billroth's paper and pages 150-153 describe the work, Coronado Press (1981).

111   George A. Otis, "The Medical and Surgical History of the War of the Rebellion," published in multiple volumes from 1866 to 1872.

112   Karel Absolon, Volume II, page 63.

113   HR Ranke, "Die Backterien-vegetation unter dem Lister' schen Verbande," *Centralblatt für Chirurgie* 1:193-4 (1874).

114   C Schimmelbusch, "The aseptic treatment of wounds," HK Lewis, London. (1894).

115   Roy Porter, page 374.

11

Medicine, bacteriology and infectious diseases

LISTER, JENNER, AND FLORENCE NIGHTINGALE USED PRACTICAL MEASURES to deal with microorganisms they could not see and, indeed, had no proof that they existed. The microscope opened a window on this world of unseen threats, but it took the work of the early bacteriologists to make sense of it and apply the knowledge they gained to human health. Girolamo Fracastoro, in 1546, had proposed the cause of infectious diseases as *seminaria contagiosa*, "disease seeds" that were carried by the wind or communicated by contact with infected objects. Francesco Redi, in 1699, boiled broth and sealed it in containers proving that maggots did not develop in meat protected from flies and putrefaction did not occur without contamination. This should have disproved spontaneous generation, but John Needham, in 1748, repeated the experiment and saw "animalcules" in the broth, which must have appeared spontaneously. The debate about spontaneous generation continued for a century. In 1835, Agostino Bassi, manager of a silkworm estate, conducted an experiment with a silkworm disease, muscarine. A fungus on the dead silkworms could produce the disease when healthy silkworms were incubated with it. One of Koch's postulates was established. Johann Schoenlein studied ringworm in Zurich in 1839 and showed that the fungus seen in lesions could produce the disease in healthy subjects. Jacob Henle, influenced by Bassi's observations, concluded in 1840 that a living agent that acted as a parasite caused infectious diseases. He wrote, in *Pathologische Untersuchungen* ("Pathologic Investigations"), "The substance of contagion is not only organic but living, and endowed with a life of its own, which has a parasitic relation to the sick body." He proposed measures to test the theory that anticipated Koch. The organism should be found in the sick patient, it should be isolated from mixed specimens and it should be capable of reproducing the disease in animals by transmission of the purified parasite. The concept of miasma persisted, however, until Pasteur.

PASTEUR AND BACTERIOLOGY

Louis Pasteur, the son of a tanner who was a veteran of Napoleon's army, was educated at Ecole Normale Superieure. He developed a particular interest in chemistry, which ultimately led him to biology as described in the last chapter. His interests focused on fermentation of sugar to alcohol and the souring of milk. By 1860, he was convinced that fermentation was a biological phenomenon, rather than purely chemical. The advocates of spontaneous generation had a religious, or rather anti-religious, motivation as they tried to upset the concept of creation by a supreme being. A solitary source of life was uncomfortably close to creation and spontaneous generation served the purposes of the rationalists and scientific rationalism. This made its refutation more than a scientific matter.

Pasteur devised a set of elegant experiments that began with drawing air through a wad of gun cotton (nitrocellulose) in a flask. The gun cotton was then dissolved and microscopic organisms were visible in the solution. Air then contained the organisms of fermentation. Next, air that had been heated was drawn into the flask, into a sterile solution, and the organisms were not present. They were alive and could be killed by heat. Next, he showed that a sterile solution could be left exposed to air if the neck of the flask was curved down to prevent particles from falling into the flask. The organisms, or at least the particles carrying them, had weight and responded to gravity. Then, he tested the distribution of organisms in the air and showed that pure mountain air contained fewer organism carrying particles than did the air of Paris. The controversy between Pasteur and the advocates of spontaneous generation reached the Academie des Sciences which, possibly responding to the religious concerns of conservatives, ruled in Pasteur's favor.

Pasteur worked on problems of the wine industry and proved that *Mycoderma aceti* was the microorganism responsible for souring wine. Furthermore, he demonstrated that heating wine to fifty-five degrees centigrade, which did not damage the wine, killed the organism and prevented the souring. Eventually, the principle was applied to beer and milk and the term "Pasteurization" became a common one. The Pasteurizing process has virtually eliminated the risk of tuberculosis from milk without affecting its quality. Henle had argued that fermentation, putrefaction, and disease were related and Pasteur had demonstrated microorganisms, which produced these phenomena, in the air. The connection was there to be explored.

The next step was study of another silkworm disease, pebrine, which was producing serious problems for the industry. Pasteur demonstrated that the cause was a living organism, a protozoan, and discovered its life cycle from moth to egg to chrysalis. On February 19, 1878, he appeared before the French Academy of Medicine to present the germ theory of disease. Later that year, he, with Jules Jobert and Charles Chamberland, published a report developing this theme and predicting that specific organisms would be found to produce specific diseases and that vaccines, similar to that which prevented smallpox, would prevent those diseases. In 1879, he studied chicken cholera and anthrax. Taking samples from an old, "stale" culture of the cholera organisms, he injected chickens and found that the disease did not develop. The stale culture was the result of a lab accident, but he quickly recognized the significance of the observation. Subsequently, he took samples from a fresh "strong" culture and injected those same chickens and another "naïve" group of chickens. The disease did not develop in the chickens that had first been inoculated with the "old" culture, but did appear in the chickens not exposed to the first inoculum. He had succeeded in immunizing chickens against the cholera.

KOCH

Anthrax was a common disease in cattle that occasionally infected human agricultural workers with a condition called "woolsorters' disease," pulmonary anthrax. The condition had for years been attributed to a rural miasma and caused severe losses because fresh cattle could be infected from fields that had previously contained infected cattle. Surely, this was a good argument for the existence of miasma. Some research had already been performed with evidence of microorganism involvement. Franz Aloys (1800-1879) and Casimir Davaine (1812-82) had seen microscopic bacilli in the blood of dying cattle. Robert Koch (1843-1910) had been studying anthrax as well. Koch had studied medicine in Gottingen under Henle and served as a surgeon in the Franco-Prussian War of 1870. He was appointed to an office as district health officer in Posen, in modern Poland. Anthrax was endemic in Posen and Koch set up his own laboratory to study the disease. He learned that anthrax formed spores, which were resistant to heat and could revert to the bacillary form and produce the disease. This explained the appearance of anthrax in fresh cattle grazing in infected fields.

Pasteur used samples of Koch's *Bacillus anthracis* to conduct experiments on attenuation of the virulence of the organism. Finally, he was able to produce a "weak" form that could be used to produce a vaccine. On May 5, 1881, he injected twenty-four sheep, a goat and six cattle with the attenuated strain of anthrax at a public demonstration. A similar group was left unexposed. On May 17, a second injection, using a stronger culture, was given to the test animals. On May 31, all animals, inoculated and naïve (the control group), were given an injection of virulent anthrax. By June 2, all the sheep and the goat in the control group were dead and the cattle were sick. The inoculated group was all healthy. The era of vaccines had begun and medicine finally was able to prevent, if not yet treat, disease. It had taken nearly 100 years since Jenner to develop a second vaccine. Pasteur had been able to produce artificially the attenuated strain of an organism that nature had provided in smallpox/cowpox.

RABIES

In 1880, Pasteur, aided by Chamberland and Pierre Roux (1853-1933), began to study rabies, the ancient and greatly feared "hydrophobia." He failed to find the organism, a virus too small to be seen in conventional microscopes, but persisted in trying to produce immunity. He injected the spinal cord tissue from infected individuals into rabbit brain, reasoning that nervous tissue seemed to be the site of attack. Extensive experiments produced an infection with an incubation period of six days. He called this unseen organism a *virus fixe* (virus is Latin for poison). He injected the material into spinal cords and then dried the cords for various periods trying to produce an attenuated virus that would not produce disease, or at least a mild form analogous to cowpox. After two weeks of drying, the virus seemed to be attenuated. In 1884, he was ready to test the attenuated, but still live and infectious, virus for inoculation. He set up a series of vaccines using different periods of drying to study the effectiveness of different preparations. He injected dogs with attenuated virus beginning with the "weakest" and progressing to stronger preparations. The idea was that the weaker strain would protect against the stronger until the strongest would protect against virulent rabies. After two weeks the immunized dogs, and a control group, were given virulent rabies. The immunization worked and all the test dogs remained free of disease.

Later, in further studies, he learned that, because of a long incubation period, not the six days in rabbit brain, immunization was effective even after exposure to the virulent rabies. One hundred years later, it was learned that this longer incubation period was due to the virus' route of spread to the brain; along the sensory nerves rather than via the bloodstream. In evolutionary terms, this behavior of the virus minimized exposure to the victim's immune system but it allowed the development of the therapy. The farther the site of inoculation was from the brain, the longer the interval between initial inoculation and brain involvement.

On July 6, 1885 a patient, named Joseph Meister, a nine-year-old boy, was brought to Pasteur. Two days before, the boy had been bitten fifteen times by a rabid dog. A doctor told the boy's mother to take him to Pasteur who was willing to take a chance with the untested therapy if his patient was. He began the same series of injections he had used on his test dogs. For fourteen days, Joseph was injected with daily doses of increasingly virulent strains of rabies. He did not develop the disease. Three months later Pasteur repeated the series of injections in another boy, fourteen years old this time, who had been bitten severely by a known rabid dog. This was also successful. Experimental biology had passed its first test in humans. Over the next fifteen months, 2,000 people received the vaccine and during the next decade over 20,000 were inoculated. There was criticism because not all victims of dog bites, even if the dog seemed rabid, would develop rabies and the vaccine contained live virus that could possibly produce the disease he was trying to prevent. In 1915, a ten-year study showed that, of 6,000 people bitten by rabid animals, only 0.6 percent of those vaccinated died but of those not vaccinated, sixteen percent died. Pasteur had been dead for nineteen years when his final vindication was published. The Institut Pasteur was set up in 1888 with, appropriately, Joseph Meister, the first patient treated for rabies, as gatekeeper. Pasteur died in 1896 and was buried in the Insitut.

KOCH'S POSTULATES

Koch continued the work begun by Pasteur and established the principles which still dominate the bacteriology of disease. In 1879, he published a paper on the etiology of infectious disease which presented the first statement of what would become Koch's Postulates. Bacteria must be identified and classified, then connected to the appropriate clinical entity. The germ theory became more than a theory. In 1882, the Postulates were formalized:

1. The organism must be discoverable in every instance of the disease.

2. The organism, recovered from the patient, must be isolated in pure culture and the culture must then be subcultured over several generations to insure purity.

3. The disease must be reproduced in experimental animals from a pure culture, obtained after several generations of pure culture, and initially derived from the original sample.

4. The same organism must be recovered from the experimental animal and subcultured through several more generations

Viruses do not lend themselves to this model, although in modern times it has been possible to fulfill Koch's postulates with tissue cultures in which the viruses can be grown. Some tissue cultures have contributed contaminating viruses to confuse the issue but the principles remain the gold standard. Koch added the technique of solid culture media while Pasteur contented himself with liquid media. Koch began with potato slices as a culture medium and progressed to gelatin-broth mixtures. Eventually, he adopted Japanese *agar-agar*, a seaweed extract that remains solid at body temperature. Richard Petri (1852-1921) invented a flat round dish that lent itself to bacteriological studies.

On March 24, 1882, Koch demonstrated the organism that causes tuberculosis, *Mycobacterium tuberculosis*, before the Berlin Physiological Society, a great triumph. The next year he traveled to Egypt during a terrible cholera epidemic to seek the responsible organism. By this time, Koch and Pasteur were rivals and Roux, one of Pasteur's assistants, led a French team for the same purpose. The Pasteur team failed because there is no animal model for cholera. Koch identified the organism, *Vibrio cholerae*, in Alexandria in 1883 and confirmed this work in India the next year. He showed that the organism lived in the human intestine and was transmitted in polluted water, confirming the early work of John Snow who by now had become Britain's first anesthesiologist. Koch's report was disputed by Munich hygienist Max von Pettenkofer (1818-1901) who was a miasma and spontaneous generation diehard. He requested, and received from Koch, a flask of culture medium containing *Vibrio cholerae*, which he proceeded to drink! He suffered no ill effects, probably a result of very low gastric Ph (high acid concentration) which is protective, and reported himself in good health. Koch's lab, notwithstanding von Pettenkofer's quibbles, proceeded to discover the organisms responsible for diphtheria, typhoid, pneumonia, gonorrhea, meningitis, undulant fever, leprosy, plague, tetanus, syphilis, whooping cough (pertussis), and the streptococcus and staphylococcus.

DIPHTHERIA

The age of vaccines began with Pasteur and continued until antibiotics were discovered in 1935. Diphtheria was the next to be tackled. The disease produces a severe pharyngitis with development of a gray membrane on the tonsils and palate. The membrane is leathery (*diphthera* is Greek for leather) and slowly blocks the airway covering the pharynx. After 1850 the disease became common in large cities and, in the 1870s, 2,000 children died of diphtheria each year in New York City. The only treatment was tracheostomy (the author's mother had a tracheostomy performed on her family kitchen table at the age of two for diphtheria). Pierre-Fidele Bretonneau, an early advocate of germ theory, provided the name of the disease in 1826 and identified its characteristics including the pharyngeal membrane. Theodor Klebs, a student of Virchow, identified the organism in 1883 and named it *Corynebacterium diphtheriae*. Friedrich Loeffler, one of Koch's assistants (Koch was by now consumed with administrative matters), succeeded in cultivating the bacteria and identified it in the secretions of healthy children, thus first discovering the existence of disease carriers.

Between 1888 and 1890, the nature of the disease process was identified by Roux and Alexander Yersin (who identified the plague organism) when they discovered that a toxin produced by the organism was actually responsible for the symptoms and the mortality. In 1890, Fraenkel, a German bacteriologist, produced attenuated cultures of the organism that could induce immunity in guinea pigs. Emil Behring and Shibasaburo Kitasato (who co-discovered the plague bacillus), working in Koch's Institute, announced that the blood or serum of an animal immune to diphtheria would protect another, non-immune animal from the disease. This anti-toxin was another step in the treatment of infectious disease and was successfully used on a child in Berlin on December 25, 1891. In 1894 anti-toxin was produced in volume and introduced into German clinics. The mortality rate of diphtheria fell. In Paris, Roux and Yersin produced large volumes of anti-toxin by immunizing horses. The French serum was introduced into England by Lister in 1895 and ten years later mortality had dropped by more than half. In New York the mortality rate peaked in 1894 at 785 per 100,000 population (not 100,000 cases) and by 1940, when sixty percent of school-aged children had been immunized, it had nearly disappeared. In 1926, a relay of dog sleds carried diphtheria anti-toxin to Nome, Alaska to treat an epidemic in that isolated town. The trek is memorialized in the Iditarod Dog Sled Race run every year from Anchorage to Nome. The diphtheria story showed that, not only live vaccine, but also cell-free serum could protect from disease. The production of serum was extended to the treatment of tetanus, plague, cholera and snakebites. There were problems as it became evident that serum varied in potency and effectiveness. Problems with the serum itself appeared. Some patients became allergic to horse serum and died of allergic reactions. Serum sickness (caused by antibodies in the serum that attacked the host) was identified, although the cause was not understood for years.

TUBERCULOSIS

Tuberculosis remained recalcitrant to all attempts at treatment of the organism, itself. Koch identified the organism after J.L. Schoenlein, in 1839, had named the disease for the tubercles visible in the microscope. William Budd (1811-1880) studied the epidemiology(although no such term existed at the time) and became convinced that it was a communicable disease. Jean Villemin (1827-1892) attempted to inoculate animals with the organism and argued that the disease was present in cattle as well as humans. Virchow got off on a wrong track by arguing that the pulmonary form and miliary (named for millet seeds which are about the same size as the tiny lesions) tuberculosis were different diseases. His skepticism about bacteriology, and Pasteur, may have led him astray here. In 1882, Koch ended the speculation with his proof of the presence of the organism and its role in the disease. Koch had been an administrator for years, leaving his assistants to do the scientific work, but returned to the lab for his final effort in the investigation of tuberculosis. It would lead to a scandal.

In 1890, Koch reported a discovery before the Tenth International Congress of Medicine. He had identified a substance that arrested the growth of the tubercle bacillus in the test tube and named it "tuberculin." The result was a sensation and the Kaiser, Wilhelm II, presented him with the Grand Cross of the Red Eagle. Koch avoided disclosing the nature of tuberculin, contrary to a German law against "secret medicines." Sir Arthur Conan Doyle, author of the Sherlock Homes stories and a well-known physician, visited Koch at this time and described a scene reminiscent of Lourdes, the faith healing center in France. Koch proceeded to administer tuberculin to thousands of patients without proper controls and, when it finally became apparent that they received no benefit, there was a violent backlash. In 1891, Koch finally revealed the composition of the material and it proved to be a glycerin extract of the tubercle bacilli. There were allegations that his recent divorce and remarriage had tempted the scientist to seek a financial windfall, and he soon vanished from Europe with his new bride leaving a debacle behind him. Eventually tuberculin proved to be useful as a skin test but it conveyed no immunity. His second great blunder was his opposition to Villemin's theory that bovine tuberculosis was similar, if not the same, as the human disease and was transmissible between the species. In time, the association was made and Pasteurization of milk was adopted.

In 1906, Albert Calmette of the Pasteur Institute and his collaborator, Jean Marie Guerin, took a strain of bovine tuberculosis and succeeded in attenuating it until the disease-producing characteristics were lost, but it would produce immunity. The vaccine was called BCG, Baccilli-Calmette-Guerin, and was first used for inoculation of calves. In 1924, its use was extended to humans and, by 1928, 116,000 French children had received the vaccine. It has remained controversial as the immunity is not perfect and it produces a positive tuberculin skin test so an uninfected recipient cannot be followed with negative skin tests after receiving BCG.

TYPHOID AND OTHER BACTERIAL DISEASES

Typhoid fever was differentiated from typhus in 1837, and the organism was isolated in Koch's lab in 1884. Immunization was introduced in 1887 but, again, there was controversy about efficacy. In the Boer War, the British Army lost 13,000 men to typhoid fever, nearly twice the battle casualties. Further investigations using the new techniques of epidemiology and bacteriology led to immunization of the army in World War I. Paratyphoid A and B (similar diseases caused by related organisms) were discovered around the same time and the vaccine combined all three organisms (the TAB vaccine). The incidence in WWI was low and the death rate minor. A similar story concerns tetanus immunization. The organism was identified in the 1880s and anti-toxin was available by 1890. In the first year of WWI tetanus became a major problem with thousands of cases and forty percent mortality. Anti-toxin was used after 1915 with a dramatic decrease in incidence. Immunization, rather than anti-toxin after injury, was practiced in WWII and there were only six cases in the US Army. In 1894, Yersin isolated the plague bacillus and proposed the rat as vector suggesting that extermination of rats would be useful as prevention. Plague vaccine proved to be of doubtful value, however, and remains so. Scarlet fever resisted the application of Koch's Postulates since a toxin causes the disease and immunity from a vaccine is not effective. Klein isolated the streptococcus from scarlet fever patients in 1887, but it will not produce the disease in animals. It is pathogenic but does not produce scarlet fever except in humans. Eventually immunity to the toxin was found in convalescent patients, but immunization or anti-toxin has never been successfully employed. The solution would come with the introduction of penicillin.

HOST RESISTANCE

Therapy in the late nineteenth and early twentieth century, aside from digitalis and quinine, was dominated by vaccines and serum treatment of infectious diseases. The French, under the influence of Pasteur, emphasized live vaccine. The Germans pioneered serum therapy, as in diphtheria. Both fields used immunity and studies of what would become immunology, to try to understand how this worked, began. Elie Metchnikoff (1845-1916) was a Russian pathologist who became sub-director of the Pasteur Institute. In 1884, Metchnikoff saw amoeba-like cells ingest other microorganisms. He then noted that white blood cells could be seen ingesting bacteria. Pasteur supported Metchnikoff but the Germans remained devoted to the serum theory suggesting, as Koch did, that the white cells might even be part of the disease. Metchnikoff called the white blood cells "phagocytes" (Greek, *phagein* – to eat). He identified macrophages and granulocytes and noted the increase in numbers of white cells in infection. Metchnikoff and the Germans were each partially correct.

By 1890, lymphocytes had been identified and were noted to increase under the stimulation of tuberculin. In 1895, two Belgian scientists, Denys and Leclef, demonstrated that immune serum increased the activity of phagocytosis. The two systems were complementary. Almoth Wright, director of the Institute of Pathology at St. Mary's Hospital, London named the components of immune serum "opsonins," because they made the bacteria more "tasty" for the phagocytes (Greek, *opsonein* – to prepare food). Immunization had some negative consequences like serum sickness, which Clemens von Pirquet studied in Vienna. He coined the term "allergy." Typhoid carriers were identified and "Typhoid Mary," an Irishwoman who infected hundreds in New York City between 1900 and 1907, became famous as an example. Eventually, it was found that the typhoid carrier's gallbladder was the site of bacterial colonization and gallbladder removal stopped the process. Immunity and resistance to disease was complicated.

PAUL ERLICH

Paul Erlich (1854-1915) became director of the Royal Prussian Institute for Experimental Therapy in 1899. Erlich had been trained in pathology at the Medizinische Klinik by Theodore Frerich (1819-1885), successor to the great Schoenlein at Charité Hospital in Berlin. Frerich had succeeded in establishing a small chemical laboratory and here Erlich worked on blood morphology. From there he moved to Koch's Institute of Infectious Diseases. He had become interested in tuberculosis when he discovered the organism in his own sputum. He tried tuberculin and spent a year in Egypt, the European equivalent of Arizona at the time.

Paracelsus had advocated chemical therapy for disease and Sydenham had hoped for more examples like the Peruvian bark, which was so effective in malaria. Willow bark had been advocated for fever by Edmund Stone, an

Anglican minister not a physician, but found little support. Finally, Felix Hoffman (1868-1946) isolated acetylsalicylic acid from the bark and, in 1899, the Bayer Company named it "aspirin." The chemical industry was part of the great industrial revolution, and eventually the production of chemical dyes led to pharmaceuticals. The color mauve (aniline purple) was isolated from coal tar in 1856 by W.H. Perkin in Britain. In 1858, E.R. Squibb began to supply medicines to the US Army and produced chloroform and ether in large volumes during the Civil War. William R. Warner invented the sugar-coated pill in 1866 and Parke, Davis invented the gelatin capsule in 1875. The tablet compression machine was invented by William Brokedon in 1843 and in the US by Jacob Denton in 1864. What was needed was something useful to put in the pills, capsules, and tablets.

Erlich's interest was focused on bacteriology by Koch, and the idea of using synthetic drugs to substitute for natural antibodies occurred to him. The variability of staining of natural fibers by dyes suggested that some tissues were attracted to certain chemicals. Wright's use of dyes to stain white blood cells, and Gram's stain for bacteria, supported this concept. Erlich believed that chemical structure was important to biological activity and coined the term "receptor" as a structure that received a dye.[116] Langley, in his studies of sympathetic nerve endings and the effects of poisons used the term "receptive substance" and is sometimes given credit for the concept, as well.[117] In 1890, Erlich proposed that each molecule of anti-toxin combined with a molecule of toxin. He also theorized that tetanus toxin attached itself to a chemical side-chain on a cell in the nervous system and inactivated some cell function. He began to look for chemical agents that were toxic for bacteria but did not harm the host. He shared the 1908 Nobel Prize for his studies of the antigen-antibody reaction (although its nature was not understood at the time). He used the term "lock and key," coined by Emil Fischer to describe enzyme action, to describe the relationship between toxin and antitoxin. He recognized that a toxin might become attenuated, as did the rabies vaccine of Pasteur, but still stimulate antibodies. Mechnikov shared the prize with Ehrlich for his discovery of phagocytosis.

MALARIA

In 1891, using quinine as a model, Erlich treated malaria with methylene blue, one of the aniline dyes. He thought he detected some effect. The Germans continued this work during World War I, because they feared that they would be cut off from sources of quinine in South East Asia. They succeeded in modifying the methylene blue molecule and finally developed a dye called "atebrin," which was extensively used by the Americans in the South Pacific during World War II. The drug produces a yellow discoloration of the skin and eyes, but is effective prophylaxis against the malaria parasite. Eventually, this work led to another drug named "chloroquin" which is more effective than atebrin and does not produce any coloring of the skin.

SYPHILIS AND "606"

Next, Erlich tried to treat the trypanosome, another parasite and the cause of sleeping sickness, with atoxyl, an arsenical drug. It was effective, but too toxic causing blindness and neurological damage in some patients. The next disease he tackled was syphilis. It had become more virulent again after a century of decline. The disease had been studied for years and the three clinical stages identified. The parasite was discovered by Fritz Schaudinn and Erich Hofman and was named *Spirochaeta pallida* (since changed to *Treponema pallidum*). August Wassermann had developed a specific blood test in 1906, but the only treatment was mercury, in use since Paracelsus. By 1907, Erlich had tested over 600 arsenical drugs. He patented one, number 606, and his assistant Sahachiro Hata retested this drug in 1909 and found it effective in syphilis. He began treatment of advanced cases with the new drug to test for efficacy and risk. All were volunteers; the first two were physicians. By 1910, over 10,000 syphilitics had been treated and the drug was named Salvarsan. In 1914, a modification called Neo-Salvarsan was introduced and was very effective although still toxic. It looked as though great progress was close, but no other useful compound was to be identified for twenty years.

116   Paul Erlich, *Collected Papers Volume I* , Ed. F. Himmelweit, Hirschwald: Berlin (1885). pages 435-438. Here he mentions the receptor and first describes his concept of the "side-chain" that was so important in his theoretical work.

117   J.N. Langley, "On nerve endings and special excitable substances in cells," *Proceedings of the Royal Society*, 78:174-176 (1906).

12

The Rise of Medicine

CLAUDE BERNARD AND PHYSIOLOGY

CLAUDE BERNARD FOUNDED EXPERIMENTAL MEDICINE AS A DISCIPLINE. Jenner and Withering had made discoveries based on observation, but Bernard went from theory to experiment. Before his time it was believed only plants could synthesize complex molecules. Fats, sugars, and proteins could be broken down, but not produced in the animal metabolism. In 1843, Bernard decided to study sugar and its utilization by the body. He fed an animal glucose, and then showed that glucose could be recovered from the portal vein, proving that it had been absorbed. He also recovered glucose from the hepatic veins showing that the sugar passed through the liver and its capillary bed. He now fed an animal with a purely meat diet, no glucose. He tested the portal vein and found, as expected, that there was no glucose in the blood. Then he tested the hepatic veins and found glucose was present! He even was able to extract glucose from liver tissue. In 1855, he concluded that glucose was produced in the liver and he called this "internal secretion."

An accident in the laboratory further clarified what was happening. He was extracting glucose from animal livers and was interrupted before finishing for the day. The second liver, examined one day after death instead of immediately, contained more glucose than the first. He repeated his experiment flushing the liver with water until no glucose could be recovered. The next day there was abundant glucose present; the liver was making glucose, or a substance in the liver was producing the glucose. Since the liver was dead, there must be a substance present that changed into glucose. In 1857, he identified the substance and called it "glycogen." Eventually the glucose-glycogen cycle was identified by Carl and Gerty Cori, a husband and wife team of biochemists. For this accomplishment they were awarded the 1947 Nobel Prize in Medicine. Another of their discoveries was the "Cori cycle" in which glucose is metabolized to lactate in anaerobic muscle metabolism. This occurs during exercise when the "oxygen debt" builds up while oxygen consumption cannot keep up with energy requirement. Lactate is the partial metabolic product which is then converted back to glucose after the oxygen catches up, a process called "gluconeogenesis." When this mechanism was first discovered, it was thought to be the principal energy source of metabolism but later studies showed that the Krebs cycle fulfills this role. Hans Krebs, at Cambridge, first described this process in 1937 and eventually the entire cycle (also called the citric acid cycle), which takes place in mitochondria, was described. Krebs and Fritz Lipmann, the latter for the discovery of coenzyme-A- important in the cycle, shared the 1953 Nobel Prize.

Bernard next studied pancreatic juice, which had been identified by Regnier Graaf, discoverer of ovarian follicles. Graaf collected pancreatic secretion from dogs in the eighteenth century, but had no idea what its function was. Another accidental observation led Bernard onto the right track. He was dissecting a rabbit that had been fed meat and noticed that the lacteals, the lymphatics in the mesentery filled with milky absorbed fat, ended well below the pylorus. Dogs, recently fed, have visible lacteals all the way to the stomach. The only difference in anatomy between these two species is that rabbit pancreatic duct enters the gut lower than it does in the dog. Bernard then suspected that pancreatic secretion had something to do with fat digestion. He next mixed crushed pancreas with fat, kept the mixture at body temperature and noted that the mixture produced a layer of fatty acid and glycerol. He next ligated the pancreatic duct in the dog and showed that fat was not digested. He observed the digestion of starch into maltose in the presence of pancreatic juice but did not realize that protein is also hydrolyzed by the juice. His preparation contained trypsinogen, not yet activated to trypsin. He studied carbon monoxide and, because of its absorption by red cells, concluded that oxygen is carried by them, as well. He studied curare, the South American arrow poison, and found that it blocked nerve impulse transmission to muscle, but did not prevent direct stimulation of muscle. His work opened the door to biochemistry, physiology and modern medicine.

THE 19TH CENTURY PHYSICIAN

The social status of the physician in the nineteenth century is illustrated by literary allusions of the time. Author George Elliot had a character in *Middlemarch*, her novel of 1872, remark, "For my own part, I like a medical man more on a footing with the servants." William Jenner (1815-98) was physician to the Royal family of England and published a report which distinguished typhoid fever from typhus in 1840. He treated the Queen's consort, Prince Albert for typhoid fever in 1860 (unsuccessfully) and the Prince of Wales for the same disease in 1871 (successfully). He ended as President of the Royal College of Physicians, but even well connected physicians had little to offer their patients until the end of the century. In Somerset Maugham's *Of Human Bondage*, written in 1915, a snobbish old lady remarks that in her youth, the 1850s, medicine was not regarded as "fit for a gentleman's son." In France, Napoleon reorganized the medical profession and was quite sophisticated in medical matters. The French medical profession had higher social status than that of England; Laennec and a few colleagues contributed genuine progress in diagnosis and classification of disease. Germany differed from both as a result of Bismark's social legislation that established a government health program in 1883 and offered government employment to doctors. Surgery and public health were the two areas of real scientific progress prior to the 1880s when bacteriology finally began to offer physicians some effective tools to treat disease.

OSLER AND DIAGNOSIS

In 1867, William Osler, a minister's son from Dundas in Upper Canada, entered the University of Trinity College in Toronto. He was destined for the ministry himself, but fell in love with natural history, a dangerous field for a minister's son since Darwin's *Origin of Species* had come out in 1859. In fact, his presence at Trinity, a small sectarian school, was intended to keep him from the godless University of Toronto. James Bovell taught at Trinity and at the Toronto School of Medicine and introduced Osler to the dangerous subject. The microscope was the lure and he spent hours examining specimens from local ponds. In 1868, he saw a slide of *Trichinella spiralis*, a parasite encysted within the muscle of the man it had killed, and was hooked. Osler kept his scholarship at Trinity for a second year but jeopardized his status severely by bringing a fetus to school, one he had obtained from the medical school. The provost gave him a tongue-lashing: "Sir, you are persistently and essentially bad-you are a disgrace to yourself, to your family, to your college, to your church, and, and, you may go now sir."[118] Medicine was to be the richer as the erstwhile divinity student made his decision. Bovell, his mentor, was pleased. The stethoscope and the thermometer and the laryngoscope had all recently appeared to give wider scope to the physician in his efforts to see into the body. Virchow's book, *Cellular Pathology*, came out in 1858, the year before Darwin's book, and the effect was of a window opening on the nature of life itself. Osler was just in time for the new age of modern medicine, which was dawning. Bovell, his mentor, encouraged his pupil,but remained himself partly in the old model. He is remembered in Canada for infusing milk into the veins of cholera victims, because he believed that milk globules turned into white blood cells, a remnant of the spontaneous generation theory. Bovell left Canada for the West Indies and ended his days as a priest, still using his microscope to study nature. Osler moved on to McGill, a better medical school in Montreal with a larger hospital than that in Toronto.

Osler did his service as a "dresser" for the surgeons, many still wearing their old blood-encrusted frock coats. He served as "clerk" for the best of the physicians on the faculty who still resorted to blood-letting in difficult cases. He wrote his first paper for the *Canada Medical Journal and Monthly Record*, in 1871, describing five cases, including one in which he performed the autopsy on a man who had died of pneumonia. This report established a trend as Osler was to learn, and to teach, medicine from the autopsy room most of his career. He chose to write his degree thesis on postmortem studies of diseased organs and, when his new mentor Palmer Howard, called by some of the students a "Canadian Sydenham," gave him a copy of Samuel Wilks's new book *Lectures on Morbid Anatomy*, Osler said that from then on "Everything was plain sailing." When he finished his degree studies, he spent a year in London, benefiting from his brother's help with $1,000 to make it possible. His first plan was to study ophthalmology, but a letter from Howard informed him that three other men were planning to settle in Montreal as ophthalmologists. The market for eye diseases would be glutted. Howard advised him to "cultivate the whole field of Medicine & Surgery," still a possibility at the time. In October of 1873, Osler moved to Germany to continue his studies. The language of advanced science then was German and Osler was a bit unusual to have spent so much time in England. He was most attracted to Virchow, then at the height of his powers and influence on medicine. He spent time at the Allgemeines Krankenhaus in Vienna and found it "swarming" with fifty or sixty American students. He found Vienna to be far less sophisticated in pathology than Berlin and complained that autopsies were "performed in so slovenly a manner, and so little use is made of the material."

Back at McGill in mid-1874, he was appointed Lecturer in the Institutes of Medicine. He had little interest in private practice, being determined on teaching and research, but his salary was only $1,129 per year and he was obliged to augment it. At the end of the first year, he was promoted to professor, but his private practice was slow in developing. His first two months netted a total of $9.25 from his new office. He further supplemented his income with an appointment as physician to the smallpox hospital in Montreal, the absolute bottom rung on the ladder of the local medical profession. Most of the patients were French-Canadians who avoided vaccination. This was dangerous work in an era before gloves were introduced and he contracted a case of smallpox in spite of vaccination; fortunately, it was mild, but a friend, a minister, died of the disease contracted by handling a corpse that no one else would touch. He recorded his attempts to treat the smallpox victims with remedies, including ergot, turpentine, lead acetate and even quinine, that had no effect, but his $600 salary from the "pest house" paid for fifteen microscopes he planned to use for a course on microscopic anatomy; an innovation in Canada. His courses on microscopic anatomy and pathology, including the 1,000 autopsies that he and his students performed at McGill, were typical of the best of medical training anywhere at the time. One autopsy that Osler had been anticipating was not available. Alexis St. Martin, Beaumont's patient, was old and near death. Osler looked forward to performing the autopsy once the inevitable took place. In the spring of 1880, the day finally came, but a telegram arrived from the village doctor who had attended St. Martin: "Don't come. Will be killed." The local French-Canadians guarded the body with rifles and the family made certain that it was hidden until decay was far advanced.[119] Aside from quinine, digitalis, vaccination, and morphine, there was no effective, non-surgical treatment of disease. They were learning physiology and pathology, though, and eventually that understanding of the mechanisms of disease would lead to effective therapy.

In 1881, he was able to travel to London again for the Seventh International Medical Congress. The presidential address was given by Sir James Paget and Osler saw Virchow again. In 1883, he was elected to the Royal College of Physicians of London, one of only three Canadians so honored. In 1882-83 the McGill students rebelled against William Wright MD, the old and incompetent lecturer on *materia medica*. One of them complained, "The older the remedy and the less used, with the greater elaboration was it dwelt on." Osler was successful in getting them back into class and negotiating improvements in the curriculum. He was always good humored and "simply laughed us into good humor," as one said. By 1884, it was apparent that he was a major star in international medicine and McGill expected to lose him. He had come very close to discovering blood platelets, investigated phagocytosis and was close to being the first to describe appendicitis. He was just too busy to follow up his discoveries and keep up with his teaching and practice. In March of 1884, he sailed again to Europe to visit Germany. Medical discoveries were being announced every month and he wanted to be closer to the action. The changes in Germany astounded him. Berlin was a "bright, well-drained (in contrast with a previous visit), bustling metropolis." He saw surgeons working inside the abdomen under stringently controlled aseptic conditions. "The entire building is lighted by Edison lamps," he marveled. He spent time with Virchow again. He met von Frerichs who had just produced a monograph on diabetes. In the ten years since his last visit, bacteriology had exploded as a science. Koch had just identified the cholera bacillus in Egypt. Carl Friedlander had just identified the pneumococcus as the cause of pneumonia. The atmosphere was much like that a century later as the human genome was deciphered. Osler had already demonstrated the tubercle bacillus in a lung lesion to his students in Canada, within a month of Koch's first report in 1882. Still, he was not sure that bacteria were responsible for all diseases. He stood somewhere between Koch and Virchow. He did write back to McGill suggesting that they fix up a room as a bacteriology lab and promised to bring back some cultures to start a department.

The Medical Department of the University of Pennsylvania, founded in 1765, was the oldest medical school in the US. The affiliated hospital, the Pennsylvania Hospital, was older, founded in 1751. Only one faculty member in the first 120 years had been both a non-Pennsylvanian and a non-alumnus. Osler was to be the second. When first approached by the board, while studying in Leipzig, Osler thought friends were playing a practical joke. Finally convinced that they were serious, Osler made his decision by tossing a coin. When he left Montreal, admitting that he left because of ambition, the students escorted him to the railroad station en masse. The Pennsylvania students were, at first, put off by his strangeness and his diffident manner. As they followed him around the wards and into the autopsy room, however, they realized they had a great teacher. They compared him to the faculty's great naturalist Joseph Leidy who, not a physician, had discovered *Trichinella spiralis* in 1846. Leidy's passion for dissecting animals extended to the dinner table. Weir Mitchell, the neurologist who wrote a monograph on head injuries from the Civil War (and created the popular "rest cure" for neurotic women), said "Never give Leidy anything that is edible and worth dissecting."[120] A skeptical student reported of Osler, "His first ward class was an eye opener. In it, he fairly frolicked in enthusiastic delight, and in a few moments had every man intensely interested and avid for more." "Before Osler came the student was prone to regard cancer as a cancer; when Osler left the student studied it as an aggregation of cells possessing untold mysteries to be unraveled."[121] Osler continued with his dead house instruction even though the huge hospital already had two full-time pathologists. He had by this time acquired *Verruca necrogenica* (cadaver warts) common on the hands of those performing autopsies and caused by tuberculosis nodules. Long exposure had made him otherwise immune and he treated them with mercury oil.

He established a private practice here, as well, and, in 1886, was called to the home of William W. Keen, the great surgeon who wrote the *American Textbook of Surgery*. Keen's wife was terribly ill, but neither he nor Osler could do anything to save her. Still, Osler's presence was a great comfort to Keen. By 1888, Osler's income rose to $7,330 and he repaid his brother for the loan which had sent him to Europe and began his climb to success. In 1885, he saw Walt Whitman as a patient and found him "a splendid old man, and [with] a room the grand disorder of which filled me with envy." In 1888, he saw him again for a series of small strokes. They saw each other a number of times and, while Whitman's poetry never appealed to Osler, Whitman concluded that Osler "gains on you," although he did complain of "the jaunty way in which he seems inclined to dismiss troubles." Doctors had few other tools but a "jaunty way," at the time.[122] Osler got involved in a bit of medical politics when he helped form the Association of American Physicians in 1885, in reaction to the provincialism of the American Medical Association. At the first meeting, June 17 and 18, 1886, he made a rare clinical misstep when he criticized William T. Councilman's paper on malaria.[123] Councilman was reporting the presence of parasites (he called them "pigmented amoeboid bodies") in the blood of victims and Osler rejected this interpretation. Osler was considered an expert on blood having written on the platelets, attributing the blood clotting function to these new structures. He had also suggested the bone marrow as the site of blood formation. Both observations were correct but he was dead wrong on Councilman's findings. Osler said that the bodies seen by Councilman were "vacuoles or hyaline spaces." Councilman's reply at the discussion was that it was odd "that vacuoles should stain with aniline colors." The following September, after more study of malarial blood (rare in Montreal), Osler ate his words and described the other forms of the parasite life cycle. He wrote further papers on the subject and never failed to acknowledge his hasty conclusion, describing it as "folly." The same meeting of the American Association of Physicians saw the first report by Reginald Fitz on "Perforating Inflammation of the Vermiform Appendix with Special Reference to Diagnosis and Treatment." This was the beginning of the recognition of appendicitis as a clinical entity.

Osler's "dead house" work tailed off in Philadelphia and he seemed to rechannel his energy into clinical work. He studied cerebral palsy and attributed it to birth injury after an extensive correspondence with Vienna neurologist Sigmund Freud. Often accused of being a "therapeutic nihilist," appropriate in most cases in this era of useless remedies, he studied anemia and concluded that iron supplements were of value in certain types. He tried nitroglycerine in epilepsy, because others theorized that vascular spasm was responsible. It did not help. The new aspirin-related compounds were effective in fever and he advocated their use although he eventually realized that they did not affect the underlying disease. These observations brought some, including Osler, to consider the role of fever in the body's defense against infection. Previously, fever had been considered part of the disease, if not the disease itself. He ridiculed faddish remedies like the use of rectal gas infusion for treatment of tuberculosis. Typhoid, pneumonia, and tuberculosis were still untreatable. In 1887, he saw a woman with jaundice and intermittent fever (two thirds of Charcot's triad) and recommended surgery for gallstones. She was operated on and nothing was found. She died three days later and, chagrined, Osler followed the body to Jenkintown to obtain an autopsy. He found a stone in the common bile duct, out of surgical reach at the time, and kept the organs for future reference. So far, his career had been an example of the best that could be found in medicine of the time.

OSLER AND THE JOHNS HOPKINS HOSPITAL

Osler had an image of the "model hospital" and medical school that would be so good European study would be unnecessary for an adequate education. Still, he was conservative in some matters continuing to recommend bleeding for certain cases of pneumonia. He thought that it might relieve the strain on the heart, but saw no beneficial effect.

The Johns Hopkins Hospital was the creation of wealthy merchant Johns Hopkins who died in 1873. Like another wealthy merchant, Peter Bent Brigham, who died the year before, he left a fortune to establish a hospital. Half his fortune was to be used for a university, but it was clear that medicine was to be the focus of both institutions. The trustees chose John Shaw Billings, director of the Surgeon General's Library and one of the great scholars in American medicine, to organize the hospital staff. Billings later founded the National Library of Medicine and *Index Medicus*. The university was organized in three years, but it took twelve years to build the hospital. William Welch was chosen as professor of pathology in 1884 and spent a year touring European clinics. Upon his return, he organized the first laboratory for experimental pathology ever established on a full-time basis.

By 1887, the hospital was under construction and many saw that it would be the greatest American medical institution of the time. Osler's name was mentioned as a prospective member of its faculty. He spent time with John Shaw Billings, the architect of the hospital, and the Penn professors began to worry saying, "We're likely to lose Osler and what in the devil shall we do?"[124] Soon enough, Billings made the offer and Osler accepted. In 1889, the Penn faculty gave him a farewell dinner and one of those attending commented that: "He is one of the most popular men I ever knew." The Johns Hopkins Hospital was designed with the benefit of current knowledge of medicine. Prevention of contagion was uppermost in everyone's' mind and it was open and breezy with sixteen buildings for its 272 beds. The twelve years spent in construction led to some anachronisms as there were no elevators or running water on the wards. The city of Baltimore did not have a public sewer system at the time and the hospital had to build its own. The organization of the staff of non-physicians, including food services, housekeeping, and laundry, was modeled, wisely, on a hotel. Nowadays we refer to these areas as the "hotel functions" of a hospital. The Johns Hopkins leaders were the first to see this. The medical staff organization on departmental lines followed the German model.

Even though the hospital had opened, the trustees had trouble raising the funds to open the medical school and there was doubt whether Osler would stay. Four women, all daughters of university trustees, formed The Women's Fund Committee in 1888 to raise enough money for the endowment. They raised $100,000 and, when the trustees still hesitated to accept their terms – admission of women to the medical school – Mary Garrett contributed another $400,000 in 1892. The medical school opened in 1893 with three of the eighteen students women.

After his arrival, Osler convinced Howard Kelly, another Penn trained surgeon, to assume the chair in Obstetrics. With Halsted, who had arrived before the hospital opened to work in Welch's pathology department, the Big Four, as they were famously called, was complete. In 1906 Mary Garrett commissioned the famous John Singer Sargent painting of them which hangs in the library of the medical school.

They proceeded to attract the greatest group of young men ever assembled in one place for medical research. None of them, including the chiefs, was over thirty-nine. Kelly was thirty-one. The graduates of this institution spread out across America to reform American medicine. William T. Councilman took over the Harvard Department of Pathology in 1892. Simon Flexner later developed the Rockefeller Institute and wrote the report in 1910 that reformed American medical education. Walter Reed discovered the cause of yellow fever and succeeded in eradicating the mosquitoes that blocked construction of the Panama Canal. In the early days of the new hospital, Osler continued his study of the malarial parasite; Councilman was still there and active as well. Amoebic dysentery was next to be identified and Osler remarked on the amazing activity of the living amoebae. He spent less time in the autopsy room now and his students carried on in his model. His ward teaching continued at the same rate and he traveled frequently to the continent.

In 1892, Osler married the widow of his friend Samuel Gross who, before his death in 1889 (the year Osler left), was the leading surgeon of Philadelphia. She was thirty-seven and childless and descended from American and British bluebloods, including Paul Revere. They had a child less than a year after their marriage, but the boy died on the fifth or sixth day. A second child survived and was named Edward Revere, after his mother's family. Revere Osler was to die in World War I, on August 30, 1917 in spite of the frantic efforts of his father's friends, the best surgeons in the world, after being hit by shrapnel. He had initially been assigned to a field hospital in the Canadian Army (he was not a physician), but requested assignment to the field artillery. His father never recovered. Six months later, Osler was described as weeping intermittently as he thought of his only son.

THE PRINCIPLES AND PRACTICE OF MEDICINE

In 1890, Osler began work on his great textbook. His accounts of the natural history of disease are still classics. The endocrine system was not yet identified, viruses could not be seen, and genetics was largely unknown. The x-ray and the electrocardiograph were not yet discovered. It did incorporate the new knowledge of bacteriology, and he explained the evolution of medical thought and controversy. The only area where confusion reigned was in therapeutics, and that of course was the problem. He complained that: "A desire to take medicine is, perhaps, the great feature which distinguishes man from other animals." Patients wanted cures and, with a very few exceptions, only surgery could offer them. He aggressively recommended surgery in patients likely to benefit. Osler's book became the most popular textbook of medicine in the world and the income from it brought financial security. In 1896, Cushing arrived at Johns Hopkins and soon became an intimate of Osler and his wife, Grace.

In 1899, Osler turned fifty and began to feel his age just a bit. He commented that he no longer jumped across a stream on the golf course, choosing instead to cross on the small bridge as befitted a man of his age. The next year, he was offered the chair in medicine at Edinburgh and was tempted, as he was clearly an Anglophile, but when he returned to

Baltimore, he faced what he called "a perfect hullabaloo." The Johns Hopkins people did not know what they would do without him and he backed down. This annoyed the Edinburgh committee, but they had only themselves to blame for they had required him to apply as a candidate and he had not yet been selected. Had they simply offered the position with no delay he would have felt obliged to accept. In a year, all was forgiven when he returned for a visit. One bit of evidence for his changing opinions with age was the famous comment about pneumonia in the 1898 third edition of the textbook. He wrote, "Pneumonia may well be called the friend of the aged." In the previous edition, he had referred to pneumonia as "the special enemy of old age."[125] His 1905 edition represents the best that turn of the century medicine could offer. Nitroglycerin was recommended for angina pectoris although amyl nitrate was preferred. Vaccination and the antitoxins for diphtheria and tetanus were effective for a few bacterial and viral diseases. Rabies vaccine was in wide use. Mercury would soon be superseded by arsenicals in the treatment of syphilis. Surgical diseases were being recognized and referred to the surgeons. Typhoid fever, the great killer of the late nineteenth century, was beyond the physician's power to stop, although it was well known that the patient must be kept on a limited diet during convalescence to avoid perforation of the bowel. Pneumonia could be treated only indirectly, by draining pleural effusions as they developed. Public health had taken great strides during the century and cholera could be largely prevented although epidemics continued, and continue to this day. Collapse therapy was useful in cavitary lesions of tuberculosis and its use would continue until modern times.

THE MAYO FAMILY

American medicine was rapidly improving in quality, even if the physicians in more remote areas could not travel to "finishing school" in Europe. The Mayo family began with humble origins and eventually reached heights beyond those of all but a very few American doctors. William W. Mayo studied medicine at the Manchester Infirmary as a apprentice and spent time in Glasgow where he met Dr Alfred Stillé, an American physician from Philadelphia. In 1845, possibly influenced by the acquaintance with Stillé, Mayo emigrated to America finding work at Bellevue Hospital in New York as a pharmacist. He moved west, to Buffalo, then, following the shore of Lake Erie, to Indiana. In 1848, he set up as a tailor in Lafayette, Indiana, but later that year resumed the study of medicine as an apprentice to another local doctor, Elizur H. Deming. A cholera epidemic in 1849 precipitated him into medical practice but when it subsided, he resumed his studies at a local proprietary medical school, the Indiana Medical

College. He received his degree on February 14, 1850. In 1851, he married Miss Louise Wright, the daughter of a mechanic. In 1853, Dr. Mayo and his wife moved to St. Louis, accompanying his partner and mentor Dr. Deming as he assumed a position with the Medical Department of the University of Missouri, a school little larger than the Indiana Medical College, which was now defunct. Finally, he and Mrs. Mayo left St. Louis to escape periodic episodes of malaria, endemic in the Missouri area. They headed north and landed in St. Paul, Minnesota.

St. Paul had a surfeit of doctors and Mrs. Mayo set up a millinery shop, while her husband scouted the new territory. Eventually, they settled on a farm in the valley of the Minnesota River, south-west of St. Paul. His medical practice was small and he earned a living doing other things, including running a steamboat on the river. Dr. Mayo became active in the new Republican Party in 1860, and his growing recognition in the territory did his medical practice no harm. When the Civil War broke out, Dr. Mayo volunteered to be a regimental surgeon but politically connected doctors from St. Paul were appointed even though one of them had not practiced for years. In 1862, the Sioux Indians attacked the settlers and Dr. Mayo accompanied the volunteer militia into territory west of his valley to rescue farm families and treat the injured. A battle with the Indians devastated the town of New Ulm and the next day the settlers and militia evacuated, traveling east to Mankato. The Sioux Outbreak was finally suppressed and thirty-nine Indians hung for rape and murder. The executed Indians were quickly exhumed by local doctors for anatomical dissection and Dr. Mayo kept the skeleton of one of them for years in his office. In 1863, Dr. Mayo was finally appointed to a position as examining surgeon of draftees for the Union Army and moved east to Rochester, a larger town on a good road to St. Paul. He became extremely busy and Rochester grew quickly with all the war-related activity. Dr. Mayo was dismissed from his examiner post in a scandal over medical exemptions from the draft, although he was never charged with any crime. He remained in Rochester, buying two lots and building a home. His medical practice continued to grow in spite of the contretemps with the Army. The railroad reached Rochester in 1864 and, in 1865, his son Charles was born in the house on Third Street.

When Dr. Mayo moved to Rochester, the town already boasted a "clinic" of sorts, a homeopathic infirmary operated by two brothers named Cross. A number of other quack practitioners were active in the town, one of whom had confined a young woman to bed for two months for "dropsy of the heart." She finally sought another opinion from Dr. Mayo who made the correct diagnosis and saw her through the rest of her pregnancy. Another opened a "Western Healing Institute" and had a busy practice, until his new young wife died suddenly. Strychnine was detected and the doctor was exposed as a "botanic doctor" from New Jersey who had lost three previous wives to sudden death. Dr. Mayo stuck to his house calls and made daily rounds with a horse and buggy in the surrounding farming community. He designed his own examination table, suited to the complete examinations he performed in contrast to many of his colleagues, and the same design was still in use in 1941 at the Mayo Clinic. In 1869, aware of new developments in gynecologic surgery, he spent a few months at Bellevue Hospital in New York to learn about the new operations for vesico-vaginal fistula and ovariotomy. In 1866, he had successfully drained a huge ovarian cyst in a patient through a small abdominal incision and he decided to expand his medical reach. In 1871, he successfully repaired a large rectocele (a hernia through the posterior vaginal wall). Gradually he increased his skill in gynecologic surgery. By 1874, he was chairman of the Minnesota Medical Society's committee on gynecology. In 1880, he performed the second successful excision of an ovarian tumor in the state in spite of rupturing what was described as an abscess associated with the mass. She recovered suggesting that the mass might have been endometriosis with a sterile abscess. It weighed more than twenty pounds. There was still no hospital in Rochester and the operation was performed on the patient's kitchen table. Her husband, a blacksmith, had fabricated several of the instruments to Dr. Mayo's design. His sons, Will and Charles, peeked through the door during the operation.

Dr. Mayo was still interested in education, although there was, yet, no medical school in Minnesota. He encouraged a pharmacy clerk in the drugstore downstairs from his office to go east to study chemistry. The boy, Henry Wellcome, took his advice and, after completing a course in pharmacy in Philadelphia, traveled to England for further study. There, he met a manufacturing chemist named Burroughs. He went to work for the older Burroughs, married his daughter and they formed a pharmaceutical manufacturing company called Burroughs Wellcome. They introduced the tablet (which they called the "tabloid"), which had been invented in the US, to England. A few years later Will Mayo, the doctor's son, had matured enough to take over the prescription clerk job previously occupied by Henry Wellcome and, when Charlie Mayo graduated from school, he also worked in the drugstore. Dr. Mayo bought a new, very expensive microscope and taught the boys to prepare and examine specimens. They began to assist their father in surgery and, after another doctor, acting as anesthetist during an operation, lost his composure, Charlie began to administer anesthesia for his father's operations. He was eighteen, although Mayo family tradition has it that he was much younger at the time. Dr. Mayo was concerned about where his sons could obtain an adequate medical education; there was never any doubt about their choice of a career.

In 1880, Will Mayo entered the new University of Michigan Medical School. It had been organized on the same pattern as Harvard, still using the old proprietary model at this stage. While there, he was exposed to the new doctrine of "Listerism," the use of carbolic acid disinfectant to prevent infection. Once infection was established, there was no treatment and would not be until 1935. Donald MacLean was a professor of surgery at Michigan and had studied with Lister in Glasgow. His adoption of antiseptic technique was superficial, in part because he was sensitive to the chemical, but Mayo at least became familiar with the principle. This was unusual in 1880 anywhere in the US, let alone Michigan. Mayo's friend and partner in the anatomy lab was Frank Mall who would become a professor of anatomy at Johns Hopkins. In 1885, Charlie Mayo entered the Chicago Medical College, which was affiliated with Northwestern University. Frank Billings, classmate of John B. Murphy at Rush Medical College seven years earlier, taught physical diagnosis after returning that year from Europe. By the time Charlie Mayo came along, Listerism had become the standard in operating rooms in Chicago. The medical college used Mercy Hospital as its teaching institution. Charles Mayo received his degree in 1888. Both sons now joined their father in practice in Rochester, although it was some time before patients would accept the younger Drs. Mayo as substitutes for the older.

The senior Dr. Mayo continued his series of ovarian surgeries with a twenty-five percent mortality rate, highly successful given the time and place. The progress of the Chicago and Northwestern Railroad into the Dakota Territory allowed an increasing flow of referrals from the western territories back to Rochester when surgery, still primarily for ovarian tumors, was necessary. In 1884, Will Mayo spent time in New York for postgraduate study. There he learned about the diagnosis of "perityphlitis" (appendicitis) from Dr. Henry B. Sands at Roosevelt Hospital. He watched a number of these abscesses being drained, early diagnosis would have to wait for Reginald Fitz and John B. Murphy. Back in Rochester in 1885, Will made the diagnosis of perityphlitic abscess in a young girl, his father disagreed and the girl's family refused permission for surgery. She died and, at autopsy, Will found the typical findings of what would come to be called perforated appendicitis. He was learning to make the diagnosis. The following June of 1885, Reginald Fitz published his paper "Perforating Inflammation of the Vermiform Appendix,"[126] finally providing evidence for the true nature of the disease. Fitz was a pathologist and it would be 1889 before Charles McBurney would provide the physical diagnostic measure (tenderness at "McBurney's point") leading to early diagnosis before perforation. In 1888, Will Mayo published his experience, still vague about the nature of the disease, "Inflammations Involving the Caecum, its Appendix or Both," read before the Minnesota State Medical Society. He was still opposing early surgery, placing himself among the older generation of surgeons in spite of his age. Later that year, Will performed his first ovariotomy on a woman whose tumor was so large that it filled a washtub. His father was planning to perform the operation himself but, when his train from St. Paul was delayed and the patient objected to waiting, the son proceeded with the surgery. The St. Paul surgeon, who was accompanying Dr. Mayo, senior on the train to assist, laughed until tears came at hearing that the son had stolen his father's big case.

The adoption of antisepsis in Rochester was delayed until about 1887, due to the old Dr. Mayo's good results without it and Will's rather sketchy experience at Michigan. Another trip to New York in 1885 and the experience of Charlie at Chicago Medical College (possibly influenced by Murphy) brought him around. Arpad Gerster, a Hungarian surgeon who learned the technique at Volkmann's clinic in Halle before emigrating to New York, was the deciding influence on Will. His book *The Rules of Aseptic and Antiseptic Surgery* was published in 1887 and many of the photographs in the book were taken while Will Mayo was attending Gerster's postgraduate course in 1885 at Roosevelt Hospital (where Halsted was also proselytizing for antisepsis). When Charlie graduated from the Chicago Medical College, he joined his father and brother in practice. Soon, he took a trip to Europe where he saw Pasteur but missed Lister. He studied the new techniques of aseptic surgery that were slowly replacing antisepsis and carbolic acid spray. He saw surgeons now scrubbing their hands and a few were even wearing gloves.

In 1887, St. Mary's Hospital opened in Rochester, an event that stimulated more controversy than might be expected today. Hospitals were traditionally associated with the poor and indigent and did not have a good reputation at the time, no doubt due to the puerperal sepsis problems of the previous fifty years. Secondly, the Midwest was home to considerable anti-Catholic bigotry and the "Know-Nothing" party, formally named the American Protective Association, a center of anti-Catholic frenzy, had been formed in Iowa, only a few miles to the south. There was considerable concern whether the largely Protestant population of Minnesota would be willing to enter a Catholic hospital. The Mayos, as supporters (not founders as has been often written) of the hospital, were even subjected to considerable suspicion. As if that were not enough, Catholics were upset that non-Catholic doctors (the Mayos) would be in charge. All this eventually subsided and the hospital has been associated with the Mayo Clinic for over 100 years. Everyone was inexperienced as the sisters had been teachers, not nurses, and neither of the Mayo brothers had served a hospital internship. Old Dr. Mayo was now seventy but he had never practiced in a hospital either. Still, they muddled through. Of the first 400 admissions to the hospital, there were but two deaths. By 1893, the hospital was paying for itself and they could afford a new set of operating room equipment from Berlin.

The Mayo brothers continued to travel to New York each year for new developments in surgery. In 1890, Will Mayo visited Philadelphia for the first time to observe Joseph Price. Price, using the Lawson Tait methods, which anticipated aseptic technique with scrupulous hand washing, but rejected antisepsis, had obtained spectacular results in gynecologic surgery, but was widely regarded as a liar by other surgeons. Price was reluctant to accept this new young visitor but, once Mayo had watched him operate, he was convinced and Will returned every year for further instruction. Price, like John B. Murphy in Chicago, had a sharp tongue and made many enemies, but was a far superior surgeon to most of his detractors. Mayo's father, now retired in his seventies, had told him, "Sometimes a good man is cussed more vigorously than he would be if he were bad. [G]o to see him."[127] The advice was sound. Another mentor to the Mayo brothers was Christian Fenger of Chicago who has been called the "father of modern surgery in the West." Fenger had nurtured John B. Murphy as an intern ten years earlier. Fenger, though a marvelous pathologist and teacher, was such a poor surgeon that Will Mayo was often inclined to tell Fenger's patient, "You poor devil," as he was wheeled into the operating room. Albert Ochsner, chief of staff of Chicago Medical College and another disciple of Fenger's, described the case of a young woman referred to Fenger who made a careful examination and then stated, "We must operate at once." "Will she get well?" asked Ochsner. "No, she will die." "But will she get well if we don't operate?" "God only knows," was Fenger's reply. Ochsner vetoed the operation but was criticized by Fenger who said, "Well, where is your diagnosis then?" Will Mayo recounted another case in which Fenger made a brilliant diagnosis of a brain tumor. He operated on the patient and removed the tumor but, as he was closing the head, the patient died. "Dr Fenger, the patient is dead," said the anesthetist quietly. There was no answer. Again, more clearly, "Dr. Fenger, the patient is dead." Still not a word. Carefully the surgeon sewed up the incision and as carefully wound the bandages around it. Then he said softly, "You damned fool, to die just as you were cured."[128] The diagnosis was the thing. Still, he was a wonderful teacher of pathology if a bit single minded.

Nicholas Senn, another immigrant from Switzerland, was an excellent surgeon and teacher, second only to Murphy in technical skill. The Mayos attended his lectures whenever they traveled to Chicago. Senn, unfortunately, was egotistical and humorless, traits that eventually led him into a feud with Murphy. Ochsner learned this harsh side of Senn when he made the correct diagnosis in a case of Senn's, contradicting the professor. He lost his job. Ochsner had studied in Germany after graduating from Rush Medical College and soon found another position.[129] He is little known today but was an outstanding surgeon in the early history of Midwestern medicine. In 1920-21 he supervised the residency training of his nephew, Alton Ochsner, and arranged for the young man to spend time in Europe with Paul Clairmont in Zurich and Viktor Schmeiden in Frankfurt. Not long after Alton Ochsner returned to Chicago, he was appointed chairman of the surgery department at Tulane University, succeeding the famous Rudolph Matas. In 1942, he formed the Ochsner Clinic, associated with Tulane, where he had trained a young resident named Michael DeBakey.

Will Mayo's trips to Chicago paid off for one patient in 1892 when the Murphy Button he brought back to Rochester from Murphy's clinic saved a life. Intestinal anastomosis was extremely hazardous prior to World War I as the proper techniques for what Halsted called "circular suture" of the intestine were still in development. Murphy's button was a vast improvement, but led to the feud with Senn. In 1894, Will traveled to the new Johns Hopkins Hospital for his annual postgraduate session. His first morning he was greeted in the hallway by Osler who then took him on rounds. He was quickly converted to the "Hopkins system" as he saw the microscope in use on the wards and the friendly relationship between the young professors and their residents (unique in America where a one-year internship was the standard). After the first visit, all three Mayos, even the old man, made frequent visits to the new institution. They learned radical mastectomy and "radical cure" of inguinal hernia from Halsted. They did not go to Europe until 1900 and avoided Berlin and Vienna, as the operating rooms were said to be so crowded with visitors that the surgeon could not be seen, let alone the patient or the procedure.

The Mayo brothers continued in general practice in the early 1890s, as the volume of surgery was still too small for an exclusive practice. To obtain

more experience with surgery they agreed to provide free surgical services to two state hospitals for the poor within a day's journey of Rochester.
They did not want official appointments, and the politics that would
entail, nor fees, but only the experience of surgery and the autopsy rooms.
Long after the need for the experience had passed, they continued the
arrangement and refused any compensation except for improvements to
the operating rooms. At home at St. Mary's, they had no opposition to
innovation and could do as they pleased. Antisepsis was the standard
from the day the hospital opened in spite of the father's skepticism. They
adopted Halsted's rubber gloves and, by 1897, were using steam sterilization and the aseptic methods pioneered by the Germans. Will gradually
became the pelvic and abdominal surgeon and Charlie spent more time
on head and neck and bone cases, although they continued to assist each
other for years. By 1905, the Mayo brothers were performing 637 gynecologic operations per year. That same year they performed over a thousand
appendectomies; two years earlier the total had been only 186. John B.
Murphy was winning his battle for early diagnosis and surgery and the
Mayos were in the forefront of new developments. They performed their
first operation for gallstones in 1890, a cholecystostomy (opening the gallbladder for stones).

In 1893, Will Mayo used a Murphy button to perform a cholecyst-enterostomy for a common bile duct obstructed by a stone. Halsted wrote about
the difficulties of operations on the common bile duct in 1897. In 1905,
they performed 324 gallbladder operations, many of them cholecystec-
tomies (removing the gallbladder, an innovation). The same year they
performed 300 radical hernia repairs, using Halsted's technique. In 1903,
Will Mayo developed a technique for repair of umbilical hernia, hereto-
fore incurable, by overlapping the fascia in what he called a "vest-over-
pants" technique. That year he and his brother performed thirty-five
such repairs with only one recurrence. In 1895, Will Mayo turned to surgery of the stomach, still fraught with high mortality. Gastroenterostomy
had been described by Wölfler in Germany and, pyloroplasty by Mikulicz
and Heineke. When faced, in January of 1895, with a case of gastric outlet obstruction, Will Mayo (given the high mortality of the Billroth operations), elected to use Mikulicz' technique (widening the pyloric channel
between stomach and duodenum) to relieve gastric outlet obstruction. It
was successful but subsequent cases of pyloric cancer converted him to
gastroenterostomy for most of these patients. He routinely used the
Murphy button for these procedures until after 1906. Diagnosis was still
the major problem. By 1906, they reported 100 resections for gastric
cancer using the Billroth II method that combined resection and Wölfler's

gastroenterostomy. The Mayos were largely responsible for the popularity of the gastroenterostomy as they had an enormous experience and made a number of modifications that reduced the complications of bilious vomiting and "afferent loop syndrome."

An American Surgical Association lecture on duodenal ulcer stimulated the Mayo brothers to look for this lesion and they were able to differentiate this disease from gastric ulcer, even prior to x-ray diagnostic techniques still in the future. In 1906, Will Mayo reported 217 operations for stomach and duodenal diseases, including the gastric cancer cases mentioned above. Total abdominal operations in 1905 were 2,157, a stupendous number for two men. Their total surgical caseload for that year was 4,000 operations. That is more than ten operations per day, every day of the year.

Charles Mayo began doing tonsillectomies in the 1890s and, by 1905, was performing about 100 tonsillectomies, combined with excision of the adenoids, per year. They saw many cases of severe varicose veins and skin ulcers among the farmers and Charles Mayo invented a set of ring forceps that made stripping of the saphenous vein much easier. German surgeon, Karl Thiersch had invented the split thickness skin graft in 1886 and Charles Mayo adopted it for closure of these varicose skin ulcers in 1893. The brothers applied the Thiersch skin graft to the Halsted radical mastectomy, as well, and performed fifty-nine mastectomies in 1905. In 1897, they treated their first case of cretinism, a five-year-old boy with classical findings. The response to thyroid extract was amazing. By 1904, they had performed sixty-eight thyroidectomies for simple goiter. In 1907, they began to use thyroid extract in the treatment of goiter and myxedema, as well. They were providing modern surgery, the equal of that in Chicago or New York, in this frontier setting. Gradually, they began to receive referrals from wider parts of the country, stimulated perhaps by the practice of welcoming visitors to the operating room to witness surgery. Dr. W. J. Mayo was appointed surgeon for the Chicago and Northwestern Railroad when St. Mary's Hospital was built and this added to the practice of the sons. In 1892, a railroad accident injured a woman from New York and Charles Mayo performed a successful craniotomy for an acute subarachnoid hemorrhage. She made a complete recovery and her husband commended the surgeons who had saved his wife. The railroad began running special emergency trains from the Dakotas to Rochester with patients needing immediate attention or bringing Dr. Will to the scene of accidents. In 1892, they began to add associate physicians after their father retired from active practice. In 1901, Henry Plummer came to Rochester to open a clinical laboratory at what would become the Mayo Clinic. Edward Starr

Judd came in 1902 to serve an internship and remained as another surgeon to assist the brothers. In 1904, the Mayo brothers began to buy property and build parks and other city facilities to improve the town of Rochester. They knew that they were going to have to recruit physicians from other areas and this would require convincing them that Rochester was a good place to live.

In 1899, Will Mayo submitted a paper to the *American Journal of the Medical Sciences* reporting the results of 105 operations on the gallbladder and common bile duct. The editor, Alfred Stengle, asked a number of Philadelphia surgeons of his acquaintance how many similar cases they were aware of in the city and found that the total experience of Philadelphia surgeons was about the same as the total from this small town of Rochester, Minnesota. He returned the paper unpublished. Others were similarly skeptical, but those who troubled themselves to go and see were convinced. In 1903, Professor Johann von Mikulicz-Radecki, originator of the pyloroplasty operation and successor to Billroth, visited Rochester to see the Mayo brothers at work. Soon, other European surgeons were visiting the small town in Minnesota. Gradually the Mayo brothers limited their practice to surgery and added younger physicians to the growing Mayo Clinic.

118   Michael Bliss, *William Osler. A Life in Medicine*, p 47, Oxford University Press (1999).

119   Harvey Cushing, *The Life of Sir William Osler*, p 178 Volume I, Oxford University Press (1925).

120   Ernest Earnest, *S. Weir Mitchell, Novelist and Physician* p 91, U of Pennsylvania Press (1950).

121   Thomas Hubbard, quoted in Michael Bliss, p 135.

122   Michael Bliss, pp 142-144.

123   William T Councilman, "Certain Elements Found in the Blood in Cases of Malarial Fever," Association of American Physicians (1886).

124   Harvey Cushing, p. 296 (1925).

125   William Osler, *The Principles and Practice of Medicine*, p511, 1892 edition.

126   Reginald Fitz, "Perforating Inflammation of the Vermiform Appendix," *Transactions of the Association of American Physicians*. June (1885).

127   Helen Clapesattle, *The Doctors Mayo*, p 275, University of Minnesota Press (1941)

128   Both stories from *The Doctors Mayo,* by Helen Clapesattle, p 281.

129   Another Helen Clapesattle story, p 283-284.

13
The New Science

MICHAEL FARADAY HAD A LIMITED FORMAL EDUCATION, BEING apprenticed to a bookbinder in 1805 at the age of fourteen. At the age of twenty-one, he obtained an appointment as assistant to Humphrey Davy on the basis of notes he had made of Davy's lectures. As Davy's assistant, he discovered two new chlorides of carbon and succeeded in liquefying chlorine gas. In 1825, he identified benzene and was appointed director of the laboratory. Davy had shown in 1807 that sodium and potassium could be isolated from their compounds by an electric current, a process he called "electrolysis." Faraday carried on with experiments in electrolysis and, in 1834, compiled what are known as Faraday's Laws of Electrolysis. Faraday continued in his study of electricity and electrolysis developing a theory that all the forces of nature: heat, light, magnetism, and chemical affinity were manifestations of a unified force. His theory was incorrect, but led him to electromagnetism. Charles Coulomb, in 1785, had first demonstrated how electric charges repel one another. In 1820, Hans Christian Oersted and Andre Marie Ampere discovered that an electric current produced a magnetic field. Faraday, because of his ideas of conservation of energy and a unified force, believed that, if an electric current could produce a magnetic field, a magnetic field should be able to produce an electric current. In 1831, he demonstrated the principle of induction with the first dynamo and provided the theoretical basis for the invention of the generator and the electric motor. He expressed the current produced in his apparatus as the number of lines of force cut by the wire. His concept of lines of force was rejected by most physicists at the time because they assumed that charges attract and repel each other at a distance without the requirement for such mechanisms. Faraday's experiments continued to demonstrate electromagnetism, however, and the theoretical basis and the mathematical formulas necessary to calculate the forces were provided by Maxwell. In 1845, Faraday demonstrated that an intense magnetic field can rotate the plane of polarized light, now called the "Faraday effect." He published his experimental work in several volumes from 1844 to 1858. At one point, in *Thoughts on Ray-Vibrations*, he stated the conclusion that "radiation [was] as a high species of vibration in the lines of force," a preview of the later trend in physics that was ignored at the time.

James Clerk Maxwell was born in 1831 and was quickly recognized as a prodigy. He presented a study of the mathematics of ovals to the Royal Society of Edinburgh in 1846 at the age of fourteen. He entered Cambridge in 1850 and was described by a contemporary: "he brought to Cambridge in the autumn of 1850, a mass of knowledge which was really immense for so young a man, but in a state of disorder appalling to his methodical private tutor."[130] He graduated with a degree in mathematics from Trinity College in 1854. In 1855, he presented the first of two papers titled *On Faraday's Lines of Force* to the Cambridge Philosophical Society, and the second in 1856. In these two papers, he demonstrated the equations that describe the behavior of electricity and magnetic fields and their interrelation. Maxwell studied the rings of Saturn and, in 1857, published a paper on the perception of color, which established the three primary color basis of color vision. In 1862 he calculated that the speed of light and the speed of propagation of an electromagnetic field are the same. His conclusion was: "*We can scarcely avoid the conclusion that light consists in the transverse undulations of the same medium which is the cause of electric and magnetic phenomena.*" Maxwell actually printed these words in italics in his book to emphasize the revolutionary significance of them.

His further work on the kinetic theory of gases showed that temperature and heat involve only molecular movement. Phlogiston was gone forever. His work changed the understanding of heat from a steady flow of energy from hot to cold to a statistical probability of molecular movement being greater from heat to cold. This did not change the thermodynamic law but used a better theory to explain observations in experimental conditions. Finally he accepted the post as the first Cavendish Professor of Physics at Cambridge in 1871. He designed the Cavendish Laboratory and opened it in 1874. His book, *Electricity and Magnetism*, appeared in 1873 and included the four partial differential equations known as Maxwell's Equations. In 1879, he published Henry Cavendish's papers in *The Electrical Researches of the Honorable Henry Cavendish*, showing that the eighteenth century genius had anticipated most of Maxwell's work one hundred years earlier. Maxwell made possible all that was to follow in studies of electromagnetism and electricity.

Max Planck, writing in 1931, stated that while neither Faraday or Maxwell "originally considered optics in connection with their consideration of the fundamental laws of electromagnetism," yet "the whole field of optics, which had defied attack from the side of mechanics for more than a hundred years, was at one stroke conquered by Maxwell's Electrodynamic Theory." Planck considered this one of "the greatest triumphs of human intellectual endeavor."[131]

Heinrich Hertz confirmed Maxwell's and Faraday's work with experiments measuring the speed of light and electromagnetic waves. He showed that the electromagnetic waves behaved exactly like light in properties of reflection, refraction and polarization and that they could be focused. The Germans took Maxwell's theory and subtracted some of his tortured ideas about how these forces acted at a distance. Gauss had already worked on the subject of static charges and the way that they act at a distance. One issue was the speed of propagation of electromagnetic forces along a wire, through a vacuum and through air. The old theory, based on Newton, was that these forces acted instantaneously. Maxwell believed that all the forces acted at the same rate, the speed of light. Hertz proved this to be true. The textbooks, which followed Hertz' publication of his work in 1888, spoke of a "revolution" in thought. The term was used in the German text studied by the young Albert Einstein, in school at Zurich. In 1920, Einstein described the revolution as, "The simplest law of this kind (mechanics) is Newton's expression: 'attraction equals mass times mass divided by the square of the distance.' In contradistinction to this, Faraday and Maxwell have introduced an entirely new kind of physical realities, namely fields of force." In his Autobiographical Notes, in 1949, Einstein added, "The most fascinating subject at the time I was a student was Maxwell's theory."[132] The application of the new physics and electromagnetism to medicine was not long in coming.

ROENTGEN AND X-RAYS

Wilhelm Roentgen was expelled from gymnasium, because he would not identify a classmate (possibly himself) who had drawn a caricature of a teacher. Because of his recalcitrance, he was barred from other Dutch and German gymnasia and could not obtain his *abitur*, his diploma. Without an abitur, he could not be admitted to university and was forced to matriculate at Polytechnic School in Zurich in 1865. For the next three years, he studied mechanical engineering rather than theoretical physics and learned to construct intricate apparatus of all kinds. His skill came to the attention of August Kundt, a professor of theoretical physics at Zurich. Kundt persuaded Roentgen to abandon mechanical engineering, although he had just obtained his degree, and accept a position as his assistant. Kundt, as a consolation prize or, perhaps, inducement, allowed Roentgen to study for his doctorate in theoretical physics at the same time. Kundt left Zurich in 1870 for a new position at the University of Würzburg and Roentgen followed him. In 1872, Kundt and Roentgen moved again, this time to the University of Strasbourg. In 1874, at the age of twenty-nine, and in spite of the missing *abitur*, he was appointed Instructor at Strasbourg and in 1876 promoted to Assistant Professor. Finally, in 1879, he accepted a full professorship at Giessen. He had married in 1872 and lived a quiet life socially. He was not popular with students and his teaching skills were weak, but he was strong in laboratory research. He studied electricity, still new with many unknown properties. He learned that when a dielectric material, like glass, is moved between two electrically charged condenser plates, a current arises.

Sir William Crookes, an English physicist, discovered thallium in 1861 and studied the effects of electrical discharges on gases. He used rare gases and, to collect and experiment on pure samples of them, he invented a structure now called a "Crookes' tube." It is a cylinder from which the air could be pumped until a vacuum exists. The cylinder contains electrodes connected to an induction coil and battery. He wanted to use the cylinder to study the effect on rare gases of an electrical discharge between the electrodes in the tube. The electrical current in such an arrangement is conducted by what came to be known as cathode rays (the electron was not yet discovered). Crookes accidentally exposed photographic plates to his tube when it was in use. He left them lying on the same table as the tube. Later, he found that the film was fogged and he wrote to the manufacturer complaining about the film cassettes, never imagining the cause of the shadows on his film. Another physicist, Phillip Lenard, noticed that slips of paper coated with barium platinocyanide salts, which had been left lying near his Crookes' tube, fluoresced when he had a current running through the cylinder. He also failed to appreciate the significance of what was occurring near the tube. Lenard noted that an aluminum sheet, which covered a window in the tube, permitted the effect of the cathode rays to pass through. He even sent one of the tubes with the aluminum window to Roentgen for further study.

In the evening of November 8, 1895, Roentgen repeated Lenard's experiments with the modified Crookes' tube and observed the passage of some of the cathode rays through the aluminum. Roentgen repeated the experiment of placing a small screen covered with barium platinocyanide crystals near the window. Again, the crystals fluoresced when the current was producing cathode rays. Roentgen then went further than Lenard had gone, reasoning that perhaps the window was not necessary for some of the cathode rays to escape. He believed that fewer of the rays would escape through the glass and he must be very careful to prevent the luminescence inside the tube from producing so much light that weak fluorescence could not be seen. He carefully covered the tube with cardboard to prevent escape of light from within the tube. He also covered the windows of his laboratory to produce complete darkness in the room. His meticulous experimental technique was about to produce a discovery that would change medicine dramatically. He tested the shrouding of the tube by charging the electrodes to see if any light escaped through the cardboard. He noticed a greenish glow in the room behind him when the electrodes were charged. It was coming, he found after he lit a match to look for the source, from a screen coated with barium platinocyanide that was lying on a bench nearby. He repeatedly switched the current to the tube on and off and observed the fluorescence flashing on when the current was on. Roentgen, unlike Lenard and Crookes, immediately realized that the fluorescence could not be produced by cathode rays (electrons we now know), which will travel only a few inches in air. The fluorescing screen was at least a yard from the tube. Roentgen then carried the screen a greater distance from the tube and it still fluoresced even when the screen and tube were many yards apart. This must be a new form of energy, a new electromagnetic wave.

Roentgen interposed a deck of cards and a two-inch thick book between the tube and the screen and the screen continued to fluoresce when the electrodes were excited. He broke away from his experiments to eat his dinner after his wife, Bertha, repeatedly called him. She was annoyed that he ate almost nothing and quickly returned to the laboratory. As he resumed his work he began to experiment with material that would not permit passage of the new ray that he had already begun to call "x-ray." He quickly realized that lead would not permit passage and most metals, depending on their density, would block most of the ray. The fact that wood would not obstruct passage of the ray prompted him to place a wooden box filled with metal weights on top of a photographic plate. The developed film showed the metal weights and only a faint shadow of the box.

In early December, as he continued his experiments, he was shocked by an unexpected finding. He held a lead pipe over a photographic plate and exposed it to the x-ray. On the developed photographic plate, he saw not only the pipe, but also the bones of two of his own fingers that had been holding the pipe. He discussed this with his wife; she had been sorely tried by his behavior these past few weeks. To prove to her that he was not imagining these things he placed her hand on a photographic plate. He energized the Crookes' tube for six minutes with her hand held in place. He developed the plate and showed her the result. She was shocked and upset at the view of her own bones on the film. Her rings are clearly visible on the film. Roentgen realized that his discovery was one of history's great scientific advances. He resolved to continue his work in secret, for the moment. Crookes' tubes were common and the discovery could be repeated if another physicist happened to duplicate his experiment. He wanted to publish his findings in the proceedings of the Physical-Medical Society of Wurzburg meeting for December. In spite of a frantic work schedule, he was unable to prepare his preliminary report until after the meeting was held. He persuaded the secretary of the society to include his paper in the journal issue that included the meeting, even though it had not been presented.

His paper, "On a New Kind of Ray: A Preliminary Communication," appeared one week after it was completed, a record in scientific publication. The journal was not widely read so Roentgen had reprints printed at his own expense and sent them to prominent physicists in Europe. He included with the reprints copies of the x-ray photographs of the box of metal weights and Bertha's hand.

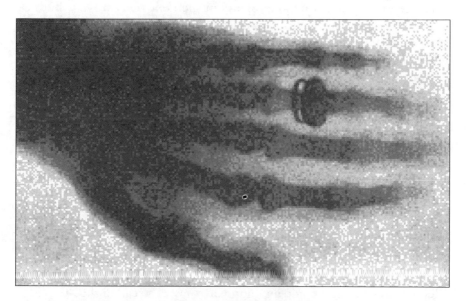

Figure 8 – Bertha's hand showing her rings.

The photographs of her hand were so startling that major newspapers picked up the story quickly and on January 6, 1896 the *Vienna Die Presse* printed a front page story.

In the first six months of 1896, x-ray photographs of many people were taken, often to their fright and dismay. By December 1896, x-ray photographs were admitted as evidence by an American judge. The case was a medical malpractice case in which a physician had missed a leg fracture. He prescribed exercises and, when the law student patient experienced severe pain with exercise, he had an x-ray performed that showed the fracture. The doctor's lawyers bitterly opposed the admission of the x-ray evidence, but were unsuccessful. Since Crookes' tubes were widely available, physicians all over the world quickly began using the new diagnostic test. Two weeks after the publication of his discovery, Roentgen was invited to demonstrate the method to the Kaiser, Wilhelm II and, after a successful demonstration, was awarded the Prussian Order of the Crown, Class II. One month later, he attended the January meeting of the Physical-Medical Society to give his paper at last. He was greeted with cheers and demonstrated the x-ray by examining the hand of a famous professor of anatomy, Albert von Kolliker, who commented that this was the most significant presentation in physical or medical sciences he had ever heard. A discussion of the possible application of the new ray to medicine followed the meeting. Everyone agreed that it would be limited to examination of bones.

Roentgen published two more reports in the next year on x-ray, but had nothing to say about medical applications. His studies all concerned the physics of the ray itself. Meanwhile, all over the world, physicians were using the diagnostic tool in hundreds of applications. He admitted his failure to demonstrate the electromagnetic nature of the ray. Seventeen years later Max von Laue won a Nobel Prize for demonstrating the refraction of x-rays by a crystal lattice. Roentgen received the first Nobel Prize in physics in 1901 for his discovery. He had declined all speaking engagements after his initial report in Wurzburg and he now declined to give a speech at the Nobel ceremony. He even willed the prize money to the university, the only Nobel laureate ever to do so. The Kaiser insisted that he become director of the Institute of Physics at the University of Munich and his research days were largely over. His life was disrupted by the war in 1914, and his wife died in 1919. Lonely and inactive he died in 1923.

In 1913, William Coolidge, an American scientist working for the General Electric Company, invented an improved x-ray tube called the "Coolidge tube," which produced a more stable beam of x-ray. This tube, rather than the Crookes tube, has been the standard design for modern radiology apparatus.[133] Coolidge's invention was the tungsten filament, used in all light bulbs, and the tungsten cathode in the x-ray tube.

RADIO-IMAGING METHODS

Not long after the discovery of the x-ray it was found, by Walter Cannon at Harvard, that bismuth salts and organic iodine were opaque to the rays and many new diagnostic techniques were developed. Evarts Graham, professor of surgery at Washington University in St. Louis, learned of a chemical that was concentrated in the gallbladder after being excreted by the liver. The chemical, phenoltetrabromphthalein, was used as an early liver function test (In the days of my training we used a similar test called "BSP retention." The chemical was BromSulPthalein). Dr. Graham had spent two years in a chemistry fellowship after medical school. He suggested to the Eastman Kodak Company, who manufactured the chemical, substituting iodine for the bromine in the molecule. The resulting compound should allow the gallbladder to be visualized on x-ray (because iodine is a heavier atom than bromine and x-rays are more completely absorbed by the heavier atoms) and stones could be identified.

Dr. Graham, and his assistant Warren Cole (later to be another professor of surgery), gave the new compound to patients with known gallbladder disease, but were disappointed when the gallbladder did not visualize on x-ray. It worked in dogs but not in patients. Fortunately, it occurred to them to give the compound to patients with normal gallbladders and these did concentrate the chemical and the gallbladder could be seen on x-ray. They learned that abnormal gallbladders had damaged mucous membrane lining that was unable to concentrate the chemical. The normal gallbladder absorbs water from bile, concentrating it and storing it between meals. The test, known as the "Graham-Cole test," has been replaced by ultrasound in recent years but, for fifty years, was the only method for visualizing the gallbladder. Gallstones are cholesterol (ninety percent are) and do not show on x-ray. They can be seen in the Graham-Cole study, if the gallbladder visualizes, as dark shadows (like ice cubes in a glass of milk) in the white gallbladder.

Cannon used Bismuth salts in animal studies and eventually changed to safer Barium for human use. Barium upper GI and Lower GI exams became common, although they are being gradually replaced by direct visualization using fiberoptic scopes. Chest x-rays required long exposures at first, limiting their usefulness. Roentgen, and others, discovered that x-rays could produce skin burns and this knowledge was turned to therapeutic uses.

THE CAT SCAN

In 1972, an English computer engineer named Godfrey Hounsfield, and a neuroradiologist colleague, devised a new technique they called computerized transverse axial tomography. Tomograms, x-rays with a thin slice of tissue clearly shown, had been performed for years with conventional x-rays by moving the film to blur all but the layer to be studied. Hounsfield used a system of narrow beams of x-ray from many angles in a 360 degree rotation of the tube. The x-ray beam was converted to digital values by receptors, in place of film, and an algorithm calculated specific images. The first applications were to the brain where the small differences in density had defeated previous efforts to establish contrast between structures. The development of the technique had taken years of experimental study using the heads of cows. Hounsfield received the Nobel Prize in Medicine in 1979 for the discovery. He shared the prize with Allan Cormack who had, in 1963, published a theoretical study using models, but no clinical subjects, human or animal. Hounsfield had been unaware of Cormack's work, which was published in a physics journal and never applied to patients.

MARIE CURIE AND RADIUM

Within weeks of Roentgen's discovery, Henri Becquerel, a French scientist, attempted to study uranium with x-rays. If barium was radio-opaque, uranium should be as well. Becquerel placed some uranium salts over an x-ray plate, which was protected by an aluminum cover. Inadvertently he developed the film without exposing it to x-ray. He found that it had darkened at the point in contact with the uranium salts. Uranium emitted x-rays, or at least rays like x-rays which penetrated matter. In addition to exposing photographic film, it would discharge an electroscope, suggesting an electromagnetic energy. He published his findings but did not pursue the matter. Manya Sklowdowski, born in Warsaw in 1867, was recognized as a brilliant student by the age of sixteen when she was awarded a gold medal for academics. Her mother had died, her father was a poor teacher of mathematics and physics and her sister, Bronya, had left home for Paris. Manya left Poland in 1891 to study at the Sorbonne and live with her sister. Soon after arriving, she changed her name to Marie. She worked diligently, surviving on a starvation regimen, and graduated in 1894 with a second place award. There she married fellow scientist, Pierre Curie. He was already Supervisor of the School of Physics and Industrial Chemistry having graduated in 1878 at the age of twenty. They were married in 1895 and both continued to work in spite of the subsequent birth of a daughter, Irene.

Having become aware of Becquerel's work with uranium, she chose this as the subject of her doctoral thesis. She studied thorium, another element that was "radioactive," the term she coined to describe the "Becquerel rays" emitted by the material. She set to work to see if any other element shared this property of radioactivity. She then noted that pitchblende, uranium oxide ore, was four times as active as uranium, leading to speculation about a new element. She announced this conclusion on April 12, 1898. Marie and her husband (who had abandoned his own researches to assist his wife), in order to isolate a new element, purified 100 grams of pitchblende and, in July 1898, announced the discovery of a new element she called polonium, after her native Poland. By November, it had become apparent that the remaining pitchblende liquid, even after refining, remained highly radioactive; there must be another new element present.

Further separation revealed a substance 900 times more radioactive than uranium. They required huge volumes of pitchblende to extract the rare element and found the source in Bohemian glass factories, which discarded the ore after extracting uranium for glass. On December 26, 1898, they announced the discovery of radium. It took another four years of frustrating and incredibly tedious work to extract one tenth of a gram of radium from a mountain of pitchblende ore and determine its atomic weight. Part of the discovery was her and her husband's conclusion that the rays were emitted as a function of the atomic structure of the element, since no electric current was necessary. At first, they were concerned that the radiation might be cosmic rays that were somehow focused by the element, but soon arrived at the correct, and revolutionary, explanation.

Both of the Curies had accidentally burned themselves during their research and, in 1901, Pierre taped a vial of radium to his arm after Becquerel told him of an accidental burn he suffered when he forgot a quantity of radium, in a glass tube, in his coat pocket for fifteen days. It took Pierre's resulting skin lesion, produced by this exposure, a month to heal. In 1904, radium was shown to destroy abnormal cells and this led to radiation treatment for cancer. They were awarded the Nobel Prize in 1904, along with Henri Becquerel, and, when Pierre was accidentally killed in a cart accident in 1906, Marie was offered his chair, the first woman professor at the Sorbonne. She suffered considerable opposition because of her sex and, in an election for the Academy of Sciences of France in 1910, she was opposed by and defeated by a male scientist, Edouard Branly, of lesser achievement. A campaign against her included an allegation that she was Jewish. The Dreyfus Affair had rocked France only seventeen years before. A brief love affair late in 1911 (after three years of widowhood) with another physicist, Paul Langevin, who was unhappily married, led to considerable public criticism and she spent some time in England and America.

In the midst of this press scandal, she received her second Nobel Prize. The French, belatedly realizing her worldwide fame after an enthusiastic reception in England, supported her work and the Pasteur Institute helped to establish her Radium Institute. In 1914, with the outbreak of war, Marie and her daughter Irene raised funds to equip twenty motor vans with x-ray machines for use in field hospitals and she trained a group of women as x-ray technicians. She and her daughter served at the front with one of the vans, called by the soldiers "*petites Curies.*" She suspended research work at the Institute until the war was over. In 1919, she returned to her lab at the Radium Institute and spent the rest of her life working there.

Enthusiasm for radiation, x-ray and radium, eventually went beyond caution and severe consequences were later encountered. In 1903, a "radium dinner" was held at MIT, which provided dinner guests with "radium cocktails" containing a small cube of low-grade radium. Many of the early researchers died of leukemia or other radiation complications. Some lost fingers. An association between skin cancer and radiation was noted as early as 1902. Radiation therapy began in France and the initial applications were to skin diseases, not all cancerous. By 1914, radium had been shown to be effective in the treatment of uterine cancer in Germany and a radium center was established in Vienna. In 1905, Robert Abbe first used the implantation of radium material into a cancer in the United States.[134] Radiation was applied to the treatment of diseases that were completely inappropriate or not diseases at all.

A radium refinery opened in Pittsburg in 1913 providing an enhanced supply of the new agent.[135] An example of the unqualified enthusiasm for the new therapy is a quote from a European physician: "At Freiburg we no longer operate, we radiate."[136] Successful treatment of uterine cancer led to treatment, with radium implants, of uterine fibroids, menorrhagia (heavy periods), and metrorrhagia (irregular periods). There was little or no understanding of the mechanism by which radiation affected tissue. In 1914, a study of the effects of radium on two cancers, a breast cancer and a sarcoma, was published showing death of cancer cells, inflammation and scarring.[137] A Canadian physician treated a patient with "neurasthenia" administering X-ray to the solar plexus and reporting that the patient went home and "slept soundly through the whole night, a thing he had not done for many months."[138] Others found that it cleared up acne and adopted radiation for this condition with enthusiasm that would last for more than fifty years. Chest x-rays in infants revealed the presence of the large thymus gland (a normal finding it was eventually determined). Radiation was applied to this structure in cases of upper respiratory disease (the only reason to perform a chest x-ray on an infant, an early example of statistical bias in research) and twenty years later many of these patients developed thyroid cancer. Until recent years, the highest incidence of leukemia in the population has been in radiologists.

On the other hand, some malignant tumors untreatable by other means did respond. In 1923, Aikens reported on the case of a young man with inoperable sarcoma of the orbit that was producing protrusion of the eye. There was no sign of recurrence of the tumor ten years later. Another patient with a "rodent ulcer" of the scalp (a basal cell carcinoma that is eroding through the skin), that had produced bone erosion exposing the brain, responded with healing of the ulcer and underlying skull. After 1920, the radiology specialty gradually took control of the use of x-ray and scientific investigation of the effects followed. Still, the inappropriate uses, including radiation of "enlarged thymus" in children, continued until the 1950s.

ABUSE OF X-RAY

Medical malpractice suits were rare prior to World War II and, in the 1920s and 1930s, most of them involved burns from misuse of x-ray machines on patients. When I was a child, most shoe stores had fluoroscope machines. The customers could stand on a small step, slide their feet with the new shoes into a slot in the machine, and push a button that turned on a fluoroscope. You looked into a viewer, somewhat like those used in old-fashioned peep show kinescopes (machines which flip cards rapidly creating a movie-like show with scenes that would seem tame on television today). You could see the bones of your foot and see how close your toes came to the end of the shoe. There was no real value to this procedure except to amuse children and sell more shoes.

In the 1940s, the major malpractice insurer in California was Lloyds of London. They insured a doctor who ran a full-time emergency clinic in a Long Beach shipyard. He had a fluoroscope and he allowed his patients to amuse themselves by looking at their hands and feet in the fluoroscope while waiting to be seen in the clinic. It was not too long before serious x-ray burns began to appear among this doctor's patients. Suddenly, Lloyds was confronted with dozens of lawsuits brought by patients with x-ray burns. Eventually, the flurry of lawsuits was settled for a total of about $500,000, an enormous sum for the time. Lloyds left the medical malpractice business.[139] They did not learn their lesson, however, and in the

1980s, many of Lloyds' "names," the individual underwriters, were bankrupted by asbestos litigation.

OTHER RAYS

Other ray types were investigated and Danish physician Niels Finsen suggested that ultraviolet rays were bactericidal. The use of ultraviolet rays for various purposes, some useful and some not, followed and even tuberculosis was treated by building sanitaria at high altitude to take advantage of the increased ultraviolet radiation at that altitude. Suntans were encouraged and much quackery resulted as was the case in radiation with x-ray and radium.

130   Peter Guthrie Tait, the *Proceedings of the Royal Society of Edinburgh* (1879-80).

131   Max Plank, "Maxwell's influence on theoretical physics in Germany," in *James Clerk Maxwell : A Commemorative Volume 1831-1931* (Cambridge, 1931), 45-65.

132   Albert Einstein, "Maxwell's influence on the development of the conception of physical reality," in *James Clerk Maxwell : A Commemorative Volume 1831-1931* (Cambridge, 1931), 66-73.

133   Michael Wolff, "William Coolidge: Shirt-Sleeves Manager," *IEEE Spectrum* (May 1984).

134   Robert Abbe, "The Therapeutics of Radium," *Canada Lancet* 47:580-94 (1914).

135   RF Robison, "The Radium 'Business' of Providing Medical Sources," *Current Oncology* 3:156-62 (1996).

136   Frederick Bryant, "Radiotherapy," *Boston Medical and Surgical Journal* 181:270-276 (1919).

137   William B Aikens and KMB Simon, "Histological and Clinical Changes Induced by Radium in Carcinoma and Sarcoma," *Dominion Medical Monthly & Ontario Medical Journal* 43:97-107 (1914).

138   Charles R Dickson, "Some Uses of the X-Ray Other Than Diagnostic," *Dominion Medical Monthly & Ontario Medical Journal* 19:72-76 (1902).

139   Howard Hassard, "Fifty Years in Law and Medicine," an oral history. "Hap" Hassard was the general counsel for the California Medical Association for 50 years. The oral history was collected in 1984.

The Development of Modern Surgery

THE SURGICAL SPECIALTIES

SURGERY PROGRESSED RAPIDLY AFTER THE DISCOVERY OF SUCCESSFUL anesthesia and Lister's work with antisepsis. The foundations for many specialties were laid early in the century, however, before anesthesia and antisepsis made the methods practical for wide use. Georg Stromeyer had successfully corrected clubfoot with division of the abnormal tendons in 1830 in Hanover. William John Little, an English surgeon who had a clubfoot himself, learned the method from Stromeyer and returned to London to open the Orthopaedic Institution which, in 1843, became the Royal Orthopaedic Hospital. In 1854, Anthonius Mathijsen developed (or rediscovered) quick drying Plaster of Paris, a boon to the splinting of fractures. Hugh Owen Thomas devised the Thomas Splint at the same time and developed a number of new devices that contributed to the progress in treatment of crippled children.

Surgery of the ear required improvements in the understanding of anatomy and Jean Itard, a surgeon in Paris, published a new textbook in 1821 that corrected many of Vesalius's errors. He became interested in deafness and developed methods of teaching the deaf. Mastoiditis was a common problem due to inadequate treatment of middle ear infections. In 1853, Sir William Wilde of Dublin, the father of writer Oscar Wilde, recommended incision and drainage of mastoiditis in his book, *Practical Observations on Aural Surgery and the Nature and Treatment of Diseases of the Ear*. James Hinton, of London, and Hermann Schwartze of Halle, jointly reported on mastoidectomy and, by 1900, it had become the standard form of therapy. It would continue to be the standard until the appearance of antibiotics after World War II.

Ophthalmology began with Gottingen who established a course of study in Vienna in 1803 and opened an eye clinic in 1812. Work on eye disease was stimulated by the experiences of French soldiers who returned from Napoleon's Egyptian campaign with trachoma and other eye conditions acquired in Egypt. The New York Eye Infirmary opened in 1820. The ophthalmoscope was invented by Helmholtz in 1851 following on the research by Frans Donders, of Utrecht, in optics and eye physiology. Albrecht von Graefe, in Berlin, became the greatest of the eye specialists and developed modern eye surgery including correction of strabismus by eye muscle revision and iridectomy (removal of a section of the iris) to relieve glaucoma. Lister provided the key to orthopedic surgery with antisepsis and Karl Koller's introduction of cocaine topical anesthesia accelerated the development of eye surgery.

APPENDICITIS AND JOHN B. MURPHY

A localized infection in the right lower quadrant of the abdomen had been described by anatomists in the sixteenth century (although the appendix was not connected with the condition) and a diagnosis had been made in a living patient by Willhelm Ballonius in 1734. Claudius Amyand, a "Sergeant-Surgeon" to Queen Caroline, performed the first appendectomy in 1756.[140] Amyand was the son of a Huguenot immigrant and a court favorite who had inoculated the children of George II with smallpox, using the method brought back from Asia by Lady Montague. He operated on an eleven-year-old boy who had an inguinal hernia that was draining fecal matter. In the hernia sac, Amyand found a perforated appendix containing a metal pin. He ligated the appendix and removed the abscess, including a portion of the omentum. He exteriorized the appendix stump (brought it to the surface of the abdomen) and his patient recovered.[141] There were other reports of foreign body perforation of the appendix but the patients died. James Parkinson described the association between the appendix and peritonitis in 1812. Robert Lawson Tait performed an appendectomy in 1880 and Kronlein did the same in 1886 (both associated with perforation), but the nature of the disease was still poorly understood. In 1884, Hall at Roosevelt Hospital in New York performed the first appendectomy in the US, also in a case of appendicitis in a hernia sac. I have seen several such cases in my own career and have actually performed an incidental appendectomy with a hernia repair.

In 1878, John B. Murphy, the son of Irish immigrants, entered the Rush Medical College in Chicago after serving an apprenticeship with a local country doctor. His attention was immediately captured by the professor of surgery, Moses Gunn, who was called "Minute Gunn" by the students, because of his speed in the operating room. Murphy was exposed to the work of Lister and became a fervent advocate of antisepsis as a student, which did not endear him to his professors, still skeptical of the newfangled theories from Scotland. At one point, the arguments among the students became so heated that Murphy threw a classmate into the pit of the operating theater; fortunately, the professor had not yet arrived. At the end of his second year, Murphy passed an oral exam and was selected for the coveted internship at Cook County Hospital. His mother objected to his spending a year in a "pest house" but he entered into his duties, along with five other "junior interns," in the 450 bed charity hospital.

Cook County Hospital in 1880 had no clinical laboratory and no microscope. Antisepsis practices had not yet appeared in Chicago and puerperal fever was rampant as interns continued to go from the autopsy room, and from dressing infected wounds, to the obstetrical wards. That ward was often closed for weeks at a time while walls were whitewashed and floors were scrubbed, but the transmission of infection by unclean hands was ignored, although not by Murphy. The young intern was powerfully influenced by Christian Fenger, the Danish physician who had studied pathology and bacteriology with Virchow, and who paid $1,000 for appointment as pathologist to Cook County Hospital. The enormous sum was paid for an appointment that paid no salary and provided no other source of income but provided unlimited opportunity to study disease. Murphy became a passionate disciple of this gifted teacher and once a week the interns, including Murphy and Frank Billings--both destined for fame--met with Fenger to study microscopic slides from the cases of the week and discuss the medical literature. Their studies complete for the evening, they would have dinner together, sharing a beer as Fenger told them, in his halting English, of clinics in Europe. Murphy became fired with the thought of study in Germany, but had no idea of how he, the son of poor immigrant parents, might do so.

Edward W. Lee, an Irish immigrant who had become a prosperous surgeon in Chicago, had originally advised Murphy to seek out Fenger and the young man now asked Lee's advice about how he might find the funds for the trip. To his astonishment, Lee offered to support Murphy for a year in Europe, if he would return to Chicago and join him in the practice of surgery. Murphy spent a year saving his money and, with the help of his mother, left for Europe in September of 1881. His first stop was Billroth's clinic in Vienna, across the square from the Allgemeines Krankenhaus, the most modern hospital in Europe. Billroth had just performed the first gastric resection for cancer of the stomach. Murphy spent a year in Europe dividing his time between Vienna, Berlin, and Heidelberg.

In 1882, he returned to Chicago to resume his practice with Lee. With Dr. Lee's help, he was appointed to a position of instructor at Rush Medical

College, but he did not have the $1,000 that Fenger had paid for an appointment to Cook County Hospital. He was busy in practice, but performing very little surgery. Again, Dr. Lee managed to procure an appointment at Cook County for his assistant. In early 1885, Murphy was called to see the daughter of a wealthy family, who was seriously ill, and he quickly made the diagnosis of typhoid fever. The young woman recovered slowly (there was no treatment except a restricted diet) under his careful supervision and she soon decided that she wanted him to marry her. Eventually, he got the idea while she concluded that he was a genius and it was her mission in life to see that he had everything he needed to achieve success. On November 25, they were married. Less than a year later, on May 4, 1886, the Haymarket Riot thrust him into the spotlight.

Nearly one hundred police officers were injured by a bomb and shooting by anarchist rioters. Murphy, who knew many of the policemen, was called to the police station where the wounded and dying had been carried. He dressed wounds and administered first aid before sending the seriously injured to Cook County Hospital. There he spent the next thirty-six hours in surgery, operating on bullet and shrapnel wounds. In the later trial of the rioters, Murphy testified as a witness for the prosecution, where he proceeded to give a scholarly description of wound surgery. The result was fame in Chicago and considerable jealousy on the part of colleagues. There were allegations that high fees had been paid to Murphy by the city, but this has been shown to be false. The publicity, of course, was priceless to his career and that was the real source of the resentment, that and his description of modern methods many of which were not followed by competing surgeons. With the help of his wife, and the large home they received as a wedding present from her parents, Murphy set up a research laboratory in his barn. The couple had little social life and eventually his wife, in order to spend more time with her single-minded husband, began to assist him in the lab.

On March 2, 1889, Murphy made the diagnosis of early appendicitis in a young man hospitalized with a leg fracture. He had read the report by Reginald Fitz, of Boston, about the treatment of peri-typhlitis, as appendicitis was called at the time. It was a well documented study and recommended early appendectomy, but Fitz was a pathologist and no one had succeeded in making a diagnosis early enough to avoid perforation. Murphy performed the first appendectomy, for acute appendicitis prior to perforation, that day, on the young laborer named Monahan. Murphy had proved Fitz right. Now, he and Lee pored over old accounts to document the course of the illness. Convinced, Murphy next had to educate the public and other physicians about early diagnosis. He performed several appendectomies on patient's kitchen tables because they could not afford to go to the hospital. He presented his findings on his first fifty cases to the Chicago Medical Society and met skepticism and even hostility from other surgeons. Fourteen years later, he presented a series of two thousand appendectomies to the same society and met no doubters, but it was a hard fourteen years. In 1905, he was invited to write the chapter on appendicitis (he had coined the term) for W.W. Keen's huge *American Textbook of Surgery* and the battle was won.

THE MURPHY BUTTON

In 1890 Murphy developed symptoms of tuberculosis and, mindful that his sister and brother had died of the disease, took off eight months in New Mexico. While there, he filled the hours by thinking about surgery. He returned with a determination to find a way to improve the suturing of intestine. He spent hours in his laboratory working on the problem. The result was the "Murphy Button," now obsolete but in common use until the past forty years. It produced a sutureless anastomosis somewhat similar to that created by present day circular (EEA) stapling devices. The metal button, which was left inside the intestine when closed to connect the two bowel loops, sloughed after healing of the anastomosis and was passed by the patient in the stool. It was a huge improvement at the time and resulted in worldwide fame.

A new hospital appointment produced competition with Nicholas Senn, an old mentor. Murphy, under attack by competitors, but confident of his ability, began to insist on accurate record keeping of results and complications. He felt that this objective information on the results of his and others' cases would overcome the still-present jealous rivalry of his colleagues. In this, he anticipated Amory Codman's work in Boston twenty years later. In both instances, the pressure for objective analysis of results produced professional resistance and resentment, usually from lesser surgeons who were threatened by the comparison. In 1894, Senn was elected president of the America Medical Association and used the occasion to attack Murphy and his button. This example of spite wounded Murphy but, relying on his wife's always-wise advice, he made no mention of it. His practice was enormous and his family was devoted. The button continued in use and dramatically increased the volume of intestinal surgery. Sutured anastomosis, which Senn advocated, had largely replaced its use by the 1930s, but stapled anastomoses, with which the vast amount of bowel surgery is performed now, use the same principle.

Not content with his two contributions to surgical technique, Murphy in 1896 reported a series of operations on the trigeminal nerve ganglion for tic doloreaux. He added nothing new to this subject but the example of his virtuosity is impressive. In 1897, he presented a series of arterial and venous end-to-end anastomoses, anticipating Alexis Carrel's Nobel Prize winning work by fifteen years. His first arterial case was the first successful repair of an arterial transection ever accomplished. In 1898, he was at last invited to address the American Medical Association and give the annual oration on surgery. The report he presented was another masterstroke as he proposed collapse therapy for pulmonary tuberculosis.

He had noticed that the development of a pleural effusion, producing partial collapse of the lung, resulted in improvement in the underlying lung lesion. He discussed his experience with the removal of lobes and then reasoned that collapsing the lung abscess would result in improvement, as was the case in any other abscess. Collapse would function much as immobilization did for joint disease, also common in tuberculosis. He injected nitrogen gas into the pleural space collapsing the lung. The nitrogen was absorbed slowly and could be reinfused every week or so for about six months. The convention received his report with enthusiasm but the Chicago carpers began immediately to complain. An extensive newspaper account of his work and the speech were attacked as self-promotion. One criticism was valid: Murphy had neglected to credit the Italian, Forlanini, who had first reported the method (although Forlanini's method, using an incision instead of a needle to insert the nitrogen gas, was clumsy and impractical for repeated use). Collapse therapy became the standard treatment of advancing pulmonary tuberculosis until the antibiotic era and Murphy, not Forlanini, had brought about the adoption.

The humiliations were not over, however. On the way home from Europe in 1899, he was invited to address the American Surgical Association, the most prestigious surgical body in the world. Such a request was tantamount to an invitation to join the association but, in the election after his address, he was blackballed. Some members doubted the validity of some of his results, because they were so spectacular. In 1902, he was finally elected after the doubters were converted. He was elected to all the major surgical societies in the world but excluded from the Chicago Medical Society for many years as old calumnies about high fees were recirculated and exaggerated. His wife struggled to force him to relax as he anticipated the term "workaholic" by a century. In 1916, after suffering from angina pectoris for a year, he died of coronary heart disease. Near the end of his career my aunt Geraldine served as his surgical nurse and her picture (while she was still a student nurse) appeared in the newspaper with one of the famous Chicago Cubs double-play combination players (Tinker to Evers to Chance), who was recovering from an appendectomy during the baseball season of 1906.

WILLIAM HALSTED

William Halsted had an indifferent scholastic record at Yale (although he was the captain of the first Yale football team in 1873), but, graduated in the top ten of his 1877 medical school class from the College of Physicians and Surgeons in New York. He may have been an early example of favoritism because of a wealthy parent, an allegation made about another Yale graduate in recent years. He served an internship at New York Hospital and then spent two years in Vienna learning scientific surgery and pathology in the best place in the world to do so. He returned to New York in 1880 to become a member of the staff at Roosevelt Hospital and Demonstrator of Anatomy at the College of Physicians and Surgeons. He had a brilliant career during the next four years in New York, introducing Listerism to a reluctant surgical community. At Bellevue Hospital, he raised $10,000 to erect a tent that became his personal operating room. The hospital's regular operating rooms were so filthy, and the other surgeons so resistant to antisepsis, that he took this extreme step to introduce sterile surgery.

Halsted's search for better ways to perform surgery led him to research on local anesthesia, cocaine, and the addiction that was to dog his life to the end. A number of the surgeons who experimented with cocaine for local anesthesia became addicts. Halsted was one, and there has been considerable speculation about its effect on his career. In the 1880s, before coming to Johns Hopkins, he has been described as a typical nineteenth century surgeon concerned with speed (even though anesthesia had reduced its benefits) and less careful of blood loss and shock. When he arrived at Johns Hopkins, he was a different surgeon, careful, meticulous about blood loss and willing to spend hours to minimize injury to tissue. The use of fine silk suture-ligatures instead of mass ligatures of catgut, as advocated by Lister, produced less tissue injury and better wound healing.

Halsted came to Johns Hopkins in December 1886, before the hospital opened, to work in Welch's pathology laboratory. There have been suggestions that his move to Baltimore may have been part of an attempt to cure his cocaine addiction. In 1889, he was appointed chief surgeon when the hospital opened and became the Professor and Surgeon-in-Chief in 1892.

Did his cocaine addiction have anything to do with his personality change? No one knows and for many years, it was believed that he had ended his use of narcotics before 1890. Since the opening of Osler's papers, fifty years after his death at the request of his will, it is now known that Halsted's addiction continued almost to the end of his life. With the assistance of his friend and colleague, Halsted controlled his addiction, substituted morphine for cocaine and continued with a brilliant career. During Cushing's subsequent surgical training under Halsted at Johns Hopkins, he presented a proposal to his chief for the study of cocaine for local anesthesia in hernia repair, one of Halsted's principle interests. Halsted was uninterested and never explained his reasons. The secret of Halsted's addiction was kept by Osler and only revealed when his papers were examined. Cushing never knew why his proposal had been turned down although he may later have suspected.

In 1894, Halsted presented a series of fifty cases of cancer of the breast for which he had devised a new operation. In ninety-three percent of these patients, there had been no local recurrence of the cancer and in seventy-three percent, there had been no recurrence of the cancer anywhere. These were dramatic results. Typical of the time, twenty-seven of the fifty women had a prognosis regarded as hopeless at the time of the surgery because of enlarged lymph nodes under the arm. In every case, there were microscopically positive lymph nodes. Previous experience with simple mastectomy by others had been uniformly bad. Billroth, the best surgeon in Europe, had local recurrence (on the chest wall or in the scar) in eighty-five percent of his cases. None of the major surgeons of Europe reported less than sixty percent local recurrence. Now Halsted, using the operation (the Halsted radical mastectomy) that would remain the standard treatment for breast cancer until the 1970s, could report only six percent local recurrence.[142] In 1907, he reported on 232 cases of breast cancer with a postoperative mortality rate of 1.7 percent and forty-two percent of the patients who could be traced were free of cancer three to five years postop. These were almost unbelievable results for the time. Sir James Paget, twenty-five years earlier had estimated the life expectancy of a woman with breast cancer at four months.[143] The Halsted radical mastectomy is rarely performed now, because we usually see patients whose cancer is in the early stages. The Halsted operation is still effective for advanced cancer although newer methods involving radiation therapy or chemotherapy, or both, have superseded its use in modern surgery.

He was the first surgeon to ligate the subclavian artery for aneurysm, opening the chest when very few surgeons could do so successfully, and led the way in methods for the gradual occlusion of aortic aneurysms, all that was available until aortic grafts were developed fifty years later. He performed the first Whipple operation for cancer of the ampulla of Vater in 1898, fifty years before the surgeon (Allan O. Whipple) whose name the operation carries performed it.[144] He drained an empyema of the gallbladder (an obstructed gallbladder full of pus) in 1882, one of the first gallbladder surgeries in the United States, on his mother at two o'clock in the morning as she lay near death! She recovered.[145] In 1881, he transfused his own sister, after a postpartum hemorrhage, with his own blood and she survived.

In 1889, he reported the successful cure of inguinal hernia. Previous experience had produced a recurrence rate of twenty-seven percent to forty percent within one year. Ignorance of the anatomy of inguinal hernia was at fault and Halsted learned how to achieve a permanent cure by repairing the critical layers of the abdominal wall. Bassini, in Italy, had arrived at almost the same operation at the same time and Halsted generously gives him credit in his own publication of his method.[146] Halsted died in 1922 of complications after a common bile duct exploration for stones and biliary sepsis.

PEDIATRIC SURGERY

Appendicitis and hernia are the two most common surgical conditions of childhood. Tracheostomy for diphtheria was another common procedure in the nineteenth century, but the use of immune serum had nearly eliminated this threat by World War I. The third most common surgical condition in children is pyloric stenosis, a narrowing of the outlet of the stomach that occurs at about two months of age. The pathology was first described by Hirschprung in 1888.[147] The usual first symptom, at about two months of age in a previously healthy child, is "spitting up" followed by vomiting of almost everything eaten. The vomiting is often described as "projectile" and no bile is present in the material vomited. The child gradually loses weight, keeping down only clear fluids, and dies by age eighteen months or two years of starvation. The development of gastrointestinal surgery in Europe offered little or no relief from this scourge (three babies per 1,000 are affected and boys outnumber girls by four to one) until Conrad Ramstedt, in 1912, discovered a successful approach.[148]

Attempts to enlarge the pyloric channel, the passage connecting stomach and duodenum, had all failed because the obstruction, unlike that of peptic ulcer, is due to tremendous thickening of the muscle of the bowel wall.[149] It is still unknown why this occurs. Early attempts at treatment included gastric lavage with a tube, invented by Professor Kussmaul in 1866 and successful in some cases of obstruction from ulcer disease, even today. Gastroenterostomy (connecting stomach to small bowel bypassing the obstruction) was attempted in 1897 by Carl Stern of Düsseldorf but the size disparity between dilated stomach and collapsed small intestine doomed this approach in most cases.[150] Nicoll tried to dilate the narrowed pylorus through a gastrotomy (opening the stomach to insert an instrument), using a forceps to stretch the channel from inside and came close to discovering the correct procedure. His dilatation of the pylorus from the inside tore open the hypertrophied muscle that was constricting the channel and, in 1904, he noted that the tearing of the thickened muscle helped to relieve the obstruction. Still, he did not recognize what was happening and used gastroenterostomy in addition to the stretching procedure. He did have six survivors in nine cases using this method.[151]

Others were not so successful and the use of Nicoll's technique lapsed. Gastroenterostomy was technically difficult when the stomach was hugely dilated and the small bowel collapsed and underdeveloped. Mickulicz attempted his procedure, in which the pylorus is incised longitudinally and the incision is closed transversely, called pyloroplasty. This procedure usually failed because the hypertrophied muscle was too stiff to close transversely and the sutures pulled out. Still, twenty-five such procedures had a sixty percent survival rate. By 1907, gastroenterostomy had resulted in fifty-three percent mortality in sixty-four operations, out of the 134 cases reported in which some attempt at correction was attempted. Ramstedt tried to treat one of his cases with a pyloroplasty, but, when the sutures pulled out, he left the muscle incision open and covered the bare layer of mucus membrane with omentum (the fatty apron suspended from the colon). The child recovered. In his next attempt, he cut through the thickened muscle, but did not open the mucosa into the bowel lumen. He left the muscle incision open again and made no attempt at pyloroplasty. This child also recovered. Today, we routinely use Ramstedt's operation for this condition. My mother's older brother, George, died of pyloric stenosis in Chicago in 1897, the year before she was born. He had lived almost two years. The cure was still fifteen years in the future.

In 1910, Dr. William E. Ladd joined the staff of Children's Hospital in Boston. Over the next thirty years, he would devise operations to correct other major surgical conditions of childhood, most of them due to failures of fetal development. They include atresia (failure of a hollow structure to fully develop) of the esophagus, in which the esophagus does not reach the stomach and, in the most common version of the anomaly, the lower esophageal segment attaches instead to the lung. In this condition, the child is unable to swallow, as the esophagus ends blindly, but the stomach is connected to the trachea allowing gastric juice to flood the lung. He classified the different forms of the condition and reported the frequency of the variations in his report of the first successful repairs in 1944.[152] The first child to survive a direct repair of the most common variation of this condition was operated upon by Haight in 1941.[153] Bob Replogle described a double-lumen catheter, used to keep the upper blind pouch of esophagus empty of saliva, in 1963 and this helped to prevent pneumonia while the child was prepared for surgery. Primary repair was quite difficult and often impossible because the two segments of esophagus were separated and pulling them together caused too much tension on the repair.

In 1966, William Snyder used the suction tube to stretch the upper pouch, by pushing down on it, until it would reach the lower esophageal segment.[154] With this innovation, repair of tracheo-esophageal fistula has had much improved results. It is now standard treatment in cases with a significant distance between upper and lower ends of the esophagus. The usual course is immediate gastrostomy to prevent aspiration of gastric contents followed by primary repair of the esophagus once the upper blind pouch has been stretched sufficiently. This takes only a few weeks to accomplish and results are good if preoperative pneumonia is avoided.

In 1928, Ladd repaired an obstructed common bile duct in an infant, a condition called biliary atresia.[155] Holmes, at Johns Hopkins in 1916, had classified the condition, first described by Hirschprung in 1888. Holmes reported that sixteen percent of cases had patent bile ducts outside the liver and could, in theory, be corrected by surgery.[156] In 1932, Ladd performed his second successful correction of biliary atresia.[157] Thirty-five years later, in Los Angeles, I took care of that patient during my internship. He had become an alcoholic and came to the Los Angeles County Hospital with jaundice, thought to be due to alcoholic liver disease. He gave the history of an operation when he was an infant but no one had ever bothered to check on the nature of that operation. I called the hospital in Worchester, Massachusetts where he was born and obtained the records. He had been Ladd's second successful repair of biliary atresia (at age two months) and we operated on him a few days later for bile duct obstruction related to the old condition.

Improvements in anesthesia, in particular, would allow increasing success in correcting these devastating congenital defects. Kasai, in 1968, described a new approach for the eighty-four percent of cases of biliary

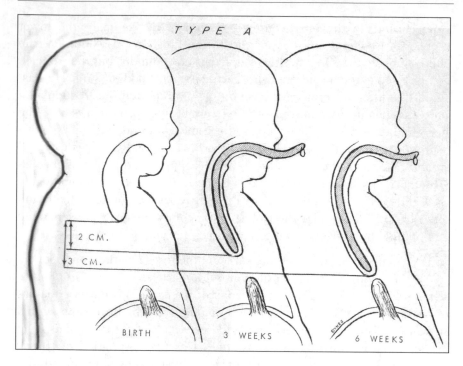

Figure 9 – Illustration from 1966 paper by Hays, Wooley and Snyder showing stretching of the upper pouch in an esophageal atresia. This anatomy is less common than the cases with a fistula connecting the lower segment to the trachea. The procedure is the same in fistula cases. From Journal of Pediatric Surgery, 1966.

atresia without adequate extrahepatic ducts.[158] His operation connects the tiny bile ducts within the liver to the small intestine; William Longmire developed a similar procedure in 1948 for bile duct injuries in adults. This is the most common surgical procedure performed in biliary atresia at present. The operation must be performed in the first months of life as the condition is now understood to be an autoimmune disease and the tiny bile ducts, if not attached to the intestine soon enough, disappear. Liver transplantation has become more popular as techniques improved and it has become apparent that the obliteration of bile ducts continues in spite of the Kasai procedure.

In 1938, Robert Gross, who had taken Dr. Ladd's place at Children's Hospital, performed the first successful division of a patent ductus arteriosus. It will be discussed in the chapter on cardiac surgery. Pediatric surgery picked up steam once the problems of caring for small children with critical illness were worked out after the Second World War.

NEUROSURGERY AND HARVEY CUSHING

In October of 1896, Cushing arrived at Johns Hopkins from Boston to be an assistant resident in surgery under Halsted. He was to remain for thirteen years as Halsted's greatest disciple and a towering figure in American, indeed in world, medicine. At first, Cushing was struck by the change in atmosphere from the Massachusetts General Hospital. Here all was quiet science instead of "the hurly, burley of the MGH." He knew little of pathology and bacteriology. Halsted was so shy and retiring that he would ask permission of the resident to examine his own patient. Elliot Cutler, a friend of Cushing's and later to be another famous professor of surgery, described Cushing's reaction to his first patient to be operated on after his arrival. It was a mastectomy and, as hours went by, Cushing began to fear the worst. MGH surgeons still operated in the old, pre-anesthetic fashion, with speed the primary concern. Halsted was meticulous, minimizing blood loss and shock, and might take five hours to perform a mastectomy, as he did this first day of Cushing's residency.

When the patient returned to the ward, Cushing was ready with the restoratives of the time, including strychnine and the Trendelenberg (head down) position for shock. As Cushing prepared to inject a syringe of strychnine, Halsted asked, "Is my patient ill? This is unusual. Let us examine her." The patient's pulse and respiration were normal. Halsted asked, "What is in the syringe?" Cushing replied, "Strychnine. It will do her good." Halsted then asked the young resident what the strychnine would do for the patient. Cushing didn't know. He was just doing what he had been taught at the MGH. Halsted asked him to read up on strychnine and added, "If your reading convinces you that strychnine is good for the patient, by all means use it." Johns Hopkins was a very different place from what Cushing was used to and he never did give the strychnine.[159]

The hospital had one of the first x-ray machines in North America and Cushing spent some time operating the machine and learning to take x-rays. On November 6, 1896, Lizzie W. was admitted with a gunshot wound of the neck. She showed paralysis on one side of her body and loss of feeling on the other, the Brown-Sequard syndrome already described in cases of spinal cord injury in which the cord is cut half-way across. This classic syndrome demonstrates features of neuroanatomy in which some spinal nerve pathways cross to the opposite side at the level they enter the cord and others continue up toward the brain on the same side. Cushing took an x-ray of her neck and demonstrated the bullet in her spinal canal. He reported this case at the May 3, 1897 meeting of the Johns Hopkins Medical Society. This was his first contact with neurosurgery. A year later, he was offered the senior residency position and wrote to his father, also a physician, that a year's experience had shown him the superiority of the Johns Hopkins system. In 1897, Cushing, himself, developed acute appendicitis and Halsted performed the operation, still new enough to be controversial. Cushing, with his characteristic thoroughness, wrote up his own medical history and composed a poem for the children on the ward who had also been subjected to ether anesthesia and the operation.

CUSHING AND KOCHER

In 1900, Cushing, having completed his residency, spent a year in Europe for further study. He was still undecided on a specialty but chose men who were working in neurology as mentors during his year abroad. He settled in Berne to work in the clinic of Theodore Kocher, whose writings on spinal cord injury had attracted Cushing's attention. Kocher became famous as a thyroid surgeon but his interests were wide. Cushing found his personality much like that of Halsted, "careful, painstaking." Kocher had attracted thousands of patients with goiter, a common affliction in Switzerland with its iodine-poor soil. Unfortunately he had discovered the parathyroid glands by removing them with the thyroid, resulting in tetany (severe muscle spasms), and was careful to leave part of the thyroid gland behind after those early experiences. He had also learned the other consequence of total thyroidectomy when one of his early patients developed myxedema. Myxedema is a condition, caused by hypothyroidism, in which the patient becomes mentally dull, slow, with coarse skin, and feels cold all the time. In children, it is called "cretinism" and results in slow growth and mental retardation. Treatment with thyroid hormone, at first a crude extract of the gland, would solve this problem.

Cushing's journal contrasts the careful, quiet Kocher with the flamboyant Cesar Roux, a more theatrical operator concerned with speed and drama. Roux was a leader in gastrointestinal surgery and developed the technique of bypass called "Roux en Y," in which a loop of bowel, rearranged in a "Y" configuration, is used to divert intestinal flow. Roux's procedure is still a standard operation one hundred years later. Cushing asked Kocher to propose a research project for his fellowship and the suggestion was a subject that would change surgery and dominate the rest of Cushing's career. He was to study, with professor Kronecker a physiologist in Berne, the effect of changes in intracranial pressure on the brain. Berne was filled with memories of other great physiologists from Haller, the greatest of the early physiologists who studied the changes in his own pulse as he died in 1777, to Helmholz and Ludwig. Kronecker's laboratory was in the Hallerianum, the institute founded by Haller. Preliminary experiments in Kronecker's lab concerned nerve-muscle physiology in a frog-leg preparation and Cushing demonstrated the effects of sodium chloride, calcium chloride and potassium. The results were published in the American Journal of Physiology in 1901. His work on Kocher's project was also successful and showed that, as intracranial pressure is increased, blood pressure increases, and respiration decreases. If intracranial pressure exceeds arterial blood pressure, the animal dies. This work established the auto-regulatory control of blood pressure and is essential in the treatment of head injury.

THE BEGINNING OF NEUROSURGERY

The treatment of head injury during the American Civil War was limited to timid attempts to remove bone fragments from skull fractures and very tentative efforts to probe for hematomas. The majority of head injuries were from bullet wounds. General Henry Shrapnel, who invented artillery shells that contained metal balls in a hollow outer shell, died in 1842. His invention, when it exploded, sent metal fragments flying through the air and into soldiers' bodies, but it was little used until World War I. Modern artillery shells do not follow his design, using a thick casing that is scored to fragment, but the term is used for these fragments and has become universal. Of 408,000 Civil War injuries described by Surgeon General Joseph K Barnes, 245,790 were from gunshot wounds. 13,000 head injuries were listed with 4,350 wounds to the skull. 220 cases had surgical opening of the skull, trephination. Of these fifty-six percent died. There were 487 survivors of some sort of surgical procedure for head injuries, not all gunshot wounds. This was the largest experience with head injury in the world since the introduction of anesthesia and, considering the general experience with surgery at the time, is respectable.[160] Cushing was to make enormous progress in the next thirty years with a scientific approach to brain surgery.

After completion of his work for Kocher, Cushing traveled to Italy where he studied a group of patients with skull defects and published another article on the regulation of blood pressure. In Venice, he visited the school of Vesalius and Fabricius and here he learned of the blood pressure apparatus of Professor Riva-Rocci. During a visit to Germany, he encountered the recent development of Teutonic arrogance, which had begun to discourage Americans from studying there. Florence Nightingale mourned the domination of the romantic and artistic Germans she loved by the Prussians who, following the 1870 Franco-Prussian War, had altered the nature of

German society in ways that would bring disaster in the next century. In 1901, Cushing spent time with Professor Sherrington, in Liverpool, who had been working on localization of functions in the brain. Sherrington was rather disorganized and Cushing's collaboration was valuable in several respects, one of which was performing a craniotomy on a gorilla so Sherrington could map its cerebral functions. In 1909, Cushing was to report on similar experiments on conscious patients who experienced sensations when areas of the temporal lobe were stimulated during craniotomy.

Cushing returned to Baltimore in September 1901, continued his studies of neurosurgery and introduced the Riva-Rocci blood pressure apparatus, with his own improvements, to the medical world. By 1903, his friend Councilman had taken the apparatus to Harvard and it was a required part of physical examination. Cushing established the "Hunterian Laboratory" of experimental surgery at Johns Hopkins and was deluged with requests from medical students who wanted to participate. One of the early topics to be studied was the use of physiologic saline solution in intravenous infusion. Sidney Ringer had shown that sodium chloride and water alone would not support muscle and nerve function. Other salts, as shown in Cushing's experiments in Berne, must be added.

By 1903, Cushing was operating on brain tumors and treating tic doloreaux by percutaneous injection of the trigeminal nucleus with good success. In 1905, W.W. Keen asked him to write a chapter on surgery of the brain for his new *American Textbook of Surgery*, the same edition that contained Murphy's chapter on appendicitis. In 1910, Cushing removed a huge meningioma from the brain of General Leonard Wood, Chief of Staff of the Army and later Governor of the Philippines. The general recovered nicely from this major operation but Cushing had made an error in replacing the bone flap of skull. Ten years later the meningioma had recurred and, during an operation to remove the tumor in 1923, bleeding into a cerebral ventricle occurred and General Wood succumbed postoperatively. Cushing was very distressed that this very early surgery in his career had failed to cure the tumor. Of course, few surgeons in the world would have been capable of performing the first surgery successfully and the realization that he should not have replaced the bone flap was the product of his enormous experience in the interval between the two operations.

By the time of his death in 1939, Cushing had personally operated on 2,000 cases of brain tumor, of which one half were then living. He kept track of his patients by asking them to send him a postcard on the anniversary of their operation each year. If he did not get a postcard, he investigated the circumstances. His records continued to be maintained after his death as the Cushing Brain Tumor Registry and established the outcome of neurosurgical procedures for the entire profession.

CUSHING AND ELECTROSURGERY

Electrical current was used by urological surgeons and others as early as 1911. The devices used were called diathermy machines and function by generating heat. The method is still in use in dermatology offices for the removal of warts and other small skin lesions. It is another form of cautery, which goes back to the Arabs and to Ambrose Paré. The problem of hemorrhage presented a barrier to removal of brain tumors from the beginning. The brain is very soft, almost the consistency of jello, and the blood vessels are correspondingly delicate. The flow of blood through the brain is high, nearly twenty-five percent of the cardiac output, and tearing one of the small, fragile vessels within the brain or in the inaccessible space beneath it, would often result in a fatal outcome. In 1910, Cushing invented the silver clip, to be applied with a forceps to the blood vessel, and which does not require tying a knot. This allowed deeper access to the brain but did not completely solve the problem. In 1925, he became interested in the use of electric current to control the hemorrhage that prevented removal of vascular brain and spinal cord tumors. At an American Medical Association meeting in June of 1925, Cushing watched a demonstration of diathermy on a piece of meat and two physicians with him suggested, in a jocular fashion, that he should apply the technique to brain tumors. Instead of laughing, he looked thoughtful. In Boston he was aware of Dr. W. L. Clark's work using diathermy to remove cancer.[161] Cushing by this time had moved to the Peter Bent Brigham Hospital in Boston and he decided to investigate the use of electrocautery in neurosurgery.

The Harvard Cancer Commission included a professor of physics from Philadelphia, W.T. Bovie. Cushing met with Bovie and invited him to develop better applications of his current generators. The devices generated two forms of current: a coagulating current with a frequency of greater than one megahertz and a cutting current, which used a resonating circuit to increase amperage. With further development, the newer devices we are familiar with use even higher frequencies close to those of radio transmission; hence, the output is called radiofrequency or "RF" current. The machines invented by Bovie used a pencil-like electrode held by the surgeon and a neutral electrode, much larger in area, adherent to the patient's skin at a location away from the surgical site. The coagulating current used higher voltage and produced more heat at the site and adjacent to it. On

October 1, 1926, Cushing brought back to the operating room a patient whose tumor had been impossible to remove due to hemorrhage at the first operation. The operation was described by Cushing as "a perfect circus" with many observers from the New England Surgical Association plus foreign observers ("four or five coughing Frenchmen"). The medical student who was present to act as a possible blood donor fainted and fell off his stool in the operating room. In spite of all this, the operation was a success. He was still worried about the effect of the device on the brain (this tumor was extra-cranial) and feared convulsions from electrical stimulation of the brain. His fears proved unfounded.

Cushing turned the device over to the Liebel-Flarsheim Company to build a commercial version. He called back all his patients with inoperable meningiomas and the pace for the next year was almost intolerable. Hugh Cairns became Cushing's resident in 1926 and averaged five hours of sleep a night for the next year. Cairns had been practicing general surgery at the London Hospital since 1921 and had some experience with neurosurgery, as many general surgeons at the time did. On September 1, 1926 Cairns had arrived in Boston on a one-year fellowship. Within two years of returning to London Cairns, because of his mammoth experience with Cushing, was the leading neurosurgeon in London and by 1937 was the first Nuffield Professor of Surgery at Oxford.[162] He deemed his year with Cushing more demanding than his service at Gallipoli as a private or, after completing his medical training in 1916-17, at the battle of the Marne in World War I. Cairns later summarized his year of experience with Cushing; the year after the coagulating current became available. Three hundred sixty-nine patients with suspected brain tumors were admitted (more than one a day). 157 cases were verified of whom 135 were discharged alive after operation and twenty-two died. Eight years later sixty-three were still alive and thirty-seven were wage earners.[163] The adoption of electrosurgery allowed a quantum leap in neurosurgical treatment.

Few surgeons are familiar with the history of the device still referred to as "the Bovie," which is used every day by every surgeon in every operating room in the world, although newer solid-state machines have replaced Professor Bovie's vacuum tubes and refrigerator-sized machine. Cairns went on to a long and distinguished career in neurosurgery, including service in World War II. In 1935, he operated on T.E. Lawrence (Lawrence of Arabia), after the motorcycle accident that eventually took his life, and in 1945, he treated General George S. Patton for a broken neck suffered in a jeep accident. General Patton had a spinal cord injury making him quadriplegic and succumbed to a pulmonary embolus within a few weeks of his injury. Cairns died in 1952 of intestinal lymphoma at the young age of fifty-six.

Harvey Cushing retired from Harvard in 1933 and returned to Yale where he continued to publish scholarly works until his death in 1939. In progress and nearly complete at his death was his biography and bibliography of Andreas Vesalius. It was completed and published by friends in 1943. In his last years, he was director of studies in the history of medicine at Yale. In addition to his enormous accomplishments in medicine he and his wife Kate produced three daughters who were among the most beautiful and famous women in the world. His daughter Betsey married James Roosevelt, the President's son, Mary Benedict married Vincent Astor of the legendary New York famly, and Barbara, known all her life as "Babe," married William Paley, founder of CBS. She is still known for her quip "You can never be too rich or too thin." Fortunately for humanity, her father did not take her advice and spent his life in service to his fellow man. A biography of Babe Paley sniffs that her father was "an eminent but not extraordinarily wealthy Boston brain surgeon." That seems to have been enough.

SURGERY OF THE CHEST

The physiology of lung function was not understood until this century. Andreas Vesalius had opened the chest of living animals and kept them alive by blowing air into the trachea through a tube. The Royal Humane Society adopted John Hunter's method of artificial respiration, which used a bellows attached to the nostrils. In 1827, Leroy demonstrated that forcing air into the lungs could rupture them and the practice of positive pressure ventilation ceased for years.[164] John Snow, in his research on anesthesia in 1858, used endotrachial tubes in rabbits, placed through a tracheotomy. A few others used endotrachial anesthesia, usually involving tracheostomy. In 1890, George Fell, of Buffalo, used an endotrachial device, designed by another physician named O'Dwyer, attached to a bellows to treat cases of diphtheria, croup, and even opium poisoning.[165] The method was used in the animal laboratory but not in surgical cases. Opening the chest was fraught with hazard because of pneumothorax (collapse of the lung), a catastrophe poorly understood.

Rudolph Matas, a well-known New Orleans surgeon, adopted the Fell-O'Dwyer apparatus for an operation to remove a chest wall sarcoma. He reported that the apparatus immediately corrected the lung collapse. In spite of this experience, positive pressure ventilation was not adopted.[166] The invention of the bronchoscope, by Killian in 1897,[167] improved the clinical diagnosis of lung diseases but therapy, at least surgical therapy, would have to wait until the surgeon learned to open the chest without killing the patient. In 1903, Ferdinand Sauerbruch, at the suggestion of his chief von Mickulicz, began to work on the problem of pneumothorax. Sauerbruch built a low-pressure chamber that would contain the patient and the surgery team with the patient's head sticking out the side of the chamber where the anesthetist would sit and administer ether. With the pressure inside the chamber approximately the same as normal intrathoracic pressure, about ten centimeters of water lower than outside atmospheric pressure, the patient's lungs would not collapse when the chest was opened. The patient, under anesthesia, was able to breathe with the head outside the chamber in normal air pressure. He tried his chamber on dogs and it was a success. Using Sauerbruch's chamber, von Mickulicz successfully removed a chest tumor.[168] The chamber, soon duplicated in hospitals all over the world, had many disadvantages although the surgeon and the other members of the surgical team had no difficulty breathing in the reduced pressure. Willie Meyer, of New York's German Hospital (today Lennox Hill Hospital) built a chamber that held fifteen people, but most were small and cramped.

The invention of the endotrachial tube, by Meltzer and Auer in 1909[169,170] (its use was limited until the direct laryngoscope) and devices for positive pressure ventilation through these tubes with vaporization of the ether for anesthesia, made the chambers unnecessary (See the chapter on Anesthesia and Critical Care Medicine) but Sauerbruch and other Europeans continued their use until World War II. The endotrachial tube continued to be a problem even though Chevalier Jackson invented the direct laryngoscope in 1907.[171] This allowed insertion of the tube under direct vision and avoided intubation of the esophagus, which had, and still has, fatal consequences. It took later developments in anesthesia before endotracheal tubes became standard. Roentgen's discovery of x-ray created a completely new field once the problems of thoracotomy were solved. The story continues in Chapter 20.

INFLUENZA AND THE EMPYEMA COMMISSION

Real understanding of the physiology of the lung came with the U.S. Army Empyema Commission, chaired by Evarts Graham, which studied the influenza epidemic that began during World War I. Many of the deaths from influenza followed drainage of empyema, a collection of pus or infected fluid in the chest around the lung. If the empyema was truly pus, open drainage, simply making a hole in the chest or placing a rubber drain to drain the fluid, was well tolerated. Sometimes, especially if the fluid proved to be thin and watery with little or no gross pus, the opening of the chest resulted in collapse of the lung and death. Thus, many mild cases of empyema died, but the worst cases survived. Why should this be?

Lester Dragstedt, later a professor of surgery at the University of Chicago, was a young Army pathologist during the War. He performed autopsies on young men who had died of influenza, usually complicated by a streptococcus empyema. He asked the surgeons why they had not drained the empyema, which seemed to be compressing the lungs, and was told that it was impossible because the patients died within a half hour of opening the chest. Finally, the Graham Commission found that, in cases of frank empyema, the lung had become adherent to the chest wall and would not collapse if the pleural cavity was opened. In cases where the fluid was not pus but only an effusion of clear serum, or if the lung was not adherent to the chest wall, it would collapse unless "water seal" was used. Water seal is a system to prevent air from entering the chest through the tube. The chest tube is connected to a long rubber tube. The long tube extends from the patient in bed to a bottle on the floor. The end of the tubing is placed beneath the surface of water in the bottle. When the patient inhales and the pressure inside the chest is less than atmospheric, water is sucked up into the tubing a short distance. When the patient exhales, the water returns to the bottle along with any air leaking from the lung or fluid draining from the chest. This simple device, once the physiology of respiration was understood, solved the problem of pneumothorax. This discovery, that the normal relative vacuum between the lung and the chest wall must be maintained, was to save many lives in coming years. Hippocrates had anticipated this phenomenon 2500 years ago.

LUNG RESECTION

In 1928, Brunn reported six cases of lung lobectomy for bronchiectasis. There were a few pneumonectomies (removal of an entire lung) for tuberculosis, but these cases involved inflammation, which obliterated the pulmonary artery, making the operation little more than debriding necrotic tissue. In the early 1930s, several cases of two-stage pneumonectomy were performed; in this operation the hilum (the "root" of the lung through which pass the vessels) was ligated, but the lung was not removed until later when it had shriveled to a small prune-like remnant. Finally, in 1933, Evarts Graham removed the first human lung, in one stage, for cancer, ushering in the new era of thoracic surgery. The patient in this first case was a forty-eight-year-old physician named Gilmore who continued his practice of obstetrics and gynecology for more than twenty years after the operation. When Graham died in 1957 (of lung cancer), his patient was still alive and attended his funeral.

Vascular Surgery

The first vascular procedures were attempts to repair injuries. John B. Murphy successfully repaired a brachial artery injury in 1897 before Carrel's research that resulted in the award of the 1912 Nobel Prize. Carrel described the circular suture technique still in use with small arteries. Prior to World War II most arterial injuries resulted in amputation although a few tolerated ligation without loss of limb. Repair was almost unknown. In World War II, the principle problem was the delay between wounding and access to surgical care. A study in the Mediterranean Theater showed that the time lag between wounding and arrival at the field hospital (put as close to front lines as possible) was twelve and a half hours. DeBakey, in his report on arterial injuries, expressed doubt that this could ever be improved.[172] He reported a sixty-two percent amputation rate for lower extremity arterial injuries and this increased to eighty-two percent when the injury was above the profunda femoris (near the groin) branch of the femoral artery. Upper extremity amputation rate was twenty-six percent. They reported only eighty-one arterial repairs in 2,471 injuries.

In Korea, the use of the helicopter in evacuation of casualties markedly decreased this critical time. Reported series from the war included 304 major vascular injuries with 269 repairs and a thirteen percent amputation rate for cases in which repair was attempted. Autogenous vein graft, using the patient's own saphenous vein, had the best results.[173] In Viet Nam, surgeons with vascular surgery training reduced the amputation rate still more. In his summary of the vascular surgery experience in Viet Nam, Norman Rich[174] reported only fifteen ligations of injured arteries in the first 4,000 cases of arterial injury. Repairs were accomplished, in the first series of 1,000 cases reported by Rich, using vein grafts in 45.9 percent, end-to-end repair in 37.7 percent and a variety of miscellaneous proce-dures in the other cases. Wounds involving the lower extremity made up fifty-seven percent of the cases and the overall amputation rate was thirteen percent including late complications. This was tremendous progress in twenty-five years.

Aortic aneurysm was recognized by the ancients and John Hunter pro-posed ligation for peripheral (in the limbs) aneurysms. Hunter success-fully performed this procedure for a popliteal aneurysm, a feat described earlier. Rudolph Matas provided a monograph on aneurysm for W.W. Keen's *American Textbook of Surgery* in 1909, and this remained the standard reference until after World War II. Early attempts at control of aneurysms revolved around ligation. Matas learned that simple ligation was not enough, one must open the sac of the aneurysm and ligate all branches entering it or recurrence should be expected.[175] This, of course, was usually not an option with aortic aneurysms and attempts to thrombose the aortic aneurysm with wire coils or other measures were the only treatment available until the 1950s. Correction of coarctation of the aorta (a congenital condition in children) by Gross and Crafoord, described later, revived interest in surgery on the aorta. In 1940, Rene Leriche described a syndrome in which a male patient has pain in the limbs with walking, commonly has atrophy of the legs and is impotent. The patients, all but one in his report males, have absent femoral pulses.[176] He recommended resection of the thrombosed segment of aorta and lumbar sympathectomy. He commented that the ideal treatment would be the interposition of a graft to restore continuity but that was impossible at the time. An English language version of his report was published in 1948[177] but there had been no progress in therapy since the original. Hufnagel[178] and Gross studied the use of homografts for aortic replacement.[179] Various synthetic grafts were studied and a few were implanted in patients with poor results until DeBakey introduced the use of knitted Dacron grafts in 1958.[180]

Buerger described a type of gangrene of the legs, in 1908,[181] which involved young people of Polish or Jewish descent and seemed to be most severe in the distal small vessels of the leg. He reported that veins were also involved and that he could differentiate the disease from arteriosclerosis. Sympathectomy was advocated for ischemic legs after a report on lumbar sympathectomy, (removing the sympathetic nerve ganglia, which interrupts the sympathetic nervous system's vasoconstriction effect) in 1924, showed that the leg was warmer after the procedure.[182,183] The practice continued until recent times but declined after reconstructive surgery became possible. In 1950, Edinburgh surgeon James Learmonth performed a lumbar sympathectomy on King George VI at Buckingham Palace. The King recovered and bestowed a knighthood on the surgeon.

There has been doubt about the clinical significance of Beurger's observations although, for many years, all peripheral gangrene was attributed to this condition. As angiography and reconstruction of peripheral vascular disease became possible, the number of cases of true Beurger's disease has declined until there is doubt that the disease exists. Occlusion in larger vessels was ignored until Leriche's papers and, in 1951, Kunlin described the use of saphenous vein, reversed and transplanted, to bypass obstruction of the femoral artery.[184] Robert Linton soon adopted this method and it remains the standard approach to treatment of leg ischemia when aortic obstruction is not present or has been corrected.

In 1964, Dotter and Judkins introduced a method of dilating the femoral artery with a Teflon balloon catheter.[185] They reported good results with femoral artery stenosis, but their technique was not widely used in the United States although it did have some vogue in Europe. In 1978, Gruntzig adapted their technique to coronary artery disease, which will be described in the section on cardiac surgery. In recent years, the technique of balloon dilatation of peripheral arteries has become popular although restenosis in the leg vessels has limited its use. The development of arterial stents, which prevent restenosis after balloon dilatation, has led to wide use of the combination of angioplasty and stent placement for treatment of iliac artery disease.

Lesions of the carotid artery were next to be approached and in 1954, Eastcott reported successful correction of internal carotid artery stenosis producing intermittent neurological symptoms.[186] This operation remained controversial well into the 1970s when the work of Strandness and others provided satisfactory noninvasive screening tests to determine the natural history of the disease.[187]

THE FOGARTY CATHETER

In 1961, I was a medical student at the University of Southern California listening to a lecture on the arterial system. Mention was made of the problem of arterial embolus. A pulmonary embolus is a clot that originates in a vein, usually in the legs, and travels up in the blood flow until it passes through the heart and lodges in the lung. Once it goes through the heart, it becomes an arterial embolus (The pulmonary artery carries dark, venous blood but is still an artery). An arterial embolus is a blood clot (rarely another object like a bullet) that travels in the arterial system, pushed along by the flow of blood. The arteries keep branching and the branches keep getting smaller until the next branch is smaller than the embolus. At this point, the clot lodges like a cork in a bottle, shutting off flow beyond that point. The embolus (except a pulmonary embolus, which is a special case) usually originates in the heart and may travel anywhere in the system, depending on the volume of flow to direct it. Clots to the brain produce strokes and there is usually nothing that can be done about them except prevention(although that may change soon). Clots that go to the legs are reachable, but in 1961, the treatment was cumbersome and ineffective. We were taught that the only chance for removal was to open an artery at the ankle below the obstruction, the posterior tibial branch, and attempt to flush the clot back up toward the femoral artery at the groin.

The femoral artery was also opened and, if the clot could be flushed out this way, there was a chance of saving the leg. If the posterior tibial artery could not be flushed or the clot had gone down another branch, the leg would be lost. This was no trivial problem as leg emboli are common.

Tom Fogarty had already invented several non-medical devices (including a motorcycle clutch) and worked as a hospital operating room technician while still in high school. Fogarty's father, a railroad mechanic, died when Tom was young and the boy began working at an early age. In the eighth grade, he got a job in the central supply department of Good Samaritan Hospital in Cincinnati, Ohio. After working his way up to operating room "tech," he watched the futile efforts of surgeons to remove leg emboli. John Cranley, later a very well known vascular surgeon, hired Fogarty as his personal scrub tech. It occurred to Fogarty that a thin catheter, with a small balloon at the tip, could be inserted into the artery above the clot, pushed through the clot with the balloon deflated, then, with the balloon inflated, pulled back bringing the clot with it. He arrived at this concept while still a medical student at the University of Cincinnati and actually made a few crude prototypes using ureteral (thin) catheters and small balloons made from cut-off rubber glove fingertips. He tied the glove tip to the catheter using fly-tying methods and practiced pulling a blood clot out of a test tube.

He began an internship at the University of Oregon in 1960, but returned to Cincinnati for a year of fellowship with Dr. Cranley in 1961. For a year, Fogarty made his own catheters, working on the rubber balloon especially, and Cranley used them on his patients. In 1963, they reported this new device in the surgical literature and revolutionized vascular surgery. The first report was rejected by several surgery journals and finally published in the *Journal of Obstetrics and Gynecology*, in a section called "Surgeon at Work." Three years later, with further experience, the next paper was accepted by a major journal.[188] In 1962, Fogarty returned to complete his surgical residency at Oregon and, after encountering considerable difficulty in persuading device manufacturers to make his catheters, he was introduced to Lowell Edwards. Edwards had started a company to make heart valves. (See Chapter 19). His company began to make Fogarty catheters in 1963 and the revolution followed. Now, it was possible to remove arterial emboli with a high degree of certainty that the leg would be saved. Over the next twenty-nine years, millions of these catheters were used and new applications of the concept would be devised all over the world. His was the first of the balloon catheters in vascular disease. Others would not be long in coming. Fogarty, after a research fellowship at the National

Institutes of Health, moved on to Stanford in 1969 for training in cardiac surgery.[189] He remains a clinical professor at Stanford today.

ERNEST AMORY CODMAN AND MODERN SURGERY

Amory Codman was a classmate of Harvey Cushing's at Harvard and participated in the development of the anesthesia record. He also became, shortly after graduation from Harvard, one of the first American "skiagraphers," as early radiologists were called. Codman and Cushing experimented with one of the first Roentgen tubes in North America at the Massachusetts General Hospital, prior to Cushing's move to Baltimore. Codman obtained a larger Roentgen tube in 1896, after Cushing left, and began cooperation with Walter Cannon, the great Harvard physiologist. Two years later, he published his work in the pioneering of x-ray application to patient care.[190] Much of his work concerned the function of joints. Over the next ten years, Codman became interested in shoulder disorders and modern orthopedics began here with his systematic studies. In 1900, for example, he published the first analysis, with a system of classification, of Colles' (wrist) fracture based on x-rays. He did not limit himself to orthopedics and the first detailed description of duodenal ulcer was another of his projects.[191]

In 1902, he began a series of works on what came to be known as the "End Result Method," a study of the outcome of treatment by various means. Florence Nightingale and John Snow had pioneered epidemiology and the statistical study of infections. Codman now applied the same methods to the results of surgery. This subject was to cause him enormous trouble, as other surgeons were very resistant to systematic analysis of the results of their operations. Florence Nightingale had preceded Codman in the concept of outcomes research (as we now call it) with "A Proposal for Improved Statistics of Surgical Operations." Codman was the first surgeon to take up her suggestion.

Medical education at the turn of the century was without any uniform standards and hundreds of medical schools, supported by tuition and lacking in scientific approach, covered the United States. In 1909, there were 155 medical schools in the United States and Canada. Only fifty of them required any college education of applicants and only sixteen of those required at least two years. In 1911, Abraham Flexner, mentioned in the section on polio, visited every North American medical school and published a report on their curriculum and academic standards. He recommended that only thirty-one medical schools remain in business. Codman fully supported Flexner and extended his concerns to the performance of surgeons in hospital practice. He recommended that every patient admitted to the hospital be followed to determine the results of any surgical procedure performed. This suggestion was unpopular with his colleagues.

Codman became interested in the theories of Frederick Taylor, an efficiency expert on industrial plants and manufacturing, who founded the field of "Systems Engineering." Frank Gilbreth was another pioneer in what came to be called "time and motion" studies. In a bit of self-promotion Gilbreth named the basic unit of performance a "therblig," his own name spelled backwards. A therblig is the most elementary movement which, when combined with all the other steps, constitutes an action or a process. Gilbreth began his studies with an analysis of bricklaying, the movement of material and the minimizing of excess effort. He used photographs of work activity to study the steps of a process. The Charlie Chaplin movie "Modern Times" parodies the Gilbreth system as the little tramp spends his days tightening a single nut on thousands of machines passing by on an assembly line. Time and motion studies were overdone in manufacturing but the idea of analyzing surgical procedures and studying better ways to do things began with Codman. This has become, in recent years, a major concern of quality improvement methodology and Codman's name has gained great deference for his pioneering work.

In 1912, a group of surgeons, including Codman, formed the American College of Surgeons. Franklin Martin, a gynecologic surgeon in Chicago, was one of that group and in 1905 he began the journal *Surgery, Gynecology, and Obstetrics*, which became the journal of the college in 1912. In 1910 the first Clinical Congress, of what would become the American College of Surgeons two years later, was held in Chicago and 1,500 surgeons attended. The governance of the College of Surgeons was composed of two committees. One, chaired by Franklin Martin, was to continue the organization of the college and put on the annual Clinical Congress; the other, chaired by Codman, was called the "Committee of Standardization of Hospitals." The American Medical Association formed a similar committee the same year and the American Hospital Association began to study hospital standards. The Carnegie Foundation became interested in Codman's work and, in 1913, the Foundation plus the three committees formed the "Committee on Standardization of Hospitals."

In 1911, in an effort to collect statistics and record the outcome of surgical procedures, Codman opened his own hospital. He met considerable resistance to his efforts from his colleagues at the Massachusetts General Hospital and, in his own hospital, he hoped to attract a like-minded group of physicians who would not object to collecting the results of their work and publishing them. He did his cause no good when, on January 6, 1915, he presented a cartoon to a meeting of the Suffolk (Boston) District Medical Society ridiculing doctors who were afraid to know the results of their efforts. The meeting, and the cartoon, became the subject of extensive newspaper coverage and Codman resigned from the medical society. The uproar hurt his surgical practice and the entry of the US into World War I in 1917 doomed his hospital. Actually, the closing of his hospital was precipitated by an unselfish act typical of Codman. On December 6, 1917, after a collision in the harbor of Halifax, Nova Scotia, a French ammunition ship blew up with the largest explosion in the history of the world. Not until the atomic bombs in 1945 would an explosion exceed its force. The north half of Halifax was flattened and 3,000 people were killed. On hearing the news, Codman, familiar with Nova Scotia from fishing trips, left Boston for the accident scene. His hospital closed in his absence, never to reopen. On returning to Boston, Codman was drafted into the US Army Medical Corps. He had actually enlisted in the Canadian Army in 1917, but the entry of the US into the War changed matters for him. He was not sent to France, but assigned to a recruit unit at Fort Riley, Kansas. Here, a few months later in March 1918, the great influenza pandemic began. Within a week, 500 soldiers were ill with influenza. By the fall of 1918, twenty percent of American soldiers in the US were afflicted. Codman continued his studies of the End Result System and applied the same methods to the analysis of influenza treatment.

The formation of the American College of Surgeons, in which Codman played such a significant role, was part of a larger effort to overcome the provincialism of American medicine. Osler had hoped that the founding of the Johns Hopkins Hospital would provide a teaching atmosphere of sufficient quality that it would no longer be necessary for a young physician to travel to Europe to acquire a complete medical education. The Clinical Congress would allow surgeons in practice to gather each year to learn new developments in a field that was changing rapidly, more so than medicine which was still limited in effective therapy. In 1913, John B. Murphy, another controversial figure like Codman, began to publish his results as *The Surgical Clinics of John B. Murphy MD, at Mercy Hospital, Chicago*. This was stimulated by interest in his clinical presentations to visitors who watched him perform surgery. The Saunders Company began publication and they were an immediate success. Typical of the jealousy of Murphy's Chicago colleagues, the appearance of the journal prompted yet another complaint to an ethics committee, this time of the American Medical Association. The December 1914 issue included photographs of Murphy's office and this was attacked as advertising. After a hearing, the matter was dropped but it was yet another example of the intense resentment toward more successful colleagues. After Murphy's death, the series continued as the *Surgical Clinics of North American* and was soon imitated by most other medical specialties. If surgeons resisted Codman's efforts to look at their results, at least they showed enthusiasm for education to improve them.

THE END RESULT METHOD

Eventually, Codman resigned as chairman of the Committee on Standardization of Hospitals but the work went on, as the committee became the Joint Commission on Accreditation of Hospitals. He published the results of care in his own hospital in 1915 and established the system of analysis of surgical results. In 1965, the Massachusetts General Hospital was still using his system which graded outcomes as: "E-s Errors of technical knowledge or skill; E-j Errors of judgment; E-c Errors of care or equipment; E-d Errors of diagnosis; P-d Patient's disease; and P-r Patient's refusal of care." Everyone who read his 1915 report was astonished at his honesty. After the War ended, Codman returned to Boston but, with his hospital closed and many of his colleagues still angry about his "snooping" into the results of their treatment, times were difficult. Eventually he returned to his interest in bone diseases and formed a registry of bone sarcomas. In 1922, he reported the first results of his work.[192] This was the beginning of the tumor registry system that is now used to follow cancer cases and determine the outcome of treatment. It is particularly important for rare cancers like bone sarcomas in which individual physicians or even large medical centers are unlikely to see a sufficient volume of patients with the disease to analyze outcomes.

He spent the rest of his career studying bone sarcoma and diseases of the shoulder. He even reconciled with the Massachusetts General Hospital in 1925, ten years after the notorious cartoon. In 1934, he published (at his own expense) his classic book *The Shoulder*, the first systematic study of this joint and its diseases. In it, among other pioneering work, is a complete description of the "rotator cuff injury," called by Codman the "musculo-tendinous cuff." His first journal publication describing this injury appeared in 1911[193] and a later publication by another author credited Codman, who had now been working on the shoulder since 1906, with the concepts.[194] Codman first described the modern examination of the shoulder including "Codman's paradox," in which the shoulder may be in either complete internal rotation or complete external rotation with the arm held over the head, depending on how the patient raises the arm. Many orthopedic surgeons who treat shoulder problems are unaware that Amory Codman described these problems, and their treatment, as early as 1906.

The recent intense interest in improving medical quality as the pressure of economics and managed care increases has revived interest in Codman as a pioneer in honest evaluation of the efficacy of medical care.[195,196]

MODERN ORTHOPEDIC SURGERY

In 1965, fractures were treated at the Massachusetts General Hospital on the General Surgery Service. Orthopedics, in Boston at least, applied to the correction of bone and joint abnormalities, many of which were either congenital, like clubfoot, or due to systemic diseases like rheumatoid arthritis. Fractures were the business of the general surgeon. Tuberculosis caused many joint problems prior to the antibiotic era and Lister was stimulated to seek a method of preventing infection to improve his results with operations for tuberculosis of the wrist. Joint surgery goes back to 1845 when Amédée Bonnet, of the Lyon school, wrote a treatise on joint effusions.[197] He described the findings with rupture of the anterior cruciate ligament. In 1875, Georges K. Noulis (1849-1919) wrote a thesis on *Knee Sprains* which described the functions of the knee ligaments. The test he described is now called the Lachman test. The first repair of a cruciate ligament occurred in 1895, by A.W. Mayo Robson who repaired the anterior and posterior cruciate ligaments with an excellent result.[198] After several failed attempts, Harrey B. Macey, of Rochester, Minnesota, in 1939, successfully replaced the anterior cruciate ligament with a tendon graft from the semitendinosus muscle.[199]

THE HIP

Hip surgery began in the nineteenth century with procedures to release a fused tuberculous hip and allow the patient to resume walking. Girdlestone, between 1921 and 1945, developed a method that was fairly successful in restoring the ability to walk. The cup arthroplasty, a cup shaped device placed over the head of the femur in the hip joint, was invented by Smith-Peterson in the 1930s but, while it reduced the pain of arthritis and reduced the collapse of the femoral head in cases of aseptic necrosis (where the femoral head died in place), its function was only fair.[200] His first cups were made of glass but, after Vitallium alloy was adapted to surgery in 1937, he switched to the more durable material and had better results.

Hip fracture is a common injury in the elderly, where fragile bones are easily broken and a trivial fall can result in this serious injury. Hip fractures often convert a functioning elderly individual to a bed ridden invalid. In 1960, treatment was limited to attempts to stabilize the fracture with metal rods or pins across the fracture line into the upper bone fragment. This was successful if the break did not interfere with the blood supply of the smaller bone fragment. There are two sites at which hip fractures occur, one is at the point where the neck of the femur takes off at an angle to the hip. Strong muscles attach here at the greater and lesser trochanters, knobs of bone that protrude for muscle attachment. These fractures are called "inter-trochanteric" (between the trochanters) and heal well with fixation by pins or rods. The second site is at the point that the neck attaches to the ball portion of the joint. If the fracture is across the "neck" of the femur, at the point that the ball-joint enters the joint capsule, the ball portion of the joint is often cut off from its blood supply and does not heal. In 1940, Austin Moore reported the use of a device that replaced the upper end of the femur (the neck) and the femoral head.[201] It was useful in cases of non-healing hip fracture although it was not very successful in restoring the ability to walk.

In the 1960s, John Charnley, in England's Manchester Royal Infirmary, developed a prosthesis that replaced the entire hip joint.[202] A plastic cup is attached to the pelvis with methyl-methacrylate cement. A metal ball and stem replace the head of the femur with the stem lodged in the marrow canal. He kept working on the device until he had a reliable joint replacement system that allowed normal pain-free walking.[203] Part of his innovation was the adoption of a new operating room system that reduced the risk of infection by maintaining positive pressure in a smaller, inner operating room, almost like Sauerbruch's chamber in reverse, and having the surgeons dressed in "space suits" that diverted exhaled air to the floor through full-face masks and hoses. This avoided the devastating complication of infection of the total hip prosthesis, which would not heal until the device was removed. Hospital operating rooms were equipped with "greenhouses" that provided a more sterile environment. The greenhouse was constructed inside an older operating room and was pressurized to ensure that airflow was from the more sterile area inside to the less sterile outer room. The air entering the greenhouse passed through a sterilization process and the system became known as a "laminar flow room."

In 1970, John Insall developed a prosthesis to replace the knee. Bioengineers were intimately involved in the design of these new devices as the strains of weight bearing and walking required sophisticated design. In 1971, Insall began to implant these new devices and a few years later the procedure became common.[204] Total ankle replacement followed and great advances in engineering improved results in fracture treatment, as well.

THE KÜNTSCHER NAIL

In 1945, American prisoners of war began to be repatriated from Germany. Some of them carried evidence of a major advance in the treatment of long bone fractures. Fractures of the femur and the tibia required long periods of immobilization for healing. The femur fracture was treated with traction for six to eight weeks and it might be months before the patient resumed walking. The tibia fracture required a long leg cast and there was a significant risk of non-union, a failure of the bone to knit properly. Some American POWs had been treated for fractures with a revolutionary technique that solved many of the problems of healing. In 1940, Gerhard Küntscher described a new technique for repairing fractures of the femur. He inserted a metal rod, with a "V" or "U" cross section, down the marrow cavity of the bone.[205] Rush had used a smaller rod for a fixation method with ulna and femur in the 1930s, but the method was controversial.[206] Critics feared that damage to the bone marrow would result in blood problems. It requires skill and experience to maneuver the rod down the marrow canal, across the fracture site without exposing it, and into the other end of the bone. German surgeons became the world experts at fracture therapy in the midst of a world war. At the end of the war, the method was quickly adopted throughout the rest of the world. The fears of bone marrow damage were groundless and Küntscher's technique remains the standard of care fifty years later. It was ironic that prisoners of war would receive better orthopedic care from the Germans than similar injuries would receive from our own Medical Corps.[207]

THE SPINE

In 1911, Joel E. Goldthwait described a case in which manipulation of the spine, for suspected "sacro-iliac displacement," resulted in severe pain followed by paraplegia. The patient had been seen for back problems for several years and previous manipulations had been performed. X-rays of the spine were still very new and supposed displacement of the sacro-iliac joint was frequently diagnosed. The patient suffered severe pain and paraplegia, including bowel and bladder incontinence, for six weeks after which Harvey Cushing performed a decompression procedure, removing the arches of all lumbar vertebrae. No cause for the paraplegia was found but the patient recovered over the following eight months and was walking with a cane when Dr. Goldthwait's account was published in the *Boston Medical and Surgical Journal.* [208]

In 1928, Charles Ellsberg, in a description of spinal tumors causing neurological symptoms, listed twenty-four cases of "chondroma" arising from the intervertebral disc. One of the "chondromas" he described was lying free in the extra-dural space unattached to any other structure. We would recognize that as a fragment of ruptured intervertebral disc.[209] Seven of the "chondromas" were firmly attached to the intervertebral disc and would now be recognized as herniated nucleus pulposus (the spongy core of the disc). In 1934, William Mixter finally established the true nature of the problem.[210] He recognized that the cases of "chondroma" described by Ellsberg and others were, in fact, examples of herniated intervertebral disc. He described the classical clinical syndrome and pointed out that the lesions seen on lipiodol (an oil and iodine solution that visualized on x-ray) myelograms are not tumors but bulging, or ruptured discs. He advocated a surgical approach using removal of only one vertebral lamina (laminectomy) on the symptomatic side, to avoid weakening the spine, itself. He listed nineteen patients treated with thirteen patients having good or complete relief of the neurological symptoms. Two were not subjected to operation, one of which had a malignant spinal tumor, the other had pernicious anemia causing the symptoms. One patient developed a wound infection and died as a consequence, two remained paraplegic with no improvement. Two others died of unrelated causes, one with relief of neurological symptoms. This report began the modern era of spinal surgery with recognition of the common condition of herniated intervertebral disc with sciatica.

Several new devices assisted the treatment of difficult fractures in the 1950s. Unstable cervical spine fractures had been treated with a half body cast extending from mid chest to the patient's chin and ears. The condition, a "broken neck," must be firmly immobilized to avoid spinal cord injury. My grandmother fell down a flight of stairs and was treated with a "Minerva jacket" for a neck fracture in 1953. In 1958, Vernon Nickel and Jacqueline Perry, at Rancho Los Amigos Hospital in southern California, introduced the halo splint for neck fractures.[211] The halo, instead of using a plaster cast over the entire chest and neck, used a metal ring (the halo) which was fixed to the skull with four sharp setscrews. The ring was then fixed to the shoulder harness by metal rods, holding the neck stretched and stiff, but allowing airflow and washing of the area covered by the old cast devices. In the 1960s, a new device improved the treatment of scoliosis, the curvature of the spine seen in adolescents. Paul Harrington developed a system of metal rods that attached with hooks to the spine and provided better fixation for bone grafts.[212] The spine could be straightened, and then held in place by the rods until healing occurred.[213] The technique was used initially for paralytic scoliosis only (many of them polio cases), but was later adapted to the adolescent form.

ARTHROSCOPY

The first successful arthroscopy was performed by Professor Kenjii Takagi of Tokyo in 1918. He used a cystoscope to examine the knee joint of a cadaver. He was looking for a way to improve the care of tuberculous infections of the joint. By 1936, he had been able to take color photographs and even motion pictures of the joint through the arthroscope.[214] Eugene Bircher examined the knees of twenty-one live patients with a Jacobeus laparoscope, beginning in 1919. In 1922, he published his results with what he called "Arthroendoscopy," but problems with equipment prevented acceptance of the technique until after World War II.[215] In the 1960s, a device that would revolutionize orthopedics was developed in Japan. Dr Masaki Watanabe, a former student of Takagi, developed a practical arthroscope, a thin telescope-like device that permitted examination of the joint through a small tube with better lenses, in 1959. He performed the first arthroscopic procedures, including a partial meniscusectomy, and published an Atlas of Arthroscopy in 1957.[216]

The "type 21" arthroscope was brought to North America by Robert Jackson in 1965[217] and, in 1968, the first arthroscope was introduced in the United States by Leonard Peltier at the University of Kansas. In 1974, repair of a torn meniscus (cartilage) in the knee by arthroscopic surgery was reported and a new era began.[218] By the 1980s, arthroscopy had replaced open surgery on the knee.

140   Claudius Amyand, "Of an Inguinal Rupture, with a pin the the Appendix Coeci, incrusted with Stone; and some observation on Wounds in the Guts," *Philosophical Transactions of the Royal Society* (October 1756).

141   Philip G. Creese, "The First Appendectomy," *Surgery, Gynecology and Obstetrics,* 97:643 (1953).

142   William S Halsted, "The Results of Operations for the Cure of Cancer of the Breast Performed at the Johns Hopkins Hospital from June, 1889, to January, 1894," *Annals of Surgery* 20:497-555 (1894).

143   James Paget, "On diseases of the mammary areola preceding cancer of the mammary gland." *St. Bartholomew Hospital Reports*, London, 10: 87-89. (1874) Reprinted in *Medical Classics*, 1: 75-78 (1936).

144 William Halsted, "Contribution to the Surgery of the Bile Passages, Especially to the Common Bile Duct," *Johns Hopkins Hospital Bulletin* January (1890).

145 Rudolph Matas, "William Stewart Halsted. An Appreciation," in *The Surgical Papers of William Stewart Halsted,* The Johns Hopkins Press (1924) page xx.

146 William Halsted, "The Radical Cure of Inguinal Hernia," *Bulletin of the Johns Hopkins Hospital* iv: 17-24 (1893).

147 H. Hirschprung, "Falle von angeborenen Pylorus Stenose," *Jb Kinderheilk*27:61 (1888).

148 Conrad Ramstedt, "Zur Operation der angeborenen Pylorus-Stenose," *Medicine Klinik* 1701-1705 (1912).

149 Mark Ravitch, "The story of pyloric stenosis," *Surgery* 48:1117-1143 (1960).

150 Harold C. Mack, "Hypertrophic Pyloric Stenosis and Its Treatment," *Bulletin of the History of Medicine,* 12:595-615 (1942).

151 James Nicoll, *British Medical Journal,* 2:1148 (1904).

152 William E. Ladd, "Congenital atresia of the esophagus," *New England Journal of Medicine* 230:625-637 (1944).

153 C. Haight and H.A. Towsley, "Congenital atresia of the esophagus with tracheoesophageal fistula. Extrapleural ligation of fistula and end-to-end anastomosis of esophageal segments," *Surgery, Gynecology and Obstetrics* , 76:672 (1943).

154 Daniel M. Hays, Morton M. Woolley and William H. Snyder, Jr., "Esophageal Atresia and Tracheoesophageal Fistula: Management of the Uncommon Types," *Journal of Pediatric Surgery* 1:240-252 (1966)).

155 William E. Ladd, "Congenital atresia and stenosis of bile ducts," *JAMA* 91:1082-85 (1928).

156 J.B. Holmes, "On congenital obliteration of the bile ducts," *American Journal of the Diseases of Childhood* 11:405-431 (1916).

157 William E. Ladd, "Congenital obstruction of the bile ducts," *Annals of Surgery,* 102:742 (1935).

158 M. Kasai, et al, "Surgical treatment of biliary atresia," *Surgery* 3:665 (1968).

159 Elliot Cutler, "The art of surgery," *The Aesculapian* 31:3-18 (1940) Quoted in *Harvey Cushing. A Biography* by John F Fulton, Charles C Thomas (1946).

160 Howard H Kaufman, "Treatment of head injuries in the American Civil War," *Journal of Neurosurgery* 78:838-845 (1993).

161 WL Clark "Oscillatory desiccation in the treatment of accessible malignant growth and minor surgical conditions. A new electrical effect" *Journal of Advanced Therapeutics* 29:169-180 (1911).

162 Tipu Zahed Aziz and Christopher B.T. Adams, "Neurosurgery at the Radcliffe Infirmary, Oxford: A History," *Neurosurgery* 37:505-510 (1995).

163 John F Fulton, *Harvey Cushing. A Biography,* pp 537-538 (1946).

164 J Leroy, "Recherches sur l'Asphyxia," *Journal of Physiology and Experimental Pathology,* 7:10 (1827).

165 G Fell, "Fell Method – Forced Respiration – Report of Cases Resulting in the Saving of Twenty-eight Human Lives – History and a Plea for its General Use in Hospital and naval Practice." Section of General Medicine, 1st pan American Medical Congress, (1890) p. 309.

166 FW Parham, "Thoracic Resections for Tumors Growing From the Bony Chest Wall," *Transactions of the Southern Surgery & Gynecology Association,* 11:223 (1899).

167   G Killina, "Uber Directe Bronchoskopie," *Munchen Med Wochenschraft* 45:844-7 (1898).

168   F Sauerbruch, "Über die Ausschaltung der schädlichen Wirkung des Pneumothorax bei intrathorakalen Operationen," *Zentralblatt Chirurgie*, 31:146 (1904).

169   SJ Meltzer and J Auer , "Eine Vergleichung der 'Volhardschen Methode der Kunstlichen Atmung' mit der von Meltzer und Auer in der Kontinuelichen Bewegungen Verwendeten Methode," *Zentralblat Physiologie* 22:442 (1909).

170   S.J. Meltzer and John Auer,"Continuous Respiration Without Respiratory Movements," *Journal of Experimental Medicine* 11:622-625 (1910).

171   Chevalier Jackson, *Tracheobronchoscopy, Esophagoscopy and Gastroscopy* (1907).

172   Michael DeBakey and Fiorindo Simeone, "Battle Injuries of the Arteries in World War II," *Annals of Surgery* 123: 534-579 (1945).

173   Carl W Hughes, "Arterial Repair During the Korean War," *Annals of Surgery* 147:555-561 (1958).

174   Norman M. Rich, Joseph H. Baugh and Carl W. Hughes, "Acute arterial injuries in Viet Nam," *Journal of Trauma* 10:359-69 (1970).

175   Rudolph Matas, "Traumatic Aneurysm of the Left Brachial Artery," *Medical News* 53:462 (1888).

176   Rene Leriche, "De la resection du carrefour aortico-iliaque avec double sympathectomy lombaire pour thrombose arteritique de l'aorte. Le syndrome de l'obliteration termino-aortique par arterite," *Presse Medicale* 54-55, 48:601-604 (1940).

177   Rene Leriche and Andre Morel, "The syndrome of thrombotic obliteration of the aortic bifurcation," *Annals of Surgery*, 127:193 (1948).

178   CA Hufnagel, "Resection and grafting of the thoracic aorta with minimal interruption of the circulation," *Forum for Fundamental Surgical problems*, American College of Surgeons (1948).

179   RA Gross, et al, "Methods for preservation and transplantation of arterial grafts," *Surgery, Gynecology and Obstetrics,* 88:689 (1949).

180   ME DeBakey, DA Cooley, ES Crawford, GC Morris Jr., "Clinical application of a new flexible knitted Dacron arterial substitute," *Archives of Surgery*, 77:713 (1958).

181   L Buerger, "Thromboangiitis Obliterans: a study of the vascular lesions leading to presenile spontaneous gangrene," *American Journal of Medical Science,* 136:567 (1908).

182   Norman D Royle, "The treatment of spastic paralysis by sympathetic ramisection," *Surgery, Gynecology and Obstetrics*, 39:701 (1924).

183   WA Adson and GE Brown, "Treatment of Reynaud's disease by lumbar ramisection and ganglionectomy and perivascular sympathetic neurectomy of the common iliacs," *JAMA* 84:1908 (1925).

184   J Kunlin, "La traitement de l'ischemie arteritique par la greffe veineuse longue ," *Revue Chirurgica* Paris 70:206 (1951).

185   Charles T Dotter and Melvin P Judkins, "Transluminal Treatment of Arteriosclerotic Obstruction," *Circulation* 30:654 (1964).

186   HH Eastcott, GW Pickering, CG Rob, "Reconstruction of internal carotid artery in a patient with intermittent attacks of hemiplegia," *Lancet* ii:994 (1954).

187   GO Roederer, YE Langlois, L Luisani, KA Jager, JF Primozich, RJ Lawrence, DJ Phillips, DE Strandness, "Natural history of carotid artery disease on the side con-

tralateral to endarterectomy," *Journal of Vascular Surgery* 1:62 (1983).

188 Krause RJ, Cranley JJ, Strasser ES, Hafner CD, Fogarty TJ., "Further Experience with a New Embolectomy Catheter," *Surgery* Jan;59(1):81-7 (1966).

189 W. Andrew Dale MD, *Band of Brothers. Creators of Modern Vascular Surgery,* pages 219-229 (2002).

190 Amory Codman, "Experiments on the Application of the Roentgen Rays to the Study of Anatomy," *Journal of Experimental Medicine,* 3:383-391 (1898).

191 Amory Codman, "The Diagnosis of Ulcer of the Duodenum," a four part series, *Boston Medical and Surgical Journal,* 161: 767-784, 816-822, 853-857, 887-891 (1909).

192 Amory Codman, "The Registry of Cases of Bone Sarcoma," *Surgery, Gynecology and Obstetrics,* 34:335-343 (1922).

193 Amory Codman, "Complete Rupture of the Supraspinatus Tendon. Operative Treatment With Report of Two Successful Cases," *Boston Medical and Surgical Journal,* 164:708-710 (1911).

194 P.D. Wilson, "Complete Rupture of the Supraspinatus Tendon," *JAMA,* 96:433-438 (1931).

195 A. Donabedian, "The End Results of Health Care," *Milbank Quarterly,* 67:233-235 (1989).

196 Donald M Berwick, "E.A. Codman and the Rhetoric of Battle," *Milbank Quarterly,* 67:266 (1989).

197 Amédée Bonnet, *Traité des maladies des articulaires,* 2éme edition Balliere, Paris (1845).

198 A. W. Mayo Robson, "Ruptured cruciate ligaments and their repair by operation," *Annals of Surgery* 37:716-718 (1903).

199 Harrey B. Macey, "A new operative procedure for repair of ruptured cruciate ligament of the knee joint," *Surgery, Gynecology and Obstetrics* 69:108-109 (1939).

200 MN Smith-Peterson, "Evolution of mould arthroplasty of the hip," *Journal of Bone and Joint Surgery,* 30B:59-73 (1948).

201 Austin T Moore, "The self-locking metal hip prosthesis," *Journal of Bone and Joint Surgery,* 39A:811-827 (1947).

202 John Charnley, "Total hip replacement by low friction arthroplasty," *Clinical Orthopedics,* 72:7-21 (1970).

203 John Charnley, "The long term results of low-friction arthroplasty of the hip performed as a primary intervention," *Journal of Bone and Joint Surgery,* 54B:61-71 (1973).

204 John N Insall, "Total Knee Replacement," In *Surgery of the Knee,* Ed. JH Insall. Churchill-Livingstone (1984).

205 Gerhard Küntscher, "Die Marknagelung von Knochenbrüchen," *Archiv fur klinich Chirurgie,* 200:443-455 (1940).

206 L.V. Rush and H.L. Rush, "A Technique for Longitudinal Pin Fixation of Certain Fractures of the Ulna and of the Femur," *Journal of Bone and Joint Surgery* 21:619-626 (1939).

207 Robert Soeur, "Intramedulary Pinning of Diaphyseal Fractures," *The Journal of Bone and Joint Surgery* 28:309-331 (1945). This was the first English language account of the war-time developments.

208 Joel E. Goldthwait, "The Lumbo-sacral Articulation. An Explanation of many cases of 'Lumbago', 'Sciatica' and paraplegia.," *Boston Medical and Surgical Journal,* 164:365-372 (1911).

209   Charles A. Ellsberg, "Extradural Spinal Tumors-Primary, Secondary, Metastatic," *Surgery, Gynecology and Obstetrics* 46:1-20 (1928).

210   William Jason Mixter and Joseph S. Barr, "Rupture of the Intervertebral Disc With Involvement of the Spinal Canal," *New England Journal of Medicine* 211:210-215 (1934).

211   VL Nickel, J Perry, A Garrett, M Heppenstall, "The halo: A spinal skeletal traction fixation device," *Journal of Bone and Joint Surgery*, 50A:1400-1409 (1968).

212   P.R. Harrington, "The history and development of Harrington instrumentation," *Clinical Orthopedics* 93:110 (1973).

213   C Bonnett, JC Brown, J Perry, et al. "Evolution of treatment of paralytic scoliosis at Rancho Los Amigos Hospital," *Journal of Bone and Joint Surgery*,57A:206 (1975).

214   Kenji Takagi., " Arthroscope," *Journal of the Japanese Orthopedic Association* (1939).

215   JS Parisien and DA Present, "Dr. Michael S Burman. Pioneer in the Field of Arthroscopy," *Bulletin of the Hospital of Joint Diseases and Orthopedic Institute* 45:119-126 (1985).

216   Masaki Watanabe, "Memories of the early days of arthroscopy," *Arthroscopy* 2:209-214 (1986).

217   Robert W Jackson, "The introduction of arthroscopy to North America," *Clinical Orthopedics* 374:183-6 (2000).

218   RL O'Conner, "Arthroscopy in the diagnosis and treatment of acute ligament injuries of the knee," *Journal of Bone and Joint Surgery,* 56A:333-337 (1974).

15
Blood

IN FEBRUARY OF 1665, RICHARD LOWER TRANSFUSED BLOOD FROM ONE dog to another. He was four months short of his Doctor of Medicine degree. He used quills to connect three dogs' vessels, bleeding two into a third, after first having bled the third almost to exsanguination. The third dog survived with no ill effect. He was unaware that his experiment succeeded because dogs do not have the isoagglutinins that so complicate human transfusion. Samuel Pepys mentioned the experiment in his diary later that year and suggested the further experiment of infusing the blood of a Quaker into an archbishop to see what the effect might be. In November 1667, Pepys reported the transfusion of sheep's blood into a failing student named Arthur Coga who he described as "crack brained." Jean Denis, physician to Louis XIV, reported several animal to human transfusions, but his third (some say fifth) patient, Antoine du Mauroy, died and the widow sued him for damages. Monsieur du Mauroy was receiving the transfusions at the suggestion of his newlywed wife because of bizarre behavior that sounds like bipolar disorder. After the second transfusion he suffered pain and vomiting followed by passage of black urine. This was probably a classical transfusion reaction from which he recovered. Two months later, his behavior turned maniacal again and the wife requested another transfusion. Before it could be given he died. The case was confused by an allegation that the man was actually poisoned by the widow, but the result was an end to such experiments. Although the court acquitted Denis, it placed a ban on transfusion.

One hundred years later, James Blundell resumed trials of transfusion in cases of hemorrhage in childbirth, but practical problems prevented any real attempts to use this method. Another physician suggested that the blood of one species might not be of benefit to another. Dr. Blundell then carried out a series of experiments in cross-species transfusion. He transfused dogs with the blood of other dogs and they recovered even though they had been bled to near death when the transfusion was commenced. When the same was attempted with sheep's blood, the dogs all died. In

1818, Dr. Blundell reported a transfusion from several human donors to an incurably ill patient.[219] The patient survived for several days and died of the basic affliction, not the transfusion as far as could be determined. A number of similar procedures were carried out using a syringe and funnel and pump. The invention of the hypodermic syringe, by Alexander Wood, in 1853 removed a number of technical problems. In 1863, Doctor J.H. Aveling used a device of his own design to transfuse a young woman dying of postpartum hemorrhage. She recovered temporarily and the donor, her coachman, suffered no ill effect.

The problem of clotting was finally addressed by Braxton Hicks, an obstetrician at St. Bartholomew's Hospital (who also named the slow uterine contractions of late pregnancy). He suggested the use of sodium phosphate as an anticoagulant, but his four cases, while not experiencing clotting, all died. Sodium phosphate was probably a poor choice because it is toxic. Sir Thomas Smith, in 1873, suggested the use of defibrinated blood to avoid clotting but the process was slow and damage to the blood cells may have reduced the usefulness of this method. In the 1880s saline infusion largely replaced transfusion because of the clotting problem and theoretical questions by physiologists. The same debate would occur in the US during the Vietnam War eighty years later and lead to problems in the treatment of military casualties. In 1885, William Halsted transfused his sister with his own blood after she suffered a postpartum hemorrhage and she recovered.

THE DISCOVERY OF BLOOD TYPES

In 1907, J. Jansky, at the Sbornick Klinicky in Prague, identified four blood groups. The four became the Jansky I, II, III, and IV types, no longer familiar to us, and his discovery was confirmed in 1910 by W.L. Moss at Johns Hopkins. Karl Landsteiner, an early immunologist in Vienna, is also given credit for this discovery and he actually determined that the four types were based on two antigens on the surface of red blood cells. His investigations began in 1900 as he tried to understand why blood transfusions failed. In 1875, Landois had reported that, when man is given transfusions of the blood of other animals, these foreign blood corpuscles are clumped and broken up in the blood vessels of man with the liberation of hemoglobin. Landsteiner concluded that the same reaction in human-to-human transfusions results from antigens that differ within the species. He identified two red cell antigens, A and B. When the serum from a patient with one type was mixed with the red cells from another type, the red cells clumped together. During further investigations, he noted that some patients had no antigens on their red cells and did not clump with other serum; these he named type O. Another set of patients had red cells that clumped with the serum from either of the other types, even O. In 1902, Decastrello and Sturli called this type AB and Landsteiner concluded that they had both A and B antigens on the red cells. The antibodies in the serum he named anti-A and anti-B. Type O had both antibodies and type AB had none. Type AB, since they have no antibodies, are the "universal recipient" and can be transfused with any type including O.

Europeans tend to give Jansky credit for the discovery and Americans, perhaps because Landsteiner emigrated to New York to continue his research, credit Landsteiner. In 1919, in the aftermath of the war, he left Austria and then left Europe to come to the Rockefeller Institute where he also worked on polio. In 1930, the Nobel committee awarded Landsteiner the Prize in Medicine for the discovery. In 1907, Hektoen suggested the practice of cross-matching blood between donor and recipient to improve the safety of transfusion. Reuben Ottenberg performed the first blood transfusion using cross matched blood, observed the "Mendelian inheritance" of blood groups and, since type O had no antigens, he suggested it could be transfused into all patients with no reaction; thus, type O is the "universal donor."

BLOOD TRANSFUSION

In the US, George Crile, one of the great figures of early twentieth century surgery, began to study shock. This condition is the consequence of severe injury or major surgery and treatment was ineffective. It remains, one hundred years later, a challenge to surgeons and intensive care specialists. In 1872, shock was described by Samuel Gross, the leading surgeon of Philadelphia and friend of William Osler, as a "rude unhinging of the machinery of life," a definition which has stood the test of time. In 1895, Crile spent a year at University College, London, studying shock and the physiology of circulation. By 1898, he was convinced that blood was more effective than saline in the treatment of shock. I will describe his work on shock more completely in the chapter on critical care (See Chapter 20). Technical problems barred development of practical methods of transfusion until Alexis Carrel described arterial anastomosis techniques in 1903. In 1908, Carrel reported a case in which he used this technique to save the life of a boy, using his father (a friend of Carrel's) as a donor. In 1912, Carrel would receive the Nobel Prize in Medicine for his discovery of arterial suture.

Crile returned to transfusion as a treatment of shock. The result in his first case was described as "midnight resurrection" in his 1906 publication and, in 1909; he reported a summary of his work on shock and transfusion. By 1910, transfusion was in use in large hospitals in several American cities. Direct transfusion was used, a cumbersome technique that required an anastomosis between the donor's artery and the recipient's vein (using Carrel's technique) to avoid clotting. Between 1891 and 1914, many possible anticoagulants were tried and sodium citrate was finally chosen for its safety. So long as the total citrate infused did not exceed five grams, the preparation was shown to be effective and safe. In 1915, Richard Lewisohn reported on the use of citrate anticoagulant in transfusion and established the proportions that continue to be used.[220] The same year R. Weil reported the refrigerated storage of citrate anticoagulated blood making blood banks possible. The syringe method continued in use and would be the preferred method until the Second World War.

A Canadian physician serving an internship at Bellevue Hospital in New York learned the technique and brought it back to Canada in 1913. The British medical profession, in keeping with its resistance to many new developments in surgery at the time, opposed the use of transfusion and the *British Medical Journal* reported in 1907 that "surgeons, we imagine, will find no good reasons given here (after acknowledging good results in cases of shock) for abandoning the safe and simple method of saline injection." In 1916, even after the beginning of the War, the *Lancet* and the *British Medical Journal* ignored his transfusion work in articles reviewing Crile's other accomplishments.

Once the war started, the Royal Army Medical Corps (RAMC) set up field hospitals called Casualty Clearing Stations (CCS) and it soon became clear that shock from artillery wounds was going to be a major problem. The stations adopted the French concept of *triage* (dating back to Baron Larrey) meaning that fresh casualties were put into one of three classes: walking wounded, immediate surgery, and hopeless, later called "expectant." The third class were sent to a facility that came to be called the "moribund tent," called by some "the resurrection tent" since the only survivors were likely beneficiaries of God's intervention. The casualties in the "moribund tents" were kept comfortable with morphine until they died.

RESUSCITATION

It soon became apparent to the young surgeons assigned to the CCS's that many in the moribund category of casualties were suffering from shock. They would not tolerate surgery because of low blood pressure and unstable vital signs and there was no time to give saline infusions. Initially deep abdominal wounds were categorized as hopeless and sent to the moribund tents. By 1915, it was becoming common to evacuate the injured rapidly from the front but, when they arrived at the CCS, they were often already in shock from blood loss. The *Lancet* in 1915 reported that most early fatalities were due to shock.[221] In the Boer War surgical treatment of abdominal wounds was uncommon and most were treated with "positioning, cleaning, and diet." For the rest nature took its course.[222] Edward Archibald, surgeon at the Canadian CCS #1, had spent time with Crile in Cleveland. In 1916, he observed that the usual practice of young surgeons in the CCS, when dealing with an abdominal wound case in shock, was to apply hot water bottles and give hot saline rectal infusions in an attempt to warm the patient. If the patient survived for an hour or two under this regimen, they would proceed with laparotomy (abdominal exploration and repair of bowel injury).

If this seems archaic, in early World War II, battle casualties were given a "Murphy drip," a rectal infusion of strong coffee, as part of resuscitation from shock. At the Battle of Midway in 1942 John Ford, the movie director (and a Navy Reserve Commander), after filming scenes of Japanese bombing on the island, made himself useful by brewing strong coffee for Murphy drips. Archibald noted that the appearance of shock was more common in the CCS than at the front lines immediately after wounding. The conclusion drawn was that something was happening during the time between the occurrence of the wound and arrival in the CCS. Ernest M Cowell, a young British surgeon, studied casualties, performing frequent blood pressure measurements between the time of wounding and arrival at the CCS. He confirmed the impression of progressive deterioration. He coined the term "wound shock" to differentiate it from "shell shock," a psychiatric reaction to fear and stress.[223] By the battle of the Somme (in which the British would suffer 60,000 casualties on the first day), the young surgeons were determined to save more of these men.

The official history of the British Army noted that the results of a huge trial of saline infusion for casualties were "most disappointing," One week after the battle of the Somme, the *British Medical Journal* finally broke its silence on blood transfusion for hemorrhagic shock, as wound shock was increasingly shown to be.[224] The article was written by a Canadian doctor in the British Army. By 1917, citrate treated blood was being widely used in casualty stations after missionary efforts by Canadian surgeons succeeded. In 1918, the Americans arrived with transfusion as standard practice and they are often given credit for the introduction of this life-saving therapy. Crile and a team from Harvard had arrived in 1917, and

Crile's memoirs recount his unfavorable impression of the British treatment of shock cases. Over the next year, the practice was changed with a "resuscitation ward" taking the place of the "resurrection ward" and transfusion using the citrate method became common. One of the great advantages of this method was the use of a needle inserted into a vein to draw and administer the blood. No dissection of the vessels or vascular anastomosis was necessary.

BLOOD BANKS

Oswald Hope Robertson came to England from the Rockefeller Institute where he had worked with Peyton Rous (discoverer of the first virus shown to cause cancer) in red cell preservation. Robertson, assigned to the British Army, set up the first blood bank (or depot, as they were called), collected red cells and preserved them, then transfused casualties with his preserved red cell solutions. In 1922 Geoffrey Keynes, a British surgeon and the brother of the economist John Maynard Keynes, wrote *Blood Transfusion*, the book which became the standard between the wars and gave the history of its origin in the Great War. The Canadian contribution was neglected but they had, in fact, learned from the work of Crile. In 1937, the world's first "blood bank" was established in Leningrad using Robertson's methods of blood preservation. The same year Bernard Fantus, director of therapeutics at Cook County Hospital in Chicago, established the first American blood bank, a hospital laboratory that could preserve, cross match and store blood, and coined the term.

PLASMA

In 1940 Edwin Cohn, a professor of biochemistry at Harvard, developed a method of separating plasma components by cold fractionation. He was able to separate plasma into albumin, with osmotic properties similar to plasma itself, and other fractions, including gamma globulin and fibrinogen.[225] In 1941, while treating casualties at Pearl Harbor, Isador Ravdin, a surgeon and professor from Philadelphia, used Cohn's albumin in treating shock. Albumin and plasma became widely used in World War II for treatment of shock since storage was easier than for blood. The Army developed a plasma product that was dried and could be reconstituted with distilled water. The dried plasma could be stored for five years and used in battlefield conditions.[226]

In 1943, J.F. Loutit and P.L. Mollison introduced acid-citrate-dextrose, a far superior preservative solution for blood, and blood transfusion became more common on the battlefield in time for the Normandy invasion. The first case of hepatitis transmitted by blood transfusion was reported the same year by Beeson, anticipating an increasing problem for the future. In 1945, Coombs, Mourant, and Race described the use of antihuman globulin to identify antibodies producing red cell damage and hemolytic anemia. By 1950 red cell freezing had become possible and the familiar plastic bag was beginning to be used to collect and transfuse blood although bottles were still in common use in 1970.

A NEW GENETIC DISEASE

Landsteiner continued his research and, in 1939, reported the existence of another blood type. Phillip Levine and Rufus Stetson had described a patient with a peculiar reaction to a transfusion. The woman had suffered a miscarriage and, because of hemorrhage, was given a transfusion of her husband's blood. Both were type O and there should have been no problem. Instead, she had a severe transfusion reaction and her husband's red cells clumped in the presence of her serum. Levine and Stetson tested her serum with other donors, all type O, and the red cells of four fifths of them clumped. She must have an antibody to an unknown red cell antigen that her own red cells lacked. They concluded that her husband, and presumably the fetus, had the unknown antigen along with four fifths of the population of New York.[227]

It had been learned, by Pasteur and others, that antibody production was stimulated by repeated exposure to antigen and the reaction to a second mismatched transfusion was more severe than the first. The mother had presumably been immunized to the unknown blood group by the fetus's red cells, perhaps in the placenta, and, when she received the transfusion from her husband, the reaction was severe. What would happen when she became pregnant again? How could this new antigen be identified? Landsteiner had been testing cross-species transfusion and found that anti-rhesus monkey antibodies produced by rabbits and guinea pigs would clump, not only the monkey red cells but those of six out of seven white New Yorkers.[228] He named the new antigen "rhesus factor" and the red cells of those with the antigen, Rh positive or Rh +. Those without the antigen, who were capable of being immunized against the factor, were Rh negative or Rh X. It also became apparent that Rh negative people did not have anti-Rh antibodies unless they had been exposed to Rh positive red cells. Levine and Stetson recognized the implications for pregnancy and fetal health.[229] The condition called "hemolytic disease of the newborn" must be caused by an Rh incompatibility between fetus and mother.

The original description of this syndrome, called "erythroblastosis fetalis," and the beginning of understanding, came in 1932 when Louis Diamond described the association between several newborn abnormalities, including "universal edema of the fetus," "icterus gravis neonatorum" (severe jaundice in newborns), and "congenital anemia of the newborn." All of these conditions had been observed for centuries but he recognized that they were manifestations of the same condition, severe anemia. He could not determine whether the anemia was the result of destruction of normal red blood cells or an abnormality of red cell maturation (somewhat like pernicious anemia in adults). He leaned toward the latter cause and named the condition for the symptom, erythroblastosis (presence of immature red cell forms in the blood).[230] Landsteiner and Coombs' work would finally show the correct source of the anemia.

The Rh test was developed and the implications for pregnancy eventually became clear. An Rh negative woman could be immunized by the red cells of an RH positive fetus, but this did not always occur. The Rh factor was dominant so, if the father was Rh positive, at least half of his babies (in an Rh negative mother) would be the same. The first pregnancy of such an Rh incompatible couple usually succeeded. The first baby survived. With each succeeding pregnancy, unless the baby was Rh negative (one chance in two if the father was Rr. Since the Rh factor was dominant the mother would always be rr.), the condition called "erythroblastosis fetalis" developed. Only with Coombs' description of autoimmune hemolytic anemia in 1946 was the mechanism understood. The baby's red cells would be clumped and destroyed by maternal antibodies, which leaked across the placental membrane. Why did the first pregnancy survive? The fetal red cells do not usually cross the placenta. The period of labor and delivery, with separation of the placenta, was eventually recognized as the time when the mother is exposed to fetal red cells. The second pregnancy encountered maternal antibodies and each succeeding pregnancy stimulated higher levels, or titers, of antibody. The first baby made it, the second often survived, but required transfusions, the third and later babies were lost. Still, as the mechanism of immunization was understood, therapy became possible.

In 1957, Diamond described his experience with exchange transfusion via the umbilical vein. This procedure removed free maternal anti-Rh antibodies from the infant's circulation, restored the hemoglobin and, it was soon realized, removed high bilirubin levels that had resulted in brain damage in those cases with severe jaundice.[231] Intrauterine transfusions were attempted in the 1960s and eventually succeeded as obstetricians realized that the fetus would absorb red cells infused into its peritoneal cavity. It was not necessary to inject the blood into a fetal vein. A long needle was inserted through the mother's abdominal wall and, using the new imaging methods, the needle was passed through the wall of the uterus, through the fetus' abdominal wall, into the fetal peritoneal cavity. Blood was then injected and the needle withdrawn. It could be repeated as necessary. Finally, the development of immune serum with anti-Rh antibodies allowed the "mopping up" of fetal red cells in the mother's circulation after childbirth and avoided or minimized the stimulation of the maternal immune system. This was an invention of Vincent Freda MD after basic research by Cyril A. Clarke, and Ronald Finn. They shared the 1980 Lasker Award with William Pollack and John G. Gorman for the work. This product is called "Rhogam" and is given to all Rh-negative mothers who deliver Rh-positive babies.

HEMOPHILIA AND CLOTTING

A disease involving abnormal bleeding has been noted for centuries. In the Talmud, from the second century CE, circumcision is not required of male babies if two brothers have died from the procedure.[232] Albucasis, in the twelfth century, mentioned a family in which the males died of bleeding after minor injury. In 1803, a Philadelphia physician named John Conrad Otto wrote an account of "a hemorrhagic disposition existing in certain families." He observed that the disease was inherited, affected only males and traced it to a woman three generations back who had settled in Plymouth, New Hampshire in 1720. In 1828, Hopff, at the University of Zurich, used the term "hemophilia" for the first time. Queen Victoria, who ruled England from 1837 to 1901, had a son, Leopold, who suffered from frequent hemorrhages and died of a brain hemorrhage in 1868 at age thirty-one. His grandson, Viscount Trematon, the son of his daughter, died of a brain hemorrhage in 1928. Victoria's daughters married into the royal families of Europe and brought hemophilia with them. Alice and Beatrice transmitted the disease to the Spanish, German, and Russian royal families. Alexandra, Victoria's granddaughter married Nicholas Romanov, the Czar. Her son Alexei, the Tsarevich, was a hemophiliac and Rasputin, the mad monk who exercised a strong influence on Alexandra, gained his influence with hypnosis of Alexei to relieve his pain, from the typical arthritis (from repeated bleeding into joints) of hemophilia. Rasputin developed an unbelievable power over Alexandra to the point that he was dictating government policy and command of the army as Russia entered World War I. The result was the Russian Revolution after the Czar was completely discredited by a series of blunders attributable to the influence of Rasputin. The "mad monk" was murdered by Russian courtiers, but the damage was done. The entire royal family was eventually killed by the Bolsheviks.

The state of knowledge about blood clotting in 1863 is illustrated by a lecture before the Medico-Chirurgical Society of Edinburgh by Joseph
Lister. Lister relates the current theory that the fluidity of blood requires
the presence of free ammonia in the circulation. Escape of volatile ammonia results in coagulation, hence exposure to air produces clotting by
allowing "the escape of the volatile alkali." He describes blood: it "is seen
to consist of a liquid and numerous small particles suspended in it." The
corpuscles are either white or red. When blood is shed from the body it
passes from fluid to a solid form. The solid material responsible, according
to Lister, is called "fibrine." The fibrine, after clotting, shrinks and
squeezes out the serum. The question is what causes clotting?   He
describes two theories; one is called the "vital properties" theory that
requires living tissue to produce clotting. The other current theory is the
"ammonia theory," noted above. Lister accepts neither and describes a
series of observations that are inconsistent with either theory. One of his
experiments involves collecting serum, the liquid remaining after a clot
forms and demonstrating that it immediately clots fresh plasma. A second
observation points out that inflamed tissue stimulates clotting in the
absence of air or any opportunity for ammonia to escape.[233] He was unable
to explain these observations but his willingness to record facts and reject
a theory, which did not explain those facts, helps us to understand why he
was a great scientist.

Forty years later, Osler's textbook of medicine describes hemophilia and
its hereditary nature. He clearly describes the inheritance, writing that the
mother does not contract the disease but passes it to sons. He describes
the arthritis associated with the disease and mentions that there is no
abnormality of the blood except that produced by anemia. He advises
transfusion in a few cases but mentions no change in the bleeding tendency resulting. He says that venesection (bleeding) has been used for
hemophilia (although he offers no information about why this should be of
benefit), but does not recommend it.

The cause of hemophilia was unknown until very recent times. The discovery of blood platelets by Alfred Donné in 1842 (he called them "globules") led to suspicion of these structures as the culprit. Osler published
an extensive study of platelets and their function in 1874 and saw no relationship to hemophilia but confirmed that they were important in clotting.
Georges Hayem, in 1878, learned how to count platelets and observed that
they congregated at the site of injury in a dog's jugular vein. He did not
believe that they had any role in clot formation and their clotting function
was finally described in 1882 by Giulio Bizzozero who also provided the

name by which they have been known since then. The cause of hemophilia still evaded investigation. Finally, in 1937, Patek and Taylor, physicians at Harvard, found that the clotting defect in hemophilia could be corrected with a plasma component they named "anti-hemophiliac globulin" (We call it AHG). This followed the work of Cohn in separating plasma components, described above in the section on blood transfusion. In 1944, Pavlovsky, a physician in Buenos Aires, Argentina, discovered that blood from one of his hemophiliac patients could correct the clotting defect in another. There were two forms of hemophilia with two different factors involved. In 1952, the two forms of the disease were named Hemophilia A, in which factor VIII is missing or decreased, and Hemophilia B, caused by deficiency of factor IX. Hemophilia B is also called "Christmas disease" because that was the last name of Pavlovsky's patient. Still, neither observation fit the prevailing theory of clotting.

THE DISCOVERY OF THE CLOTTING FACTORS

For fifty years the classical theory of blood coagulation involved four clotting factors; thrombokinase (or thromboplastin), derived from damaged tissue, prothrombin and fibrinogen which are present in normal plasma, and ionized calcium, which is removed by citrate solutions used to prevent clotting in blood transfusion. Blood in the normal circulation remains fluid (according to the theory) because prothrombin and fibrinogen are stable. With tissue damage, thromboplastin enters the blood and reacts with prothrombin in the presence of calcium to form thrombin. Thrombin, in turn, reacts with fibrinogen to form fibrin, which is insoluble and forms the clot. These substances, at least thromboplastin and thrombin, were assumed to be enzymes because fragments of fibrinogen had been isolated.

In 1935, Quick introduced a one-stage prothrombin time test that was based on the four-factor theory. The thromboplastin used for the test was brain extract, which had been found to be a potent stimulant to clotting. The test, while clinically useful, demonstrated puzzling discrepancies. Quick soon identified the first complication: the prothrombin time lengthens with storage of the plasma. Did the prothrombin decay? The prothrombin time could be restored to normal with addition of fresh plasma, even plasma from a patient on coumadin whose own prothrombin time is prolonged. There had to be another factor, which diminished with time-a labile factor, plus a factor that was stable and affected by coumadin. The labile factor was in fresh plasma and was not affected by coumadin anticoagulants. Rather than abandon the four-factor hypothesis, Quick called the two factors prothrombin A and B. In 1947, Owren described yet another clotting factor which he called "factor V" since it was one more than the four that had been identified for fifty years.

The problem with this theoretical explanation for coagulation was that there was no room for hemophilia. Research focused on the explanation for the effect of coumadin (to be told below), but no one could explain why hemophiliacs bled. The clotting time by the Lee-White method (tilting a glass tube filled with fresh blood until it clotted) was markedly prolonged in hemophilia but the prothrombin time of Quick was normal. The thromboplastin seemed to take a shortcut and missed the hemophilia defect. The Quick prothrombin time was then performed using tissue from hemophiliacs as thromboplastin; it was still normal. Why did hemophiliac blood not clot in glass tubes, and more important, in wounds? Several possible explanations preserved the four-factor theory (although, it was tottering from other blows). Maybe platelets, which were important for clotting in the clinical situation, were abnormal in hemophilia. The problem with this was that hemophiliac platelets functioned normally in non-hemophiliac blood and the correction of hemophiliac clotting that had been observed after addition of normal platelets was due to the plasma that accompanied them.

This is when Pohle and Taylor showed that concentrated globulin from normal plasma corrects the clotting time of hemophiliac blood in vitro and clinically.[234] Eventually, it became obvious that normal plasma contains a factor lacking in hemophilia and which did not correspond to any of the factors of classical theory. This had been suspected for a long time but the theory got in the way. By 1947, it was becoming impossible to relate the facts to the theory and by 1953 it had been shown that clotting, activated by contact of the blood with glass, occurred after a three minute delay. Then thrombin production proceeded on a steep curve that was not altered by the use of thromboplastin. The thromboplastin reduced the three-minute delay but, once the thrombin started to appear, the rate of production was the same. In hemophiliac blood, the delay phase was markedly prolonged and addition of anti-hemophiliac globulin reduced the delay with the time reduction proportional to the amount of AHG added.

Pavlovsky's 1944 case was analyzed and the two forms of hemophilia studied. Finally, a new test called the "thromboplastin generation test" was devised in which individual clotting factors, including prothrombin, could be removed and their effects studied. At this point "Christmas factor" was identified and its deficiency differentiated from classical hemophilia. New clotting factors were discovered as the process was analyzed. The new test allowed quantitative analysis of AHG and, by 1957, AHG concentrate, initially from cattle, was produced. By 1964, human AHG was becoming available with the use of cryoprecipitation techniques (This later became a problem with hepatitis and HIV). Christmas factor was isolated and found to be more stable than AHG but clinical trials were less successful than those with AHG concentrates. By 1957, at least twelve clotting factors had been identified and a Roman numeral system adopted to identify them

CLOTTING INHIBITORS

HEPARIN

Heparin was discovered in 1916 as an incidental finding during experiments in the purification of thromboplastin. In 1915, Jay McLean traveled from San Francisco to Baltimore to attend the Johns Hopkins Medical School. Finding his place already taken by another, he spent a year doing research in physiology with William Howell, chairman of the physiology department. Howell gave him the task of analyzing the clot stimulating properties of brain extract, later to be called thromboplastin. Howell believed that cephalin, a brain phospholipid, was the substance in the extract that caused the clotting. After months of work, McLean proved that cephalin was, indeed, a powerful clotting agent. Then he performed similar extractions of heart and liver, looking for thromboplastin activity but discovered that some of the extracts actually inhibited clotting.[235] He repeated his experiments until he was certain that the liver extract contained an anticoagulant. He went to Dr. Howell and found him skeptical of the finding. McLean had a lab assistant collect a beaker of blood from a cat and added the liver extract. He asked Howell to tell him when it clotted; it never did. McLean presented his findings with cephalin and the new liver extract in February 1916 at a meeting of the Philadelphia Medical Society. Professor Howell was convinced and soon developed improved methods of producing the new substance, which he named "heparin."[236] The new anticoagulant was difficult to use because it caused fever and other reactions with intravenous injection, no doubt due to impurities. It was not absorbed by mouth so the impurities prevented its use. Charles Best, co-discoverer of insulin, then began work on purification of heparin and, by 1933, a potent drug, free from impurities, was available. In 1935, studies of the use of heparin in man began and, in 1937, Erwin Chargaff and Kenneth Olson discovered that protamine neutralized heparin, providing the antidote and increasing safety.[237]

In recent years it has been fractionated and the smaller molecular fractions have proven to be as effective, or more so, than the original molecule. It continues to be the essential anticoagulant in cardiac and vascular surgery, and the fact that it is effective in inhibiting activated thrombin makes it the only useful therapy for clotting that is under way, as in deep vein thrombosis and pulmonary embolism.

COUMADIN

"In February 1933 a Wisconsin farmer, reportedly disgruntled because he could not find a state veterinarian, brought a dead heifer, a milk can of unclotted blood, and 100 pounds of spoiled sweet clover hay to the Agricultural Chemistry building of the University of Wisconsin. In the halls he met Karl Paul Link."[238] The farmer's cattle had developed a swollen abdomen and weakness that was eventually traced to anemia and heart failure. The anemia was due to spontaneous bleeding and the clotting of the cows' blood was abnormal. The hay was not directly the cause. Improperly cured sweet clover hay is infected with a mold, which produces a blood clotting inhibitor. Four years later Link published his first report on the cause.[239] The bleeding disease of cattle had already been described years before by two veterinarians and they had associated the disease with spoiled sweet clover hay. Link and his graduate students isolated the hemorrhagic substance, which they named "dicoumarol." About 100 analogues were tested and number forty-two was called "Warfarin." The Wisconsin Alumni Research Foundation had supported the investigation of this disease of cattle and the drug name is an acronym for the foundation's name. Better curing methods for hay resolved most of the veterinary problem but the drug produced by the mold was patented and put to use as a rat poison (since no one could think of any other practical use for it). Eventually the ease of use in humans, because it was effective orally, for clotting inhibition was demonstrated, but there was resistance to using a "rat poison" on people. Link, with a wry sense of humor, once asked why doctors would "give their patients cow poison but didn't want to give them rat poison."[240] He subsequently discovered the enhanced anticoagulation with the combination of aspirin and coumadin (patients on coumadin should not take aspirin) and then, in 1944, he and his students discovered the antagonism of vitamin K to the coumadin effect.[241] An oral anticoagulant, and its antidote, would make the treatment of abnormal blood clotting possible in future years. Heparin prevents clotting in a test tube and works almost instantaneously; Warfarin takes several days to affect clotting and has no effect in vitro (in a test tube). They obviously act by different mechanisms and the study of these actions added to the understanding of blood clotting itself.

GENETICS AND DARWIN

In 1814, Joseph Adams, a British physician, described what was known about heredity at the time. For centuries, it was observed that certain features of individuals were passed from parent to child. How this was accomplished was unknown. Some diseases, like gout, were thought to be inherited. Adams distinguished between familial diseases, which he defined as being confined to a single generation and hereditary diseases that were passed from generation to generation. Charles Darwin, in 1838, while trying to make sense of his observations on the voyage of the Beagle six years earlier, speculated on how inherited characteristics were passed from one generation to another. Why did male animals, and men, have nipples? Did all creatures begin as hermaphrodites and differentiate into sexes? He consulted dog breeders on pedigrees. He studied Hunter's lectures on physiology and his speculations on the creation of monsters. He read Malthus' *Essay on the Principles of Population*, published in 1798. This gave him the basis for natural selection, the force to procreate and perpetuate the race. If some new characteristic appeared that aided survival, for example longer legs or longer claws, it gave the individual possessing the trait an advantage in the Malthusian battle for survival. It did not help on the topic of how these desirable characteristics were passed from parent to child.

In the midst of all these speculations about sex and procreation, in January 1839, Darwin married Emma Wedgwood, a cousin. The Darwin and Wedgwood families had extensively intermarried, a fact that might have worried Darwin if he knew more about genetics. After his marriage, he continued his researches into crossbreeding and inheritance. In 1839, he published his journal of the voyage and became famous. Publication of his controversial conclusions about natural selection was still years in the future. The birth of a child, William Erasmus Darwin, in December 1839 brought an opportunity to observe the natural history of human development, and he studied his child as he had studied finches. In time, he discovered bees and began to consider plant reproduction.

In 1840, geology was rapidly progressing in Europe and Swiss geologist Agassiz who proposed that glaciers had once extended much further than they did now and were responsible for geologic features, extended Charpentier's earlier work on ice movements. This was revolutionary stuff for British geologists and influenced Darwin's consideration of evolution. He was shocked in 1844 to read a book by Robert Chambers, a journalist, titled *Vestiges of the Natural History of Creation*, which included a version of Darwin's theory of transmutation of species in a sort of circular cycle of evolution. The book was a sensation and Darwin was depressed. It was what would now be called popular science and, while attacked as atheistic, it went into multiple printings and was translated into German. The attacks concerned Darwin as they represented what he himself faced if he published his own, even more controversial, book. He spent the next few years studying barnacles in an attempt to understand sexual reproduction and was astonished to discover one species in which the female barnacle (previously thought to reproduce asexually) kept two tiny vestigial males in a pouch solely to produce sperm. This was at a time when sperm were still considered "animalcules," which carried a miniature intact human, at least by some. Sexual reproduction seemed to be universal the more he studied natural history.

In 1844, he published his work on barnacles and moved on to other aspects of heredity. He returned to the study of bees and wondered how members of the family of garden peas continued to breed true when they were all mixed together in his garden. Twenty years later Gregor Mendel was to explain this phenomenon. Finally, in 1859, he published his great book, *The Origin of Species*, still ignorant of the mechanism by which hereditary information is passed from parent to child.

MENDEL AND INHERITANCE

In 1866 Gregor Mendel, a monk in the abbey of Brunn, Austria, published a study of the propagation of sweet peas.[242] He worked in the garden of the abbey and became aware of the persistence of certain characteristics of the plants in their progeny. Tall plants did not always produce tall peas from their seeds but, when he crossed a strain of short peas with the tall strain, nearly all the resulting plants were tall. Eventually he isolated a tall strain and a short strain; all the plants growing from the seeds of the tall strain were tall and all those growing from seeds of the short strain were short. When he crossed the tall with the short strain, three quarters were tall. He then concluded that some "hereditary factor" was responsible for height and that it must be doubled since the crossing of strains produced a reproducible proportion of short and tall plants. He concluded that the tall strain (T) was dominant over the short strain (t). Thus, crossing the two strains allowed four possible combinations: TT, Tt, tT, and tt. T was dominant because the combinations TT, Tt, and tT were all tall. Only tt was short. Furthermore, of the tall peas, only one third bred true when crossed with another tall strain. These must be TT. The Tt and tT strains must contain a factor for shortness and, even when crossed with another tall strain, produce some short plants. Now we would refer to the strain that bred true as homozygous and that which produced both tall and short as heterozygous. (If one strain is all TT and T is dominant, then all progeny of a mating will be tall even if the other strain has both T and t.) He spent ten years working on his research before his paper was published and then it was ignored for another thirty-five years. Finally, in 1905, William Bateson, who was working on sweet pea hybridization at Cambridge, gave Mendel's hereditary factor the name "gene."[243] Bateson had spent years trying to reconcile Darwin's theory of continuous variation with his own observations of the discontinuous nature of hereditary variation. When he discovered Mendel's work, he realized that here was the model for discontinuous variation.

In 1897, Archibald Garrod was interested in alkaptonuria, a disease that turns urine dark and produces arthritis in some cases.[244] The current theory was that it was caused by a bacillus but Garrod concluded that it arose from an "error of metabolism" that was congenital. He studied four families affected by the disease. In three of the four families, the parents, while free of the disease, were first cousins. The children of these consanguineous marriages had the disease, suggesting a mechanism similar to that observed by Mendel (although Garrod was ignorant of this work). Garrod, like Mendel, was only appreciated in retrospect when later work proved their prescience.

SICKLE CELL ANEMIA

Sickle cell anemia was first reported by J.B.Herrick, a Chicago physician (and cardiologist described elsewhere) in 1910.[245] "Sickling" was studied seven years later by V.E. Emmel who reported the case of a black woman with severe anemia and leg ulcers. Her red cells, at least a high percentage of them, formed a sickle shape. Her father, who was not anemic, also had sickled red cells, but not so many. Both showed increased sickling in cell cultures. In 1923, J.G. Huck explored the family pedigrees of patients with sickle cell anemia and demonstrated its hereditary nature. In 1949, Linus Pauling, who would win a Nobel Prize in 1954 for his description of the chemical bond, discovered the cellular abnormality and opened the door to molecular biology. The hemoglobin molecule in individuals with sickle cell anemia, or the milder sickle cell trait, has a different structure. Pauling predicted that the abnormality would be found in the globin molecule and that proved the case as a single amino acid in the protein of sickle-cell hemoglobin differs from that in other forms of hemoglobin. With this start, the structure of hemoglobin and its metabolism were uncovered. Other hemoglobin structures were found including fetal hemoglobin with a difference in its oxygen affinity that conveys an advantage in intra-uterine life.

Thalassemia, another hemoglobin abnormality, which produces anemia and is hereditary, was soon identified and studied. The fact that both sickle cell disease and Thalassemia are found predominately among populations native to malaria-infested regions and that the abnormal hemoglobin conveys resistance to the parasite, raised the issue of an evolutionary influence. Genetic mutations, subject of Darwin's studies, may be perpetuated or eliminated by evolutionary pressure. If the mutation is beneficial, it may improve the potential for survival and propagation of its hosts. If it is harmful, and certainly anemia is harmful, it should disappear. Perhaps the benefits of hemoglobin S, as the sickling hemoglobin molecule is called, outweighed the harm. The individuals, like the father of the first patient studied, who have the trait, or mild form, may be less subject to malaria infection. Molecular biology, genetics and tropical medicine would attempt to answer that and other, similar questions.

219   James Blundell. "Experiments on the Transfusion of Blood by the Syringe." *Medico-Chirurgical Times.* 9: 56-92 (1818).

220   Richard Lewisohn, "Blood Transfusion by the Citrate Method," *Surgery, Gynecology and Obstetrics* 21: 37-47 (1915).

221   Cuthbert Wallace, "The early operative treatment of gunshot wounds of the alimentary canal." *Lancet* ii: p 1336-46 (1915).

222   Peter Kurt Bamburger, "The adoption of laparotomy for the treatment of penetrating abdominal wounds in war," *Military Medicine* 161: p 189-96 (1996).

223   Cowell, "Wound shock in front line areas," *Official History* I: p 57-78   ed. McPherson, et al.

224   L. Bruce Robertson, "The transfusion of whole blood: A suggestion for its more frequent employment in wartime," *British Medical Journal,* ii: p 38-40 (1916).

225   Edwin J Cohn, "Properties and Functions of the Plasma Proteins, With a Consideration of the Methods for Their Separation and Purification," *Chemistry Review* 28:395 (1941).

226   Major Douglas B Kendrick, "The Procurement and Use of Blood Substitutes in the Army," *Annals of Surgery* : 1152-1159 (1942).

227   Philip Levine and R.E. Stetson, "Unusual Case of Intra-Group Agglutination," *JAMA* 113:126 (1939).

228   Karl Landsteiner and Alexander S. Weiner, "An Agglutinable Factor in Human Blood Recognized by Immune Sera for Rhesus Blood," *Proceedingsof the Society for Experimental Biology and Medicine,* 43:223 (1940).

229   Philip Levine and Eugene M. Katzin, "Isoimmunization in Pregnancy and the Varieties of Isoagglutinins Observed," *Proceedings of the Society for Experimental Biology and Medicine,* 45:343-346 (1940).

230 Louis K. Diamond, Kenneth D. Blackfan, and James M. Baty, "Erythroblastosis fetalis and its association with universal edema of the fetus, icterus gravis neonatorum and anemia of the newborn," *Journal of Pediatrics* 1:269-309 (1932).

231 Louis K. Diamond, "Erythroblastosis Fetalis or Haemolytic Disease of the Newborn," *Proceedings of the Royal Society of Medicine* 40:546-550 (1946-47).

232 Fred Rosener, "Hemophilia in Classic Rabbinic Texts," *Journal of the History of Medicine and Allied Sciences,* 49:240-250 (1994).

233 Joseph Lister, "On the coagulation of the blood," *The Collected Papers of Joseph Lister,* Classics of Medicine Library, 1: p 109-134 (1979).

234 F.J. Pohle and F.H.L. Taylor, "The coagulation defect in hemophilia. The effect in hemophilia of intramuscular administration of a globulin substance derived from normal human plasma," *Journal of Clinical Investigation.* 16:741 (1937).

235 Jay McLean, "The Discovery of Heparin," *Circulation,* 19:75-78 (1959).

236 WH Howell and E Holt, "Two New Factors in Blood Coagulation – Heparin and Pro-antithrombin," *American Journal of Physiology,* 47:328 (1918).

237 Erwin Chagaff and Kenneth Olson, "Studies of the Chemistry of Blood Coagulation. VI Studies on the Action of Heparin and Other Anticoagulants. The Influence of Protamine on the Anticoagulant Effect In Vivo," *Journal of Biological Chemistry,* 122: 153-167 (1937).

238 C.E. Ballou, "Karl Paul Gerhardt Link 1901-1978," *Advances in Carbohydrate Chemistry and Biochemistry* 39:1-12 (1981).

239 WL Roberts, KP Link, "Precise method for determination of coumarin, melilotic acid and coumaric acid in plant tissue," *Journal of Biological Chemistry,* 119:269 (1937).

240 R.F. Schilling, "Karl Paul Link and the hemorrhagic agent in spoiled sweet clover," *Journal of Laboratory and Clinical Medicine* 109:617-18 (1987).

241 RS Overman, JB Field, CA Baumann, KP Link , "Studies on the hemorrhagic sweet clover disease. IX. The effect of diet and vitamin K on the hypoprothrombinemia induced by 3,3 methylenebis (40hydroxycoumarin) in the rat," *Journal of Nutrition,* 23:589 (1942).

242 Mendel, Gregor.. "Versuche über Pflanzen Hybriden." *Verhandlungen des naturforschenden Vereines in Brünn,* 4:3-47 (1866).

243 Bateson, William, " Problems of heredity as a subject for horticultural investigation," *Journal of the Royal Horticultural Society,* 25:54-61 (1900).

244 Garrod, Archibald E. "The incidence of alkaptonuria: A study in chemical individuality," *Lancet,* ii:1616-1620 (1902).

245 JB Herrick, "Peculiar elongated and sickle-shaped red corpuscles in a case of severe anemia," *Archives of Internal Medicine,* Chicago, 6: 517-521 (1910).

16
The Structure of DNA

IN 1846, EDUARD SEGUIN DESCRIBED A CONDITION CALLED "FURFURACEOUS idiocy." The condition included unusual facial features, slow growth, short stature, and mental retardation. In 1867, J. Langdon Down suggested that these findings were somehow related to a Mongol racial throwback. A century later his term, "Mongoloidism," was dropped in favor of "Down's Syndrome." In the 1950s, improved cytology and study of cell structures revealed that these children had an extra chromosome. The genetic material itself had been discovered by biochemist Friedrich Miescher in 1869 who noted the same material in the nucleus of every cell. Miescher's discovery has not been given the credit it deserves and has certainly been overshadowed by the later work of Watson and Crick. Prior to Miescher, no one knew what nuclei did. In Virchow's *Cellular Pathology*, he quotes Schleiden and Schwann who believed that the nucleus is a cell precursor and forms from the "blastema." Virchow rejects this theory and states that the nucleus is necessary for life, but goes no further in discussing its function. Miescher collected human pus cells to study by accumulating dirty bandages in the Tubingen clinic where he was a student. He learned to separate the nuclei from the pus cells and succeeded in extracting and purifying the material, which he called "nuclein." Miescher's professor, Hoppe-Seyler, refused to publish the paper until he, himself, had repeated Miescher's work. When it was published in 1871, Miescher was able to have the date of 1869 included to protect his priority in this great discovery. In 1889, after he had succeeded in separating the protein from the nucleic acid, Richard Altmann first used the term "nucleic acid." Albrecht Kossel, the biochemist, further analyzed the nucleic acid and identified purines and pyrimidines, for which he received a Nobel Prize in 1910.

NUCLEIC ACID

Chromosomes were first described in 1882 by Walther Fleming when he noted tiny threads in salamander egg nuclei that were dividing. Subsequently, in 1888, W. Waldeyer named Fleming's threads "chromosomes" because they stained deeply. In 1903 William Sutton, an American biologist, proposed that genes are located on chromosomes, the microscopic clusters of nucleic acid. In the 1920s, two distinct forms of nucleic acid were discovered, ribonucleic acid (RNA) and deoxyribonucleic acid (DNA). The two forms were distinguished by the ribose sugars discovered in 1909 (deoxy-ribose actually took another twenty years) by Phoebus Levine. The structure of DNA was simple and repetitive, unlikely to be capable of carrying complex information, so attention turned to the proteins associated with DNA in chromosomes as the carriers of genetic information. In 1900, Emil Fischer postulated chemical crosslinks of amino acids in proteins and genetics took a blind alley for a few years. In 1910, Thomas Hunt Morgan, experimenting with fruit flies, a useful experimental model with rapid reproduction allowing many generations in a short study period, discovered that some traits are sex-linked. He also confirmed that genes reside on chromosomes although his work did not produce any evidence about the protein vs. nucleic acid debate. In 1926, biologist Hermann Muller, still working with fruit flies, showed that x-rays can cause genetic mutations.

Finally, in 1944, Oswald Avery, Colin Macleod, and Maclyn McCarty demonstrated that DNA and not proteins carry the hereditary material in most living organisms. They had been studying pneumococcus and the discovery came during this research. This saga began with the observation in 1927, by Fred Griffith a British physician, that a killed suspension of virulent pneumococcus could transfer virulence to a live culture of harmless pneumococci injected into the same mouse. How could this be? The "harmless" species killed the mice and Griffith could not understand how the transfer of virulence took place. He referred to a "Pablum" (the name of a popular baby food) that somehow transformed the harmless bacteria.[246] He could not explain why the transformation was permanent and subsequent subcolonies of the transformed organisms continued to be virulent. Pablum, if that meant a favorable culture medium, should not change the genetic makeup of the organism.

In 1931, Griffith's observations came to the attention of Oswald Avery, a Canadian-born physician at the Rockefeller Institute. Avery had been working on the biochemistry of pneumococcus capsules, a major feature of the organism that contributes to virulence. The capsule is made up of specific polysaccharides and Avery, and colleague Michael Heidelberger, discovered that there were four types, each a different polysaccharide. The types differ in virulence, one of the first examples of macromolecules producing different biological properties. Avery's associates repeated

Griffith's experiment in the test tube, showing that virulence was transferred in a culture, not a living animal host. Avery, Macleod, and McCarty formed a team to study what they called "transforming material" and quickly identified DNA present in it. They chose the DNA fraction for further study and spent years learning to purify their DNA preparation of any of the protein residue from the chromosome (bacteria have only one). They were working to overturn the standard perception that protein carried the genetic material. Avery had been through this before when he tried to convince colleagues that the capsule was polysaccharide, not protein. Part of their success was due to the identification of an enzyme that specifically hydrolyzed DNA and the observation that transforming material was destroyed by this enzyme.

Griffith was killed in 1941 by a bomb during the London Blitz and Avery put a photograph of Griffith on the wall in his office until he retired. In December 1943, Avery presented his results to the Institute and, in February 1944, published the results in the *Journal of Experimental Medicine*.[247] The concept faced opposition from biochemists who could not be convinced that the simple molecule could carry the complex genetic code. Alfred Mirsky, a Rockefeller Institute biochemist, was adamant in opposition and, in 1946, his denial of any possible role of DNA convinced the Nobel Prize committee in Stockholm to defer an award of the prize to Avery and his colleagues. Avery became depressed at this reception to his twenty years of work and retired to his brother's farm in 1948. The story gets worse, because Erwin Chargaff, a Columbia University biochemist (who had discovered protamine), read Avery's paper in 1944 and immediately concentrated his work on DNA chemistry. In 1949, he published the first report of a one-to-one ratio between purines and pyrimidines in DNA.[248] In 1953 Watson, Crick, and Wilkins described the structure of DNA as a double helix and credited Chargaff's study as of critical importance in their work. They did not mention Avery.

CHROMOSOMES AND TISSUE CULTURE

In 1952, the "Dark Ages" of cytogenetics ended with the introduction of the "Hypotonic Era" of study. Until this point, what progress there was had been made through tissue culture techniques, invented by Ross Granville Harrison in 1907. Harrison was a brilliant student who was already an associate professor of biology at Johns Hopkins before graduation from medical school. His field was embryology and, in attempting to study frog nerve cells, he dissected out a frog medullary tube (the embryonic origin of the brain) from an embryo and placed it in a solution of frog lymph on a slide, then sealed the preparation with a cover slip. In his paper,[249] he reported keeping such preparations alive for up to four weeks. His observations showed that the nerve fiber was part of the cell itself and grew, behaving in an amoeba-like fashion at the tip, about twenty-five microns in a half hour. He subsequently became a professor of zoology at Yale and studied amphibian embryology for many years. He was considered twice for Nobel Prizes, but was not selected and his major discovery, tissue culture, was not appreciated until the 1940s.

In 1910, Alexis Carrel studied with Harrison and learned the tissue culture method. Two years later Carrel received his Nobel Prize and, because of his worldwide fame, some thought that it was granted for tissue culture work. Carrel was publicity conscious and conducted an experiment with a culture of chicken heart cells that became very famous ("the immortal heart"),[250] although the lab methods were quite crude. Harrison's work was eclipsed. Late in his life, Harrison had the satisfaction of learning that his tissue culture technique had enabled John Enders to grow poliovirus in cell culture. In 1949, Enders reported his success[251] and, in 1953, when Salk reported the clinical success of a killed virus vaccine, and again in 1954 when Enders, Weller, and Robbins were awarded the Nobel Prize in Physiology or Medicine, Harrison, in his eighties, is reported to have been totally delighted at this great triumph based on his seminal work forty years earlier.[252]

Until T.C. Hsu used the hypotonic technique to study nuclei, it was universally believed that human cells had forty-eight chromosomes. In 1952, he began to use a solution with a lower sodium concentration than intra-cellular fluid. Actually, the solution was based on Galveston (where he worked) tap water, which was a brackish mixture of fresh and seawater. The result was an influx of water into cells, and the nuclei, which spread the chromosomes widely apart, permitting better observation. Hsu, himself, actually studied animal cells, not human tissue but in 1956, J.H. Tjio and A. Levan began to use Hsu's hypotonic method on human cells. The correct chromosome count, forty-six, quickly followed.

The next stage of cytogenetics is called "the Trisomy Period" when patients with Down's syndrome and other congenital anomalies with chromosome abnormalities were studied. The trisomy 21 genotype was the first to be identified because the Down's syndrome patients were so common. Trisomy 13, Patau Syndrome, and trisomy 18, Edward Syndrome, came next. Klinefelter's Syndrome, with an XXY genotype and a tall, sterile male phenotype, and Turner's syndrome, with XO genotype and short sterile female phenotype, were identified as the first of the sex chromosome abnormalities. Eventually, the Philadelphia Chromosome (a small #22 chromosome) in chronic myelocytic leukemia was discovered. It is now known that most cancers have chromosome abnormalities.[253]

THE DOUBLE HELIX

During this period, the molecular structure of DNA was worked out using x-ray crystallography. Max von Laue had made the discovery of crystal diffraction of x-ray in 1912. William Bragg, working at times with his son William Lawrence Bragg, observed that the x-ray images were specific for each crystal and, eventually concluded that they gave information about the crystal structure on a molecular level. In 1944, Maurice Wilkins was working on uranium isotopes in the Manhattan Project, when he read of Avery's research. In 1947, he joined John Randall at King's College, London in England's first biophysics laboratory. Since Randall had invented the cavity magnetron, the heart of the radar transmitter, before the war, England was willing to do almost anything to reward him. He asked Wilkins to be his deputy at the biophysics lab and agreed with him that DNA structure was going to be an important topic. They chose for their source of material the head of the sperm (squid sperm, which is large), a fortunate choice because of the concentration of the nucleic material.

Raymond Gosling, a doctoral student, was asked to work on x-ray crystallography, a subject he knew little about. Another physicist, Alex Stokes, gave him a crash course in crystallography and Gosling got to work. He was having trouble with old equipment and poor images so he asked Wilkins for some additional DNA. Wilkins had received a very pure sample from Rudolph Singer, a Swiss physicist, and gave some to Gosling. Wilkins then took an interest and began to work with Gosling. Others had done preliminary work on x-ray crystallography of DNA and another physicist named Furberg had even hypothesized about a helical structure in 1947. In 1950, Gosling and Wilkins obtained some excellent images and that spring they recruited Rosalind Franklin, a skilled x-ray crystallography expert, for a three-year fellowship. They were amateurs and it was time for a professional in this arcane field to join them.

Their next step was to obtain a better x-ray machine from Birkbeck College where a German refugee scientist, Werner Ehrenberg, had invented a device called a microfocus generating tube. This would provide the very narrow x-ray beams, which would be necessary to obtain diffraction diagrams from single DNA strands. They also obtained a microcamera to collect the images. Rosalind Franklin arrived in 1951 and stepped into a controversy. Wilkins thought that he would be the chief investigator with

Franklin and Gosling providing the images for him to interpret. Randall had written Franklin a letter telling her that she would be in charge of the crystallography project. Rosalind Franklin was destined to die young, at thirty-seven, and was determined to become a respected scientist. The controversy, aided somewhat by her personality, would lead to tragedy. She and Wilkins immediately developed an antipathy for each other that became a feud. In the words of her biographer, Ann Sayre, "the history of molecular biology might be rather different today if Rosalind and Maurice Wilkin had not hated one another at sight."[254] Gosling had no trouble with her and they worked well together. Gosling recalled in later years that she often neglected radiation precautions and this might have contributed to her ovarian cancer, which appeared at the age of thirty-five. Later in 1951, Wilkins presented a slide of DNA x-ray crystallography to a conference in Naples attended by James Watson, a post-doctoral fellow from Indiana.

Watson was instantly convinced that this was the answer to understanding the genetic code. Watson knew nothing of crystallography, but sought out Wilkins the next day and managed to obtain a fellowship at the Cavendish Laboratory at Cambridge in the fall of 1951 to learn crystallography under John Kendrew, a well-known biophysicist. Kendrew was studying hemoglobin and myoglobin and Watson stayed long enough to learn the method, and then moved on to his own project. Also present at the Cavendish was Francis Crick who was knowledgeable about x-ray crystallography. Crick, however, was not interested in DNA, at least before Watson convinced him otherwise. Watson convinced Crick to become Wilkins' competitor in research. Linus Pauling had just announced the helical structure of protein in the US adding a further stimulus to Watson. This information, plus the comments of Wilkins to his friend Crick that DNA was probably helical, added to his interest. Through Wilkins, they were kept informed of the results of Rosalind Franklin's research.

Pauling had used molecular models using colored plastic balls to illustrate the results of crystallography. Watson and Crick adopted this method, as well. In November of 1951, Watson requested an invitation to attend a presentation by Franklin of her latest results. Wilkins obliged, but Watson did not take notes and the model that he and Crick constructed based on her lecture was incorrect. Franklin was scathing in her criticism of their efforts. A few days later, the lab director requested that Watson and Crick stop their model building efforts. The director believed that they were intruding into Wilkins' research and were not doing enough of their own work. During 1952, they stopped model building, but continued their interest. Pauling had now turned his attention to DNA.

Rosalind Franklin had her own problems understanding the structure and used a dry crystal form of DNA, rather than the moist gel-like form that actually represents biological systems. She could not see the helical form in the dry DNA structure and came to believe that the structure might not be helical after all. This comment is from Watson and may not be an accurate representation of her opinion since he was justifying himself long after the 1953 publication. In the spring of 1952, she obtained a photograph, later to become famous as photograph #51, which clearly showed helical structure in moist DNA obtained from squid sperm. She did not disclose this photo to the others for some reason.

In late 1952 Randall asked Franklin to leave because of the friction (or she chose to look for another position for the same reason) and, when she turned over her materials to Wilkins, he immediately recognized the significance of photograph #51. Had she shared this photo with Wilkins earlier they, and not Watson and Crick, would have made the discovery. Instead, Wilkins showed the photograph to Watson. Watson and Crick recognized the significance of this proof of the theory they had been working on with models. They approached Bragg, the lab director in February of 1953, for permission to resume their work on DNA structure. They told Bragg that Pauling was also working on the DNA structure and it had become a race between England and the USA, not just an intra-lab competition with Wilkins and Franklin. Using Franklin's data, they worked on the purine-pyrimidine bond. Her results suggested that the chains ran in opposite directions and that the bases were on the interior of the chain with the ribose backbone on the outside. Their lack of biochemistry knowledge was another hindrance, as Jerry Donohue, a Medical Research Council biochemist, pointed out. On February 28, 1953, they stumbled on the correct arrangement. The purine, guanine, joined to cytosine, a pyrimidine. Then adenine, another purine, mated with thymine, also a pyrimidine. The two chains fitted together perfectly.

By early March, they had assembled the correct model. At this point, March 1953, Franklin was leaving and Wilkins, not knowing that they had solved the problem with the help of his hints, proposed cooperation. In reply, they sent him a copy of the paper they were submitting to *Nature*. On April 25, *Nature* published simultaneous reports from Watson and Crick, Wilkins, Stokes and Wilson, and Franklin and Gosling.[255] The fact that Watson and Crick's article appeared before the others in the single issue, produced the appearance of priority for the first paper. Worldwide fame followed.

The Watson and Crick article is written in clear prose and is short (800

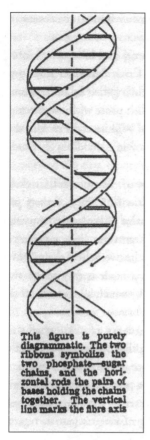

This figure is purely diagrammatic. The two ribbons symbolize the two phosphate—sugar chains, and the horizontal rods the pairs of bases holding the chains together. The vertical line marks the fibre axis

Figure 10 – Odile Crick's illustration in Nature, 1953

words) while the other two are more detailed and more difficult to understand. A simple diagram, drawn by Crick's wife, aided in understanding the results.

Thirdly, Crick added a remark that the base pairing suggested a copying mechanism, a concept recognized by all scientific readers as a major consideration. The Watson and Crick article, and another published five weeks later, did not include a reference to Avery's work. They also made the suggestion that, in a long molecule like DNA, the sequence of base pairs might contain the code of genetics. They were absolutely correct but had no evidence. Nonetheless, they were given credit for other men's (and a woman's) work which did in fact support these guesses. Watson and Crick made their discoveries without touching a molecule of DNA or conducting a single experiment. All the experimental work was done by others who received little or no credit. Their lucky guesses were confirmed in 1958 by Matthew Meselson and Franklin Stahl who used elegant experimental techniques to confirm the structure.[256] Brenner and colleagues discovered messenger RNA that year and then in 1961 Crick and Brenner confirmed the general nature of the genetic code. The 1962 Nobel Prize was awarded to Watson, Crick and Wilkins. Rosalind Franklin had died in 1958 and the Prize rules forbid a posthumous award. She worked on valuable projects right up until the time of her death at the age of thirty-seven and was just at the threshold of honors and recognition. A year before her death she met a man she cared for very much and might have married but it was too late. She has been forgotten.

246   Fred Griffith, "The Significance of Pneumococcal Types," Journal of Hygiene, 27:113-159 (1928).

247   Oswald Avery, C.M. MacLeod and M. McCarty, "Studies on the Chemical of the Substance Inducing Transformation of Pneumococcal Types," Journal of Experimental Medicine 79:137-158 (1944).

248   Erwin Chargaff, et al. ,"The Composition of the Deoxypentose Nucleic Acids of Thymus and Spleen," Journal of Biological Chemistry 177:405-416 (1949).

249   R.G. Harrison, "Observations on the Living Developing Nerve Fiber," Anatomical Record No. 5, *American Journal of Anatomy* 7: I (1907).

250   Meyer Friedman and Gerald Friedland, *Medicines 10 Greatest Discoveries*, Yale University Press, p 142 (1998).

251   JF Enders, TH Weller and FC Robbins, "Cultivation of the Lansing Strain of Poliomyelitis Virus in Cultures of Various Human Embryonic Tissues," *Science* v 109:85-87 (1949).

252   Meyer Friedman and Gerald W Friedland, p 152.

253   *Harrison's Principles of Internal Medicine*, 14th Edition, pages 402-403, McGraw-Hill (1998).

254   Anne Sayre, *Rosalind Franklin and DNA*, Norton, p 95 (1975).

255   J.D. Watson and F.H.C. Crick, "Molecular Structure of Nucleic Acids. A Structure for Deoxyribose Nucleic Acid," *Nature* 171:737 (1953).

      M.H.F. Wilkins, A.R. Stokes and H.R. Wilson, "Molecular Structure of Nucleic Acids. Molecular Structure of Deoxypentose Nucleic Acids," *ibid.* :738.

      Rosalind F. Franklin and R.G. Gosling, "Molecular Structure of Nucleic Acids. Molecular Configuration in Sodium Thymonucleate," *ibid*: 740.

256   M.S. Meselson and F.W. Stahl, "The Replication of DNA in Escherichia coli," *Proceedings of the National Academy of Science*, 44:67 (1956).

17
Fleming, Florey and Penicillin

IN 1875 JOHN TYNDALL, AN ENGLISH PHYSICIST, WAS STUDYING THE distribution of bacteria in the air, much as Pasteur had done ten years earlier. To conduct his experiment, he set out one hundred open tubes of broth, spaced a standard distance from each other. If bacteria are uniformly distributed in the air, the broth tubes should have a uniform distribution of positive cultures. Tyndall's experiment demonstrated that bacteria were not evenly distributed in the air, some tubes' broth remained clear after twenty-four hours. Tyndall also observed the presence, in one of his tubes, of a *Penicillium* mold that he described as "exquisitely beautiful," growing on the surface of the broth. He noted that; "in every case where the mold was thick and coherent, the bacteria died or became dormant and fell to the bottom as a sediment." The mold was *Penicillium notatum* and it was making penicillin, which killed the bacteria, probably staphylococcus. Tyndall commented on the antibacterial properties of the mold, but his principle interest was in the atmospheric distribution of bacteria (yet to be associated with disease by Koch seven years later) and other particles. He did not mention his observations to any physicians and passed on to other matters.[257]

In 1896, A.E. Duschene, a French medical student, commented on the antagonism between *Penicillium* mold and bacteria when injected together into experimental animals. The animals injected with both fared better than those injected with bacteria alone.[258] Again, there was no follow-up of the observation. In 1906, Paul Erlich discovered Salvarsan but the *Penicillium* mold and its effect on bacterial culture was ignored for another twenty years. In 1925, D.A. Gratia, of the University of Liege, reported that a substance produced by *Penicillium* could dissolve anthrax bacilli. Again, there was no follow-up. Alexander Fleming was born in Lochfield, Scotland in 1881, attended the University of London (which he chose for its swimming team) on a scholarship and entered St. Mary's Medical School. He graduated in 1906 and remained on the staff there as an assistant in the inoculation department. He continued his association with the hospital until his retirement in 1955. During the entire time, some forty-nine years, he served as the assistant director under Sir Almroth Wright, who had described the staining of white blood cells. Not much upward mobility in that department! Fleming became one of the leading experts in England on the treatment of syphilis and, despite the lack of promotion in his position at St. Mary's, acquired a sizable fortune through his private practice.

THE DISCOVERY

In 1928, a serendipitous observation led ultimately to the discovery of penicillin as a drug and to the era of antibiotics. Fleming was working with *Staphylococcus* and, the day before he left for a vacation, he smeared a culture sample onto a petri dish then left the dish on the workbench instead of placing it into the incubator. He was going to be gone for two weeks so he decided to leave it at room temperature. The culture would grow enough at room temperature over two weeks for his purposes (attempting to determine if temperature affected the color of the bacterial colony; Staph aureus is gold, Staph albus is white). A laboratory on the floor below Fleming's was conducting experiments with molds and happened to be growing *Penicillium notatum*. They were studying the effect of mold on children's asthma attacks and had collected samples from all over London. When Fleming returned from vacation in early September 1928, he found his *Staphylococcus* culture growing, plus a colony of *Penicillium notatum* surrounded by a zone of clear agar. The *Penicillium* had, almost certainly, come from spores that drifted through the building from the lab on the floor below. Fleming had only opened the cover on the petri dish for a few seconds. *Penicillium* does not grow at body temperature so, if the petri dish had been placed in the incubator, the colony would not have formed and Fleming would never have seen the effect. In another freak occurrence, a London heat wave broke the day he left. The room temperature during the heat wave (long before air conditioning) was close to body temperature and would have inhibited the growth of the mold. The coincidence was extreme and Fleming was unable to duplicate his discovery later.

In 1970, Hare showed that the London weather had provided a unique circumstance. The heat wave broke the day Fleming left for his two-week holiday. Two days before he returned, London had two more hot days. The mold had grown during the unseasonable cool weather then, just before Fleming returned, two hot days stimulated the *Staphylococcus* colonies to grow. This combination was responsible for the phenomenon he observed.

When he attempted to duplicate the circumstance of simultaneous growth of *Penicillium* and *Staphylococcus* on a culture plate, he could never again get the temperature right. Years later, Hare checked the 1928 weather records for London, duplicated the sequence, and reproduced Fleming's finding.[259] Unlike Tyndall fifty years before, Fleming decided to investigate this phenomenon. Prior to his discovery of penicillin, Fleming had studied lysozyme, a bacteriocidal component of tears. Lysozyme produces clear zones on bacterial culture plates, like penicillin, and his previous experience may have helped him to recognize the effect he was seeing.[260] He had trouble collecting enough human tears for his study (prompting a cartoon of him whipping medical students and collecting their tears) and he dropped the matter. Years later, other sources of lysozyme were discovered, including intestinal secretions and egg white, and research resumed.[261]

Fleming first decided to test the *Penicillium* for inhibition of other bacteria. He quickly learned that a substance, which could be recovered from the broth the mold was floating on, produced the inhibition. He named this unknown material "penicillin" and found that it was soluble and would pass through a bacterial filter. He also discovered that the material, penicillin, accumulated gradually in the broth and it took eight days of mold growth to reach a maximum concentration. His technique for testing bacterial strains for sensitivity to penicillin was similar to (actually the reverse of) the modern technique used to test one bacterium for sensitivity to multiple antibiotics. He cut a trough in an agar plate and filled it with penicillin-containing broth. He then applied samples of bacteria to the plate in streaks beginning at the canal and extending to the periphery of the plate. He knew that the penicillin would diffuse through the agar some distance from the canal and inhibit sensitive bacteria near the canal. He found that penicillin killed *Staphylococcus*, *Streptococcus*, gonococcus and meningococcus. He also learned that tuberculosis, typhoid and influenza-like organisms were not inhibited. Inexplicably, he did not test the spirochete that causes syphilis against penicillin. He was England's top expert on syphilis but did not think about testing this organism, perhaps because he knew it was not a bacterium. Had he done so, he would have learned that it is exquisitely sensitive to penicillin. Salvarsan required eighteen months of weekly intravenous injections but one or two injections of penicillin is sufficient to eradicate the disease.

He tried other *Penicillium* species and learned that they had no antibacterial effect; another evidence of the incredible serendipity of his discovery. He tested the filtrate of *Penicillium* broth in a rabbit and a mouse and found no evidence of toxicity. He tested the broth in an infected human eye, an inflamed maxillary sinus and an infected leg amputation. The infection cleared in the first two and no harmful effect was seen. He published his results in 1929 and another paper in 1932.[262,263] Unfortunately, Fleming did not attempt any experiment on the in-vivo effect of penicillin. He did not attempt Duchesne's experiment: inject an animal with both a virulent strain of a sensitive bacteria and the penicillin-containing broth. Had he done so, he would have seen the effect and could not have failed to see the significance of his discovery. His superior, Wright, believed, as many did at the time, that "antibacterial drugs are a delusion."[264] Still, Wright had adopted salvarsan when Erlich discovered it and suggested Fleming try it on his syphilitic patients. Fleming never tried penicillin as anything but a topical agent and, in his 1929 article, compares it to carbolic acid. Years later, Fleming stated that he abandoned the study of penicillin because his preparations quickly lost potency. The services of a biochemist might have enabled Fleming to extract the drug from the broth as a pure crystalline substance but Wright would not accept a biochemist in his inoculation department. Fleming went on to other subjects after 1932.

A bacteriologist named Paine read Fleming's article and obtained a sample of the *Penicillium notatum* from him. Paine made broth cultures and applied the broth to four babies and one adult with infected eyes. Three of the babies and the adult responded to this application within 48 hours; two of the babies had gonococcus infections, which have severe consequences for vision. The bacteriologist reported his results to Howard Florey, professor of pathology at Sheffield University, but Florey did not pursue it at the time. Harold Rainstruck, head of the New London School of Hygiene and Tropical Medicine, obtained a sample of *Penicillium* from Fleming in 1931 and had it analyzed by an American mycologist who identified it as a variant form of *P. notatum*, one more example of the fantastic luck involved in Fleming's discovery. Standard *Penicillium notatum* does not produce penicillin. Rainstruck's group, in continuing their study of penicillin, attempted to purify their material by evaporating an ether solution of it and found that the activity was lost. They stopped their investigation of the substance after this failure. An American graduate student began a study of penicillin in 1935 and discovered that it did not dissolve bacteria but inhibited their growth. He asked his faculty advisor if he could pursue the matter for his doctoral dissertation and was refused permission. The student, R. D. Reid reported his findings but was unable to continue his research.[265]

THE SULFA DRUGS

The dam was breached in 1935 when Gerhard Domagk reported the anti-bacterial effects of Prontosil. Paul Erlich had been convinced in 1906 that aniline dyes would have biological properties, because of the variable staining of cotton and other natural fibers. His one effective discovery, salvarsan, was, unfortunately, not one of them, being an arsenical. He was right about the principle, however, and the proof came in 1932, after I.G.Farbenindustrie obtained a patent for several azo dyes including Prontosil Red. Before Prontosil, a dye called scarlet red had been shown to have weak anti-bacterial properties and was used to saturate gauze that was then applied to wounds. It was unclear if this property was similar to that of carbolic acid, a general antiseptic, or a specific inhibition of some bacterial metabolic function. Prontosil was an unsatisfactory dye, producing a weak reddish color somewhat like scarlet red, and it was turned over to Gerhardt Domagk, a bacteriologist, for his research.

After extensive animal study, Domagk tried the new drug in patients with streptococcal infection. He gave it intravenously and found that it quickly cured serious streptococcal infections. The first patient was his daughter who, before he had tested the new drug in humans, developed a life threatening streptococcus infection. He had only used the new drug in mice but, with his daughter's life at stake, he chose to try it in desperation. She recovered, but he did not describe this experience until years later. It was less effective in the test tube, leading Domagk to suspect that the actual anti-bacterial effect was due to a metabolic derivative produced in the body. Examination of patients' urine recovered a more active compound called "sulfanilamide", produced by the liver, which cleaves the prontosil molecule in half. Sulfanilamide had been described in 1908 by Viennese chemist Gelmo but had never been applied to therapy. This was the first of the sulfa drugs and bacteriologists soon discovered that sulfanilamide was an analogue of para-amino-benzoic acid, a compound required for bacterial growth. The drug inhibited bacterial multiplication by competing with the active compound, PABA (another Gelmo discovery), for the essential chemical receptor, just as Erlich had predicted. Drug therapy could be effective against bacteria and the mechanism of action was specific.

Domagk was awarded the 1939 Nobel Prize in Medicine but the war had begun and the Nazi government of Germany forced him to refuse the award. Work on the sulfa drugs continued during the war in other countries after sulfapyridine was synthesized by the British company May & Baker in 1938. The drug was initially called "M&B 693," a name which came from the lab records of the company and did not mean, as many concluded, that it was the 693rd compound tested.[266] The story of Paul Erlich was still fresh and his exploration for a drug that would be effective in syphilis had recently been dramatized in the film "Doctor Erlich's Magic Bullet," starring Edward G. Robinson. The public went wild with enthusiasm, especially after Sir Winston Churchill was successfully treated for pneumonia during the war.

The discovery was important because sulfanilamide was effective only in streptococcal infection. Pasteur discovered *Streptococcus pneumoniae* (called pneumococcus) in 1881 and soon realized that it was the most common cause of lobar pneumonia. Dochez and Gillespie recognized four types with different levels of pathogenicity based on the capsule (Griffith and Avery learned that the capsule types were determined by a polysaccharide in the capsule – See Chapter 16). By 1936 anti-serum to the capsule antigens had reduced mortality of pneumoccocal pneumonia from 36 percent to 18 percent. Pneumococcus, which produced about 40,000 deaths per year from lobar pneumonia in Britain, was only weakly sensitive to the first sulfa drug. Sulfapyridine changed all this and resulted in a sharp drop in pneumonia mortality, especially in the young. By 1941, another sulfa drug, sulfadiazine, further reduced mortality to 8 percent.

This was not the end of the story of the aniline dyes and the sulfa drugs. It continues in the chapter "Twentieth Century Medicine" as they still had several major contributions to make. Domagk was finally allowed to accept his Nobel Prize after the war, in 1947. He was grateful for the recognition, but the money had been allocated to other recipients and he did not receive any monetary award.

PRACTICAL APPLICATION OF THE DISCOVERY

George Dreyer, professor and chairman of the school of pathology at Oxford, had obtained a sample of Fleming's *Penicillium* culture after the 1929 paper to see if penicillin was a bacteriophage. He was an authority on these virus-like organisms that infect and kill bacteria, discovered in 1917. He was disappointed to find that it was not a bacteriophage and discontinued his research, but kept the culture. His assistant, Miss Campbell-Renton, kept the culture growing to use for other purposes. A few years later, Dreyer died and his replacement was Howard Florey, the pathologist Paine had told about his success in using penicillin in infants' eye infections. Florey was an Australian, trained as a physiologist, a pathologist and an internal medicine specialist. Florey was enthusiastic about clinical research and assembled a team at Oxford with similar interests. One of the team members, Ernst Chain a fugitive from the Nazis, met Miss Campbell-Renton one day and accidentally learned that she had a culture of Fleming's *Penicillium*. He had read Fleming's paper and went to Florey with a suggestion that they investigate its anti-bacterial properties. Domagk had proven that drugs could be effective against bacterial infections. The objections that had been made ten years before were now disproved. The next problem was finding research funding in 1939, late in the Depression and on the eve of World War II. Florey had spent time at the Rockefeller Institute and he succeeded in getting funding for the project. They were not looking for an antibiotic; they wanted to understand the basic process by which one microorganism can inhibit, or kill, another. They chose penicillin because they had Fleming's culture growing right there at the school.

Margaret Jennings, a member of the team (twenty-seven years later she would marry Florey after his wife died), discovered that penicillin had no effect on mature organisms, it inhibited new growth. Norman Heatley, another team member, found a way to measure the quantity of penicillin in a sample and defined the unit of activity. Chain learned, early in his study of the molecule, that it was not an enzyme. It was a simple molecule and this disappointed him. Pressing on, he worked on the problem of stability; penicillin was very unstable. Finally, he solved the problem by freeze-drying it. He produced penicillin powder and found that this was the stable form. The next step was to test it for safety. Enormous doses had no harmful effect on mice. Chain began to suspect that they were really on to something. He went to Florey, who now believed that they were on the threshold of one of the great discoveries in medicine. Florey repeated Chain's experiments and then went another step that Fleming had never taken. He injected eight mice with a lethal dose of streptococci, and then injected four of them with penicillin. The four mice that received the antibiotic survived.

Excitement grew at Oxford. Chain and Florey noticed that the mice who received penicillin had brown urine. The urine was tested and was shown to contain penicillin, unchanged in its passage through the body and able to pass into all bodily fluids. Over the next three months they tested the drug for toxicity and repeated the experiment of injecting mice with bacteria; this time with seventy-five mice and three different types of bacteria. The experiment was successful. On August 24, 1940, at the darkest period of the war, the *Lancet* published their historic paper[267] The researchers decided that, if Germany invaded England, they would smuggle the mold cultures out of England to America or Canada.

PURIFICATION AND PRODUCTION

At this point, Florey had to break his promise to the Rockefeller Institute about limiting the study to biochemistry. England and the allies (after the US entered the war) would need this new drug. First, he must test the drug on patients. His first case was a cancer patient, terminally ill. He got a bad scare when the intravenous penicillin produced a high fever and chills. His first (hopeful) consideration was that the penicillin had an impurity in it that produced a febrile reaction, much as blood transfusions sometimes did. They returned to their purification process and changed to a two-step extraction. The resulting powder was now yellow instead of brown color and they hoped this would solve the problem. In order to get enough penicillin for clinical testing, Florey developed a mini-factory in the pathology department at Oxford. Heatley, the biochemist of the team, worked on this process and devised ways to increase production. Soon, his new process could obtain twelve exchanges of medium from the same mold colony instead of the original one. Later he devised an automated extraction process that was far more productive.

For years, the production of adequate amounts of penicillin was a major bottleneck, especially during a world war. Heatley next hired a group of women, known as "the penicillin girls," to assist in rolling bottles of freeze-dried solution to extract the drug. Next, they redesigned the bottles to save room and got a pottery company to manufacture them.

Human testing began with the new batch of drug by injecting everyone in the department with intravenous penicillin. There were no reactions this time. Florey did not yet have enough drug for wide scale human testing when he was asked to treat a policeman who was dying of septicemia. They used what drug they had and the policeman improved. When they ran out of penicillin, they tried extracting it from his urine but they still did not have enough to resume treatment. The policeman died and Florey decided to avoid another inadequate effort. Domagk had been very fortunate in his experience with his daughter. Four of their next five patients were children and all but one recovered. The fatality was from a septic aneurysm of the carotid artery that ruptured. The autopsy of the fatal case showed no residual infection. They published their first clinical report in August 1941.[268] After repeated requests from Florey, Imperial Chemical Industries began to manufacture penicillin and their supply increased enough to treat another 187 patients (most treated by Florey's wife). Florey measured blood levels and studied clinical results; soon he was learning what the proper dosage and indications were. He was extremely lucky that he did not test the drug on guinea pigs;

penicillin kills guinea pigs. As the news about the new "miracle drug" got to the newspapers, Sir Almroth Wright wrote a letter to the London Times claiming credit for the discovery for Fleming (after he had forbidden Fleming to pursue his early observation). The editor of the Times corrected Sir Almroth by properly attributing the discovery to Florey (acknowledging Fleming's early contribution). A controversy followed. Florey was reticent while Fleming sought publicity. Years later, Lord Beaverbrook, the newspaper owner who may have felt snubbed by the publicity shy Florey, encouraged the Nobel selection committee to award the Prize to Fleming alone.

CLINICAL APPLICATION

The first successful use of intravenous penicillin reported was actually in the United States, at Columbia Presbyterian Hospital in New York. Dr. Martin Henry Dawson obtained penicillin from mold supplied by Roger Reed. They presented their results at a meeting of the American Society for Clinical Investigation in May 1941, before Florey's clinical report. In July 1941, Florey and Heatley visited the US to seek help in producing more penicillin. They met Dr. Robert Coghill, who headed the fermentation division of a Department of Agriculture research laboratory and he suggested a new method of producing the drug called deep fermentation. Heatley traveled to Peoria, Illinois to work on the new method and there collaborated with a treacherous biochemist named Moyer. Moyer came up with an improved substrate for growing the mold but, after Heatley had left to return to Britain, Moyer attempted to patent the process. Eventually his scheme failed and he had to return his ill-gotten gains. Others, less concerned with personal aggrandizement, worked on other improvements in the process. They sought a more productive species of mold and found it on a cantaloupe purchased in a local market. The new mold was *Penicillium chrysogenum* and the discoverer, a secretary in the lab, was called "moldy Mary" for the rest of her life. American research on penicillin and its improvements were kept from the British during the war (as a military secret!) and that, plus the patent fiasco, led to considerable friction. Florey and Chain had a falling out, because Chain had advised Florey to patent the drug originally. The American improvements did increase production enormously, although the British were able to supply their own needs during the war. Fleming and Florey were knighted in 1944 and they, plus Chain, were awarded the Nobel Prize in Medicine in 1945.

OTHER ANTIBIOTICS

Fleming's discovery and Florey's clinical research inspired others to seek new therapy from microorganisms. In 1944, Selman Waksman, and his colleagues at Rutgers, announced the discovery of the second antibiotic (and Waksman coined the term), streptomycin. Waksman was a soil microbiologist and he discovered a new group of soil organisms, *Actinomyces*. Their first drug produced from a culture of this organism, Actinomycin, was effective but very toxic. It was to become, twenty years later, one of the first effective chemotherapy drugs for cancer, Actinomycin D. In 1944, Waksman discovered another species, *Streptomyces griseus,* and he isolated the drug he called Streptomycin from this culture. Streptomycin was particularly important because it was effective against gram-negative bacteria and, most importantly, tuberculosis. The development of resistance by mycobacteria limited its effectiveness clinically until William Hugh Feldman, another immigrant scientist, combined para aminosalicylic acid (PAS) and isoniazide (INH – See Chapter 22) with the streptomycin. This combination prevented the development of resistance. Waksman was awarded the 1952 Nobel Prize for his discovery.

Lederle Laboratories announced Aureomycin in 1948 and Pfizer followed with Terramycin in 1950; both are now referred to as tetracyclines and the category of antibiotics is still in use. Parke-Davis developed chloramphicol in 1949 and it proved to be the most effective antibiotic ever discovered for typhoid fever. All of these drugs are isolated from the secretions of molds and follow in the same tradition as penicillin and streptomycin. Unfortunately, the "miracle drugs" stimulated intense interest by the public and, as they became cheaper and more available, people demanded antibiotics for every minor illness. Some of this was stimulated by the scourge of rheumatic fever, a crippling disease of joints and heart valves that sometimes followed streptococcus throat infections. Every mother wanted her child's, or her own, sore throat treated with penicillin. The result was the emergence of bacteria resistant to penicillin, fortunately not streptococcus, which retained its sensitivity. With chloramphenicol, the first really potent broad-spectrum antibiotic, a rare and devastating complication appeared: aplastic anemia. If the use of the new drug had been limited to life threatening diseases like typhoid fever, the complication would have been an acceptable risk. The indiscriminate use had exposed millions to an unnecessary risk and legal trouble followed. Within a few years, the use of chloramphenicol was almost prohibited and a case of aplastic anemia, no matter how appropriate the use of the drug had been, was indefensible.

Resistant strains of bacteria continue to emerge and there has even been talk of returning to obsolete forms of therapy in some cases of tuberculosis like thoracoplasty, collapse therapy and even the use of bacteriophages. The AIDS crisis has produced a recrudescence in tuberculosis in that population and many strains are now resistant to streptomycin. New drugs have been developed but the hopeful expectations of Florey and his colleagues in 1945 have not been fulfilled. In the 1940s, penicillin supplanted sulfadiazine for pneumoccocal infections as the organism was exquisitely sensitive. Twenty years later the concentration of penicillin required to kill the organism had increased by five-fold in some strains. Resistance to penicillin increased in the 1970s and in the late 1980s, in Spain, 44 percent of *S. pneumoniae* were resistant. Multiple-drug resistant strains are now common world-wide and immunization is again becoming an important weapon in the battle against this problem.[269] Some of these problems are coming from the indiscriminant use of antibiotics in animal feed.

257   J. Tyndall, "The Optical Deportment of the Atmosphere in Relation to the Phenomena of Putrefaction and Infection," *Philosophical Transactions of the Royal Society* 166: 27 (1876).

258   A.E. Duchesne, "Contribution a l'etude de la concurrence vitale chez les micro-organismes: Antagonisme entre les moissures et les microbes," Dissertation, Army Medical Academy, Lyon (1896).

259   R. Hare, "New light on the discovery of penicillin," *Medical History* 26:1-24 (1982). This reproduces the 1970 article.

260   R. Hare, "The scientific activities of Alexander Fleming; other than the discovery of penicillin," *Medical History* 27:347-372 (1983). This article describes his lysozyme work.

261   Peeters T, Vantrappen G, "The Paneth cell: a source of intestinal lysozyme," *Gut* 16:553-8 (1975).

262   A. Fleming, "On the Antibacterial Action of Cultures of Penicillium, with Special Reference to Their Use in Silation of H Influenza," *British Journal of Experimental Pathology* 10: 226 (1929).

263   A. Fleming, "On the Specific Antibacterial Properties of Penicillium and Potassium Tellurite Incorporating a Method of Demonstrating Some Bacterial Antagonisms," *Journal of Pathology and Bacteriology*, 35: 831 (1932).

264   D. Wilson, *In Search of Penicillin* Alfred A. Knopf, New York, (1976).

265   R.D.Reid, "Some Properties of Bacterial-Inhibitory Substance Produced by a Mold," *Journal of Bacteriology* 29: 250-253 (1935).

266   LEH Whitby, "Chemotherapy of pneumococcal and other infections with 2(p-aminobenzenesulphonamidopyradine," *Lancet* i:1210 (1938).

267   E. Chain, et al, "Penicillin as a Chemotherapeutic Agent," *Lancet* ii: 226 (1940).

268   E.P.Abraham, et al, "Further Observations on Penicillin," *Lancet* ii: 177 (1941).

269   Morton N.Swartz, Áttacking the Pneumococcus- A Hundred Years' War," New *England Journalof Medicine* 346:722 (2002).

18
Twentieth Century Medicine

THE 1892 EDITION OF OSLER'S *THE PRINCIPLES AND PRACTICE OF Medicine* may be considered to comprise the state of knowledge of medicine at the end of the nineteenth century. The first section, "Specific Infectious Diseases," begins with typhoid fever and goes on for 268 pages describing infectious diseases. The sections on treatment are largely concerned with diet and other non-specific methods except for those few diseases for which specific therapy had been developed. Among those were malaria, in which quinine is effective, and smallpox, in which vaccination is preventative. Diphtheria is discussed but the anti-toxin, first used in December 1891, was not in common use until 1894, two years after publication of the first edition of *Principles and Practice of Medicine*. Rabies is treated with the Pasteur inoculation, although Osler is somewhat equivocal in his comments. For the rest, little can be done except supportive measures. The infectious diseases and the development of effective treatment have been discussed in other chapters.

THE DISCOVERY OF INSULIN

Under "Constitutional Diseases," Osler lists rheumatic fever but is uncertain of the etiology, later discovered to be an immunologic reaction to streptococcus infection. For gout, he recommends colchicine, an effective remedy since Paul of Aegina recommended it in 640CE. Diabetes is said to be "a rare disease in America." The error here is understandable and was repeated sixty years later when renal dialysis became available to treat chronic kidney failure. The anticipated demand was underestimated by several orders of magnitude. When a disease is known to be fatal and no effective treatment is available at any cost, the sufferers die quietly and their presence is unknown to the collectors of statistics. Once a cure is announced, the medical profession is always astonished at the volume of cases that went unreported. Rheumatic fever will be discussed in the history of cardiology but diabetes yielded to medical science thirty years after Osler's book was published and the seeds of the solution existed at the

286 A BRIEF HISTORY OF DISEASE, SCIENCE AND MEDICINE

time. Osler mentions the observation that removal of the pancreas in dogs produces diabetes.

In 1889, von Mering and Minkowski, in the experiment mentioned by Osler, removed the dog pancreas and produced artificial diabetes. Medical student Paul Langerhans discovered the pancreatic "islets of Langerhans" in 1869 and, by 1889, their presence had been noted in all mammalian pancreas glands examined. In 1900, Ssobolew and Schulze found that ligation of the pancreatic duct, which resulted in atrophy of the secreting areas, did not affect the islets and diabetes did not occur. The hormone, the "glycolytic ferment" in Osler's words, must be coming from the islets. In 1908, Zuelzer prepared an alcohol extract of pancreas and injected it into diabetic dogs (made so by removing the pancreas). He found that the urine glucose concentration fell. When the extract was administered intra-venously, a fever resulted. One problem in this research was the presence of proteolytic enzymes in any extract of pancreatic tissue. These enzymes destroyed any protein-based substance that might affect the blood sugar. As a result, many workers dismissed the pancreas as a source of therapy. Their extracts had no effect.

In the summer of 1921, Fredrick G. Banting and medical student Charles Best combined the approach of Ssobolew with new methods of extraction. They ligated dogs' pancreatic ducts and ten weeks later, when the enzyme secreting tissue had atrophied, extracted the remaining tissue with cold Ringer's solution. The substance extracted from the pancreas was injected into dogs whose pancreas had been removed, rendering them diabetic. The blood sugar in the diabetic dogs sharply declined after the injection of what E. Sharpey Schafer had named "insulin" in 1916. Banting and Best then used the same extraction method on organs taken from fetal calves whose pancreas has not yet begun to make digestive enzymes. The material was much more potent and in larger volume. Next, they succeeded in obtain-ing insulin from the pancreas of adult cows, a much larger and more available source. Finally, on December 2, 1921 the first human patient to be given insulin was admitted to the Toronto General Hospital.

The patient, a fourteen year old boy named L.T. (Leonard Thompson), had first been diagnosed with diabetes in December 1919. In spite of diet therapy, all that was available, he lost weight and passed increasing vol-umes of urine strongly positive for glucose. Frederick Allen had proposed diet therapy after noting that glucose levels in the blood and urine could be controlled with a diet that excluded carbohydrates.[270] The result was starvation and the diet was extremely difficult for diabetic patients to follow as they were hungry all the time. It did seem to prolong life but the patients became emaciated to a degree that would not be seen again until World War II. L.T. had no family history of diabetes (this was not unusual because, prior to the discovery of insulin, juvenile diabetics died young and had no children). On admission, he weighed sixty-five pounds and had an odor of acetone on his breath. His urine was strongly positive for glucose and ketones (acetone-like compounds produced by tissue metabolism in the absence of glucose. Without insulin, glucose could not get into the cells. Its concentration rose in the blood, but the cells could not utilize it). On January 11, 1922, the first dose of insulin was given. A weak extract was used for the first treatment and his blood sugar decreased 25 percent. Daily injections followed and his urine sugar declined significantly; the ketones disappeared from the urine. The insulin treatment was stopped for ten days in early February and his condition reverted to that on admission with a high blood sugar and glucose in the urine. The insulin was resumed. Within a month, he was discharged to his home with daily injections of insulin.

Banting and Best, together with several co-workers, reported their experience in the *Canadian Medical Association Journal*.[271] Their summer project had resulted in the first effective therapy for this fatal condition. A biochemist, J.B. Collip, improved the extraction process and contributed significantly to the project. The professor of physiology, John Macleod, who had permitted them to use his lab while he went to Scotland for a summer of fishing, returned in the fall and claimed credit for their work. In 1923, he and Banting were awarded the Nobel Prize; Best and Collip got nothing, one of several examples of misdirected credit in science history. Macleod spent the rest of his life explaining how he had really helped Banting and deserved the prize.[272] Few believed him and Best went on to a distinguished career, probably exceeding anything the others achieved in their later careers. He was Professor and Head of the Department of Medical Research, University of Toronto from 1941 to 1970 and succeeded in purifying heparin during the 1930s, allowing it to be used clinically. Banting, tragically, died in a plane crash in 1941. He had invented a new pressure suit for fliers and was on his way to England to test it when his plane crashed. The Eli Lilly Company, which had provided major assistance (unlike Macleod), quickly went into production and insulin became standard therapy within a year.

An enduring controversy resulted from Banting's anger that MacLeod had claimed credit and Best was excluded from the Nobel Prize. Seale Harris, who knew Banting and Best and who subsequently discovered hyperinsulinism, excoriated MacLeod in his book.[273] Michael Bliss, a historian-not a physician, was more sympathetic to MacLeod's claims. His book *The Discovery of Insulin* denigrates Banting as a country bumpkin without research experience and gives most of the credit to MacLeod and Collip,[274] but the Toronto Daily Star, in 1962 for the fortieth anniversary of the discovery, listed the discoverers and did not include MacLeod. Professor Collip, one of the team who helped to purify the new substance did credit MacLeod in the Star story. The controversy lives on today.

The Diabetes Oral Agents

There was a second form of diabetes but it remained largely unrecognized for many years. In 1875, Apollinaire Bouchardat wrote a book on glycosuria that distinguished between the two types of diabetes, even though the role of the pancreas and insulin was yet to be discovered. In the 1930s, Elliot Joslin, a famous Boston diabetes expert recognized that there was another type of diabetes which affected older, obese adults with a preponderance of women.[275] In the last chapter, I described the discovery of Prontosil and its derivative sulfanilamide. This, and the later derivatives of the sulfanilamide molecule, began the era of antibiotics. In 1942, Dr. M. Joubon, of the Infectious Disease Clinic at Montpellier University, was treating typhoid fever cases with a derivative of sulfanilamide, an isopropyl-thiodiazole. Several of his patients became weak and dizzy after receiving the drug intravenously. Investigation of this side effect revealed that they had a low blood sugar! Treatment of the symptom with intravenous glucose corrected the blood sugar level and abolished the symptom. A laboratory investigation followed and the effect could be reproduced in dogs. They tried several different protocols to investigate the source of this phenomenon and found that the drug had no effect *in vitro*; mix blood and isopropylthiodiazole and the blood sugar does not change. Then, they tried it on dogs without pancreases, Banting's experiment, and again saw no effect. The new effect required the presence of the pancreas. They tried it on dogs whose vagus nerves had been cut: no effect – it was not a nerve stimulation (Vagotomy, cutting the vagus nerve, doesn't cause diabetes anyway, but low blood sugar does stimulate the vagus). Finally, in an elegant experiment for the time, Loubatieres, the Montpellier physiologist, connected a pancreatic vein from one dog to a second, pancreatectomized, dog's pancreatic vein. He gave the sulfa drug derivative to the first dog and the second dog's blood sugar declined. The drug was stimulating the pancreas, the islets, to release insulin.

In 1946, after the war's end allowed more French research, the new drug was given to rabbits and it stimulated the islets in the pancreas to increase in size. Around this time, speculation about a new, second form of diabetes (the second type that Joslin had been suspicious of) that was not as severe as the long recognized childhood disease prompted screening of blood sugar. Initially, the new drugs were thought to be interesting, but useless in treatment since they required the presence of insulin secreting islet cells, cells that were missing in "classical" diabetes. When elevated blood sugar was found in individuals who were not classical, what later came to be called "juvenile," diabetics, the oral drug proved effective in lowering blood sugar and was chemically modified to increase potency. Further animal experiments prompted changes in the chemical structure until the final drug was chlorpropamide, which had a long duration of action and was more potent than the earlier versions. In 1955, the first trials were held in humans and, with the increased recognition of "adult onset" diabetes, the oral agents have become very important in the treatment of diabetes. In recent years, possibly as a result of increasing childhood obesity, younger patients are encountered and the second diabetes form is now called "type II" rather than "adult onset." Type II diabetes, and obesity, have increased substantially in the past fifty years and the reason is actively debated. We will refer to that issue again.

AUTOIMMUNE DISEASES

In 1943, Arnold Rich published a series of curious cases seen at the Johns Hopkins Hospital. A disease called "serum sickness" had been observed after treatment with immune serum for bacterial diseases like pneumococcus. Prior to the discovery of sulfanilamide, the only treatment available had been with serum produced by immunizing animals to the pneumococcus capsule. There were four types (mentioned in the story of DNA) of capsule and the serum was specific for each type. A laborious test, called the Quellung reaction, was necessary to determine which type of pneumococcus was causing the infection and the correct immune serum could then be administered. Occasionally, the patient developed a reaction to the serum with fever, elevated (or decreased) white cell count, joint pain, and a skin rash. The condition was self limited (probably by the persistence of the serum in the patient's system) and no deaths had ever been reported due to serum sickness. It seemed to develop during convalescence and was not found at autopsy of fatal cases of pneumonia.

With the introduction of the sulfa drugs, the mortality of infection was sharply reduced but some patients died in spite of the new drugs. At autopsy, a new lesion was detected in some of these cases. A disease called "periarteritis nodosa" had been described by Gruber in 1925, who associated it with some sort of allergic reaction.[276] A few cases had been described all the way back to 1892 but it was extremely rare. The disease includes an inflammatory reaction surrounding small arteries and is widespread in organs including heart and kidney. Cases of periarteritis had been associated with asthma by others but this was the first clear connection between a hypersensitivity reaction and the lesion. In 1946, Rich described the history of hypersensitivity and distinguished between the tuberculin reaction and immunization against soluble antigens such as diphtheria. He described the cases of periarteritis seen with sulfa drug-induced serum sickness and then outlined a connection between immune reactions and a group of diseases including rheumatic fever, periarteritis nodosa, and lupus erythematosis. This was the first description of the etiology of what we now call the "autoimmune diseases." He mentions Henoch-Schönlein purpura and rheumatoid arthritis as suspected members of this class of diseases. All that we know about this category of disease dates from his analysis of these reactions to the life-saving sulfa drugs.[277]

VITAMINS

Osler discusses rickets and scurvy and recommends lemon juice, discovered by Lind in the eighteenth century, as a cure and prevention. Cow's milk was advocated as a preventative for rickets, but the concept of vitamins was still unknown. Some other vitamin deficiency diseases had been recognized but the etiology was obscure. Lind thought that lemon juice cured scurvy like Jesuits' bark cured malaria. Pellagra was described in 1755 by Gaspar Casal, a French physician. It produces a peripheral .neuropathy, leading to paralysis in advanced cases, and encephalopathy. A skin eruption occurs as well. An early, and accurate, theory was that it was related to a diet of maize (corn) meal without meat or milk. It was a new disease and maize was a new cereal, introduced from the New World. A problem with this theory was that pellagra was not seen in Mexico, the origin of maize. Of course, the diet eaten by natives of Mexico was not limited to the maize meal alone, as was the case with the poor residents of Spain found to have pellagra. Osler, in his *Principles and Practice of Medicine* of 1892 attributes the disease to "diseased maize" and recommends moving the victims from the area and "better preservation of maize cereal." A US Public Health Service physician, named Goldberger, early in this century noticed that pellagra occurred in asylums among inmates (not among the staff who had a better diet) and was diminished by adding eggs and milk to the diet. In 1930, there were 20,000 cases of pellagra in Georgia alone where maize (corn) meal and lard ("fatback," not lean bacon) constituted the diet for a large share of the population.

Beriberi was a disease seen in the rice culture of South East Asia. The word beriberi means, "I cannot," in the Sinhalese language and the disease is characterized by weakness, including heart failure. By the 1890s both diseases, pellagra and beriberi, were thought to be due to deficiencies of protein (although not by Osler). In the late 1890s Christiaan Eijkman, director of a research laboratory in Jakarta, Dutch East Indies noticed that hospital chickens developed a polyneuritis when they were fed white, polished rice. When their diet was returned to the usual brown rice, they recovered. He concluded that there was a toxin in polished rice but a colleague believed he had it backwards, that beriberi and the polyneuritis in chickens were due to some diet factor present in the rice husks. They followed up on this suspicion by checking for beriberi in the prison population of Java. They found that it was a problem in seventy percent of the prisoners fed polished rice but only three percent of those fed brown, unpolished rice developed the disease. Clearly, diet was involved.

Animal experiments in the early 1900s pointed to a series of deficiency diseases including beriberi, scurvy, pellagra, and rickets. By 1912, Casimir Funk, working at the Lister Institute in London, isolated the active component of rice husks and called it a vitamine (vital amine). The final "e" was dropped in the 1920s when it became apparent that not all these substances were amines. Vitamin A was isolated from butter in 1933 and synthesized in 1947. Vitamin B was isolated from milk in 1926 and synthesized ten years later. Ricketts was unusual because it was a new disease and seemed to be found predominantly in cities. It did not occur in rural populations. Why? Eventually a factor was identified that was present in cod liver oil and, when excluded from the diet of puppies, caused a disease similar to rickets. Finally, it was shown that humans, unlike dogs, could synthesize the vitamin in the presence of sunlight. Children in cities were not exposed to enough sunlight. Additional vitamins were identified and vitamin B, initially believed to be a single substance, thiamine, was found to consist of several individual vitamins. Finally, pernicious anemia was investigated and the double vitamin combination of vitamin B12 and intrinsic factor (secreted by the stomach), necessary for absorption, was uncovered.

ENDOCRINOLOGY

Starling, in 1905, coined the term "hormone" for the type of substance released from the duodenum by hydrochloric acid. The substance itself they named "secretin." Secretin stimulated the pancreas to produce digestive enzymes. Thus, hormones were yet another method for internal communication by the body. Later, another duodenal hormone was discovered that, in this case, was produced in response to the presence of fat. Its effect was to cause emptying of the gallbladder. Bile functions as a detergent to assist in fat digestion and "cholecystokinin," the hormone, is stimulated by the presence of fat and results in its digestion. Research on hormones was to accelerate in the 1920s. The thyroid gland became the subject of an experiment by accident when Theodore Kocher removed thousands of goiters in the iodine-deprived population of Switzerland. A follow-up of his patients revealed that thirty of the first 100 thyroidectomy cases had developed a condition similar to cretinism, later called myxedema. In 1891, George Murray gave sheep thyroid-extract injections to a patient with myxedema and found that she improved. In 1895, Eugene Bauman identified iodine in thyroid hormone and led the way to the cause (iodine deficiency) of endemic goiter. In 1909, Kocher, another of Billroth's students, would receive the Nobel Prize for his work on the thyroid gland.

The reflex arc was discovered in 1823, by Marshall Hall (1790-1857) who cut a frog spinal cord between its front and back legs. The frog could still move its front legs, but the back legs were out of voluntary control. The hind legs were motionless until they were stimulated whereupon they twitched violently, only once per stimulus. One hundred years earlier Stephen Hales had decapitated frogs and produced similar results but Hall had localized the site of the afferent and efferent (as we say now) connection. The conduction of nerve impulses, since Galvani's experiments (described in the section on electrocardiography), had been assumed to be electrical. Golgi and Cajal had shown that the nerve fiber was a long extension of the neuron but how the nerve cells communicated, or if they were a syncytium (one huge cell), was unclear until Santiago Ramon-y-Cajal demonstrated synaptic clefts between neurons. Golgi and Cajal were awarded the 1906 Nobel Prize in medicine for their discoveries in neuroanatomy, but in their Nobel lectures, they disagreed on the nature of the neuron with Golgi holding out for a syncytium and Cajal insisting on the synapse!

In 1905, John Langley described the separation of the autonomic nervous system (which he had named in 1895) into the sympathetic and parasympathetic systems, determined by their effect of the heart. One slowed the heart and the other increased its rate. T.R. Elliot, working with Langley, discovered that sympathetic nerves release a substance that he called "sympathin." The substance had the same effect on the heart as an extract of the adrenal gland, which had been called adrenalin. That same year, Langley postulated that nerves work by releasing a substance, sympathin or another chemical which might work as an inhibitor, the first description of chemical transmission of nerve impulses. Others thought that the process would be too slow and held out for electrical transmission.

In 1914, Henry Dale discovered acetylcholine in the nerve endings of the parasympathetic system. He showed that the chemical produced the same inhibitory effects as stimulation of the nerves. He also concluded that there must be an enzyme, which he called cholinesterase, to inactivate the chemical. In 1921, Otto Loewi confirmed these observations (See Chapter 22) but the skepticism persisted until Walter Cannon's observations in the later 1920s.

Walter Cannon, the Harvard physiologist, described the autonomic nervous system after studying the effects of traumatic shock in World War I. He showed that stimulation of sympathetic nerves released another compound that increased blood pressure, eventually identified as norepinephrine. He coined the term "homeostasis" to describe physiological stability in animals. Secretory glands were identified as far back as Wirsung who described the pancreatic duct in 1642. The first evidence of an internal, ductless, secretion was by Arnold Berthold who, in 1849, transplanted the testes of a cock and showed that the comb did not atrophy, as it did when they were removed. The testes must be producing a substance and releasing it to the blood, even if transplanted to another site. In 1855, Claude Bernard differentiated between the external secretion of the liver, the bile, and an internal liver secretion, sugar or glucose. The same year, Addison described a series of cases of anemia with bronzed pigmentation of the skin, and destruction of the adrenal glands.[278] The next year, Brown-Séquard removed the adrenal glands and proved they were necessary for life. Addison did not understand the significance until Brown-Séquard demonstrated that the condition was not just an anemia; he concluded that they must be secreting some essential substance into the blood.

In 1896, Sir William Osler published a series of six cases of Addison's Disease, one of which he treated with an extract of the pig adrenal gland.[279] There were few reports following this, possibly because of a preoccupation with the adrenal medullary hormones, until 1927. Most adrenal cortical extracts, even as late as 1929, were contaminated with epinephrine and this made any injection of the extract potentially dangerous (from severe elevation of blood pressure and arrhythmia). In 1930 Hartman and Brownell described a simple method for extraction of the adrenal cortical hormone uncontaminated by epinephrine.[280] Finally, George Thorn, in 1936, showed that adrenal cortical an extract modified the renal excretion of electrolytes[281] and soon pure extracts containing a series of substances named "compound F, compound H, compound J" were produced. In 1937, the first synthetic adrenal cortical hormone was produced by Steiger and Reichstein. It was called desoxycorticosterone, or DCA, and allowed treatment of the salt-losing portion of adrenal insufficiency.[282] DCA did not replace all the functions of the adrenal hormones and the distinction between "mineralocorticoids," which affected salt retention, and "glucocorticoids," the stress hormones, became apparent. The entire story of the adrenal hormones is related by Thorn in the *Johns Hopkins Medical Journal.*[283]

The neural hormone story continued in the 1930s when Vittorio Erpsamer discovered another gut hormone (in addition to secretin discovered by Starling) which he called "enteramine."[284] The same compound was isolated from blood platelets by Irvine Page and Maurice Rapport in 1947 and, because it caused vasoconstriction, they called it "serotonin."[285] The compound was eventually shown to be 5-hydroxy-tryptamine and, in 1953, Betty Twarog and Irvine Page demonstrated it in brain and other tissue. This story is continued in the chapter on psychiatry.

Pierre Marie, in 1886, found that the pituitary gland was related to growth abnormalities. Acromegaly was described and then, about 1912, Minkowski reported that the pituitary was enlarged in those cases. Harvey Cushing identified the pituitary role in secretion of growth hormone and other "master hormones." The action of ACTH, the adrenal stimulating hormone that is secreted by the pituitary tumor, was discovered by Cushing. He described the association of basophilic pituitary tumors with the syndrome of obesity, high blood pressure and other symptoms of adrenal hyperfunction but did not identify the hormone, itself.[286] The identification, in 1933, of ACTH by Collip[287] proved that a pituitary tumor causes "Cushing's Disease." In 1946, Thorn and associates were able to demonstrate that ACTH (by now prepared from cow adrenals) was effective in the treatment of pituitary insufficiency.[288] An excess of ACTH (given externally after the hormone became available), or cortisone or some primary adrenal disease like cancer, produces the (Cushing's) syndrome with the same findings. In 1950, Jules Bauer differentiated between the two conditions and named the disease and the syndrome as two separate entities.[289] The syndrome does not involve the pituitary.

The sex hormones were next to be delineated when Edgar Allen, a zoologist, found that fluid from pig ovaries, when injected into spayed mice, would put them into heat (estrus). The fluid must contain a female hormone. Two German gynecologists injected the urine from pregnant women into laboratory mice and found that they also went into heat. The female pregnancy hormone was in urine as well as in the ovary. In 1929, Allen and

Edward Doisy announced the discovery of the female sex hormone estrone. By 1933, two other female hormones had been isolated, estriol and estradiol. The process of obtaining the hormones was extremely laborious; Doisy required 80,000 sow ovaries to extract twelve milligrams of estradiol. The next year progesterone was isolated from the corpus luteum, the ovarian structure present during pregnancy. Ludwig Haberlandt, a physiologist at the University of Innsbruck in Austria, demonstrated in 1931 that pregnancy could be inhibited by the administration of pregnancy hormones, but the practical application would have to wait until steroid chemistry provided a cheap source for the hormones.

Russell Marker was an eccentric chemist who developed the octane rating of gasoline while working for the Ethyl Corporation in 1926. In the 1930s, he became interested in hormone chemistry, specifically progesterone. In 1935, it took 2,500 pregnant pigs' ovaries to produce one milligram of progesterone. Marker devised a process, now called "Marker degradation," to convert a plant molecule called a "sapogenin" into a progestin. A sapogenin is a plant steroid, similar to cholesterol, which is the molecular "skeleton" of the mammalian hormones from the adrenal cortex and gonads. He learned that a popular patent medicine called "Lydia Pinkham's Compound," which was sold to reduce menstrual cramps, contained an extract of "Beth's root," a species of *Trillium* (like lilies and yams), that produces sapogenins which could be converted to progestins. The Beth's root was too small a rhizome to use for a commercial extraction process. Further research identified a Mexican yam, called "cabeza de negro," that produced a diosgenin, another type of sapogenin. He produced syrup from the tubers of this yam and succeeded in degrading diosgenin to progesterone. One five-gallon can of syrup produced three kilograms of progesterone!

In 1943 Marker resigned his university position and traveled to Mexico where he collected ten tons of *Dioscorea mexicana*, the proper name for cabeza de negro. Marker formed a Mexican corporation with two Mexican partners to produce hormones. In an old pottery shed in Mexico City the new company, with four employees, produced several pounds of progesterone, worth $300,000. They formed a new company in 1944 and called it "Syntex," a combination of "synthesis" and "Mexico," and produced over thirty kilograms of progesterone. After a falling out with his partners, Marker left Mexico to form a new company, which used a different yam with a higher yield of synthetic hormone. By 1946, the price of progesterone had fallen from $200 per gram to $5 per gram. Marker had failed to patent his process and his former partners in Syntex hired another chemist who, using a published description of the process by Marker, was able to resume production. Eventually, the government of Mexico, in 1970, honored Marker with an award, which he refused, believing that his Mexican partners had cheated him.

Syntex hired Carl Djerassi, an immigrant chemist, to develop a process to produce cortisone from the same yam. In 1951, he succeeded but Upjohn soon discovered a method of converting progesterone to cortisone using a bacterial fermentation system. Syntex wound up supplying progesterone to the other companies at the reduced price of forty-eight cents per gram. In 1955, Gregory Pincus, a biologist who had studied mammalian eggs and fertilization for twenty years and Min-Cheuh Chang, another biologist, reported the successful inhibition of ovulation by daily oral administration of synthetic progestins. The announcement was made at the International Planned Parenthood Meeting in Tokyo that year. Worldwide publicity followed. In 1956, the first large scale human trial was conducted and estrogen contamination of the progestin (from the process) was found to be actually beneficial. The first oral contraceptive preparations, therefore, included both hormones. In 1957, another progestin, norethynoderel, was approved for use as a "menstrual regulator" and then, in 1960, as an oral contraceptive. By 1969, the estrogen content was reduced in the pill and side effects, especially venous thrombosis, became much less common.

THE STORY OF POLIO

The poliovirus was the cause of a common childhood illness, somewhat on the order of measles, mumps, and chickenpox. The difference was that, unlike the other viral syndromes, it was capable of producing a devastating illness with paralysis and death in a significant number of cases. Measles has always had a known mortality rate, but it never produced the fear and anxiety typical of the summer "polio season" in the early 1950s. Prior to the nineteenth-century epidemic, paralytic polio was unknown. There are instances of paralysis of single limbs described which could represent isolated cases of paralytic polio but there are no clusters or epidemics recorded. A reason for the recent emergence of the paralytic disease may be the development of modern sanitation, which prevents the exposure of small children to the virus. A study of third world countries in the 1960s revealed that the virus was endemic and most children were found to have antibodies, although the clinical disease was uncommon. Infection in infancy seems to provide lifelong immunity with a very low risk of paralytic disease. Chickenpox has a similar pattern. Most children, prior to the introduction of the vaccine, contracted the disease around the age of two years and had a very benign course. Adults, who have not been exposed in childhood, are at great risk of severe pneumonia with a high mortality rate if they contract chickenpox.

In 1858, Vogt, in Switzerland, described the first adult case of polio. Prior to this report, the disease was considered a purely pediatric affliction and the name "infantile paralysis" reflected an uncertainty about the cause. Charcot, in 1870, pointed out the loss of the anterior horn cells from the spinal cord in a victim of the disease.[290] By 1884, the idea that this might be an infectious disease was developing in Sweden after the first epidemics, beginning in 1881, appeared. A devastating epidemic in 1905 in Scandinavia, with 1,031 cases, removed any doubt. Rural districts were ravaged while cities were spared, a fact that offered some clues to the epidemiologist. Children in remote villages had not been exposed because of the low level of contact with strangers.

Ivar Wickman, a young Swedish physician, studied the affected villages and quickly realized that there were many subclinical cases, more than fifty percent in some villages. He became the world expert on the disease just emerging, but the Stockholm Faculty of Medicine declined to appoint him professor of children's diseases in 1914; soon after, at the age of forty-two, he took his life. Karl Landsteiner provided the next great advance in knowledge of the disease. In 1908, only a few viruses had been identified; smallpox, vaccinia, rabies and foot-and-mouth disease of cattle. Tissue culture was still unknown and the viruses could not be grown except in animals as Pasteur had done. Landsteiner, and his associate Popper, in spite of these difficulties, succeeded in transferring the infection from the spinal cord tissue of a nine-year-old boy, who had died with typical polio symptoms, to two monkeys. The cultures of the spinal cord material were sterile (for bacteria) and inoculation of rabbits, guinea pigs and mice failed to produce results. Monkeys were expensive as lab animals but, fortunately, Landsteiner and Popper had made the decision to inoculate the primates. The monkey spinal cords showed the identical lesion found in the child. The disease in the monkey was identical to that in the human. Thus, they succeeded in approximating the postulates set down by Koch just twenty-four years before.

One year after Landsteiner's dramatic discovery, Simon Flexner was able to transmit the disease from monkey to monkey at the Rockefeller Institute. Unfortunately, he did not appreciate that there were differences between the monkey disease and that in man and, even though the virus was the same, this failure would retard the study of the disease and the search for a vaccine. By 1910, Flexner and Landsteiner had both reported the presence of antibodies in the serum of convalescent patients, although they did not use that term. The antibodies, called "germicidal substances" by Flexner, neutralized the virus when mixed with it and prevented infection. In 1911, Flexner published a very optimistic report suggesting that a cure for polio was coming very soon. He was mistaken. That same year the largest epidemic of polio to date took place in Sweden with 3,840 cases. Sweden acquired an unsavory reputation as the source of the disease, which was unfortunate, but it did permit a very large-scale study of the virus. One major discovery from this research was clear evidence of the route of infection (oral) and excretion of the virus (fecal), important for public health measures, and this information showed that Flexner had gone off on the wrong track with his monkey studies.

In 1916, the largest epidemic ever occurred in New York City with over 9,000 cases; the disease was winning. Eventually, several strains of the virus were isolated but there was no progress in developing a vaccine. In 1934, an epidemic with nearly 3,000 cases occurred in Los Angeles and panic ensued. This was not alleviated by the occurrence of nearly 200 cases among physicians and nurses at the Los Angeles County General Hospital Contagious Disease Unit. Fortunately, most of these cases were not paralytic and there were no deaths among the medical personnel. There has been some speculation that not all the cases represented polio and there may have been a significant incidence of hysteria. Private physicians declined to make rounds at the hospital, communicating with interns on the telephone, and doctors who had visited the hospital were not welcome in private homes.[291]

In the twenty-five years since Flexner's first reports, attempts at immunization had continued without success. Live virus vaccines conferred lifetime immunity, but were dangerous. Killed virus did not immunize. In 1931, Maurice Brodie attempted an immunization program using formalin-inactivated virus. He had tested his material in monkeys and adult volunteers. Then he inoculated twelve children successfully. In 1935 Brodie gave the vaccine to 3,000 children[292] and there were later reports that some children contracted paralytic polio as a result. The vaccine was never used again. Another trial of a similar vaccine was conducted by John Kohlmer of Philadelphia that same year.[293] Nearly 13,000 doses of the vaccine were distributed to physicians in Pennsylvania and thirty-five other states. Both Brodie and Kohlmer were severely criticized as it became clear that at least twelve cases of paralytic polio resulted from Kohlmer's vaccine, six of them fatal.[294] The hasty introduction of the two vaccines was attributed to the enormous publicity resulting from the epidemics and scientific rivalry between Brodie and Kohlmer. Another twenty years would pass before another attempt at immunization would take place. Considerable effort at rehabilitation of paralyzed polio patients occurred during the 1930s and 1940s, stimulated no doubt by the history of President Roosevelt who contracted paralytic polio in 1920.

The logjam began to break up in 1928 when vaccinia virus was first grown in tissue cultured cells. Ross Harrison had succeeded in growing cells in tissue culture in 1907 but the husband and wife team of the Maitlands, at Manchester, England were the first to grow a virus in culture, in minced hen kidney. By 1936, a dozen other viruses had been grown in tissue cultures. The discovery of sulfanilamide prevented bacterial overgrowth and progress accelerated. Albert Sabin succeeded in growing poliovirus in human embryonic nervous tissue in 1936, but this did little to develop a vaccine.[295]

In 1940, an odd figure appeared on the scene who would be extremely influential for the next two decades. Sister Kenny was an Australian nurse who had strong opinions and no reservations about expressing them. The prevailing treatment of acute paralysis in the 1930s was rigid immobilization of the limbs; at least until all muscle tenderness was gone. This had begun as an early treatment followed by physical therapy but the fashion had carried the immobilization method too far. She had been a nurse in the Australian outback when she saw her first cases of polio and she became convinced that the task was to return these patients to "normal" through exercise. Her concept of the cause of the disease, an acute viral illness, was vague at best. She met considerable resistance to her methods from American orthopedists and, at first, she brought a welcome breath of fresh air. Eventually her followers developed an almost religious attitude about her ideas and the pendulum swung too far in the other direction. The acute illness is best treated with muscle rest until the paralytic phase is over, and then rehabilitation with active physical therapy is beneficial.

There is some evidence that vigorous activity during the phase when anterior horn cells are infected by the virus may worsen the prognosis for recovery. In addition, the fixation of returning partially paralyzed patients to full, normal activity, even in some cases to running and athletics, may have increased the risk of what we now know as "post polio syndrome." In these cases, patients who had paralytic polio in childhood are developing paralysis in adult life after forty years of recovery.[296] The neurons that survived in the spinal cord (which took over the function of dying neurons according to the theory) may have been overstressed by the high activity level and are dying prematurely.[297] Sister Kenny spent her last years battling physicians and her foundation may have carried on her enthusiastic campaign to return polio patients to "normal life" to the point that it contributed to this new disease.

The next development in the laboratory opened the door to the cure and the eradication of polio. In 1949, John Enders reported that he had grown poliovirus in non-neural tissue.[298] His lab succeeded in growing all three strains of the virus and, even more important, they could recognize the microscopic changes in cells produced by multiplication of the virus. They no longer needed monkey infection as a biological marker for viral growth. Improvements in culture technique plus the use of penicillin and streptomycin to prevent bacterial contamination resulted in tremendous progress. By 1951, 13 strains of poliovirus had been isolated and typed in tissue culture. In 1954 Enders and his coworkers, Weller and Robbins, would share the Nobel Prize for their work.

THE SALK VACCINE

Jonas Salk began work on the typing of poliovirus in 1948. In 1950, he was chosen by the National Foundation for Infantile Paralysis (The "March of Dimes") to head the vaccine program. By 1953, Salk had begun testing a killed virus vaccine, using formalin to inactivate the virus, in a system similar to that used by the discredited Brodie. Progress since 1935, especially the tissue culture techniques, made this procedure much safer. By April of 1953, 5,000 children had received the vaccine. In 1954, a large field trial administered 600,000 doses of vaccine to children in the second grade and used children in first and third grade as controls. In February of 1955, newspapers heard that results of the field trial were to be announced and that the protection of the inoculated children had been 100 percent. A media sensation followed. On April 12, 1955, the news was announced in a glare of publicity. "Now at last we have a vaccine!"

Less than a month later, the Center for Disease Control reported that some children had received live virus in the trial, by accident, and some had developed polio! It turned out that the cases of polio were limited to California and Idaho and Cutter Laboratories had manufactured the vaccine batch. For a time it seemed that the 1935 fiasco might be repeated. In May of 1955, Canadian and Danish representatives reported that they had conducted similar, and even larger, field trials and no cases of paralytic polio had been observed. The California experience seemed to be a fluke. The final review found that 204 vaccine-associated cases of polio occurred, seventy-nine in vaccinated children and 105 among family contacts. Three fourths of the cases were paralytic and eleven people died. Under considerable public pressure, including a Congressional investigation, the vaccine commission decided to proceed with the national immunization program. Paralytic polio fell from 13.9 cases per 100,000 people in 1954, before the vaccine became available, to 0.5 cases in 1961.

By 1959, Albert Sabin was conducting field trials of a live, attenuated virus vaccine and in 1962 live virus vaccines for all three strains of polio were licensed. Polio has nearly disappeared as a health problem and this dramatic disappearance of a major public health problem in forty years has prompted this rather lengthy description of its history. In recent years, the Sabin vaccine has seen some cases of reversion of the type III virus to virulence in poor countries. This is a constant problem with that strain of virus and a few paralytic cases of polio have resulted. Disease from wild poliovirus has virtually disappeared except in India where Muslim children, especially in the state of Uttar Pradesh, have not been immunized. A rumor that the Hindu government had included a substance that causes sterility has led to resistance by poor Muslim families to immunization. In 2002, India had 1,509 cases of polio and 1,197 of them were in Utter Pradesh. Uttar Pradesh accounted for sixty-eight percent of polio cases worldwide.[299]

CANCER

The treatment of cancer had been limited to surgery until Marie Curie discovered radium and these two modalities, surgery and radiation, had comprised the sum total of cancer therapy until 1941. That year Dr. Charles Huggins reported that prostate cancer would shrink if the patient were castrated or given female hormones. In 1940, he had studied prostatic enlargement in dogs. Old male dogs, like old men, develop prostatic enlargement. Castration of the dog or injection of diethyl stilbestrol (an estrogenic hormone) reduced the size of the prostate.[300] In 1893, White had observed that castration improved the symptoms of benign prostatic hypertrophy in men.[301] In 1941, Huggins reported his experience with castration in cases of metastatic cancer of the prostate.[302] The patients all had advanced prostate cancer and after castration all showed improvement in symptoms, reduction in bone lesions and eight patients had reduction in acid phosphatase (shown in 1935 to be found in prostate gland and present in the blood in cases of cancer of the prostate). Diethylstilbestrol was given to the four patients who did not have complete response to castration and one showed a reduction in acid phosphatase.

In 1942, Huggins reported a series of forty-five patients with advanced prostate cancer, all treated initially with castration. Of these patients, thirty-one had prolonged improvement; estrogen therapy in the patients whose improvement was temporary, or who did not have a response, was not helpful. He did note that those who did not respond to hormones had undifferentiated cancers, a major consideration that would lead to intense interest in the biology of cancer. It would be found that an undifferentiated cancer, that is one that looks more primitive in the microscope (less like prostate and more like a sheet of simple cells), has lost some of the characteristics of the normal tissue from which it was derived. One of these characteristics is the presence of hormone receptors, which, in normal sex organ tissue, allow a response to sex hormone stimulation. The same phenomenon would later be discovered in carcinoma of the breast. Well-differentiated cancers (which looked in the microscope more like the normal tissue they arose from) would retain their ability to be stimulated by hormones and, conversely, to be suppressed by removal of hormone stimulation. The more the cancer looked like normal prostate in the microscope, the better chance that castration would provide significant response. Years later hormone analogues, much like the pyrimidine and folic acid analogues used in chemotherapy, would be used to further suppress cancers. In 1966, Huggins shared the Nobel Prize with Rous, Huggins for his work on hormone therapy of cancer and Rous for his sarcoma virus discovery.

In the discussion of Dr. Huggins paper at the 1942 American Surgical Association meeting, Evarts Graham commented that these results suggested that removal of the ovaries might be beneficial in metastatic breast cancer.[303] Cancers arising in sex organs were sensitive to sex hormones, newly discovered and still difficult to obtain until Marker succeeded in synthesizing them. In 1944, Dr. Alfred Gilman discovered that a derivative of the World War I poison gas, nitrogen mustard, caused lymphomas to regress. This was the first evidence of a non-hormone drug effect on cancer. It was discovered that this effect resulted from interference with the cell's ability to reproduce itself. The role of DNA was still a research subject at that time (See Chapter 16). In 1944, Fifty percent of all children with acute lymphocytic leukemia (the most common childhood cancer) died in two to four months. In 1947, Dr. Sidney Farber showed that a folic acid antagonist (a drug called methotrexate) caused regression in childhood leukemia. Antimetabolites (specific tissue poisons) were not limited to poison gases like nitrogen mustard but could include those that affected vitamin (folic acid) utilization. Leukemia was as sensitive as solid tumors. The successful programs used multiple drugs and added other modalities such as brain radiation for suspected involvement beyond the reach of intravenous therapy. By 1974, ninety percent remission in childhood leukemia was common.[304] These clues led to the discovery of a few other drugs between 1947 and 1954.

In 1954, the National Cancer Institute set up a program to study chemotherapy and drug development accelerated. In 1961, enough progress had been made to attempt the cure of acute leukemia of childhood. The Acute Leukemia Task Force was formed. In 1965, I saw, as a medical student, the first children who had gone five years without recurrence of the leukemia. They were cured. This was so astonishing that some families had trouble accepting that the fatal outcome they had been assured was inevitable was now gone. I saw one family who had completely spoiled their four year old after having been told to "enjoy him while you can" and who were having serious problems with a nine year old that no one in the family could handle. He had never received any discipline and I don't think that he had attended school regularly. Now he was cured and the family was asking the doctor when he would die.

Metastatic cancer is out of the reach of surgery and, for the most part, cannot be successfully treated with radiation therapy (only for pain relief, not cure). Only chemotherapy holds promise for cure. In 1957, Dr. Roy Hertz discovered that methotrexate, the same folic acid analogue used in childhood leukemia, would cure patients who had pulmonary metastases from choriocarcinoma. This tumor is a consequence of a pregnancy gone awry, a malignant placenta. It is frequently preceded by hydatidiform mole, a proliferating mass of fetal tissue shaped like a cluster of grapes (hence the name). The mole, itself, is not malignant but choriocarcinoma is a frequent consequence. Before this observation, the tumor had 100 percent mortality in a few months and the victims were young women who had been anticipating childbirth, not cancer. His first case was a young woman near death, but she responded to the drug and was discharged a healthy woman. Progress was aided by animal research, which delineated the distribution of drugs within body fluids and physiological systems. Molecular biology came from some of this work as the effects of chemotherapy drugs were investigated. Actinomycin D, found to be too toxic for antibiotic use, was useful in treatment of choriocarcinoma and was instrumental in studying the replication of DNA, which it blocks. Rapidly growing tumors were found to be more susceptible to chemotherapy drugs than slow growing malignancies because the drugs affected cell functions involved in replication. Actinomycin D interferes with DNA replication and methotrexate stops the cell division by blocking the actual separation of chromosomes. Choriocarcinoma and leukemia are very rapidly growing malignancies. Pediatric tumors like Wilm's tumor (a childhood kidney cancer) and rhabdomyosarcoma (a malignant muscle tumor) are also rapidly growing and chemotherapy sensitive.

Adult solid tumors are slower growing and correspondingly less sensitive to chemotherapy. In 1957 another drug, 5-fluorouracil (5-FU) an analogue to the pyrimidines in nucleic acid, was introduced and found to affect gastrointestinal cancers. In animal studies, some tumors incorporate these pyrimidine analogues into nucleic acid. Thymine is 5-methyl uracil and replacement of the methyl group hydrogen with fluorine allowed 5-fluorouracil to be incorporated into RNA in place of uracil, a normal component of RNA. It also inhibited the synthesis of thymine, a component of DNA. This was one of the first "designer drugs" in chemotherapy. The role of the drug in inhibition of RNA, which is constantly being created in the cell, may explain its better effect in tumors less sensitive to the DNA antagonists. The price was considerable toxicity as normal tissues are also sensitive.

I once killed a patient with 5-FU, using the hospital formulary instructions to give him a "loading dose." He was a professor of English literature with recurrent rectal cancer. He told me that he only wanted to live long enough to finish his book on poetry. I was a young first year resident and, identifying strongly with him, I decided to do all I could to give him time. Instead, the high loading dose killed his bone marrow and he died in two weeks. It was not a "mistake," I followed instructions. I did not understand the risk and took away the time he had left. I have never given a loading dose of 5-FU since that experience, although I have used the drug for many years in treating GI cancer.

THE APPLICATION OF EPIDEMIOLOGY TO OTHER DISEASES

In 1958, a missionary doctor in Africa, named Dennis Burkitt, began to see a large number of Ugandan children with a malignant tumor involving the jaws and abdomen.[305] This was at first called a sarcoma (sarcomas are more common in children than in adults), but was soon recognized as a tumor of the lymphatic system, a lymphoma. Hodgkin's disease was the only other malignant lymphoma thus far recognized, and this tumor differed in several respects. "Burkitt's Lymphoma," as the new tumor was soon called, is common in East Africa and almost unknown in the rest of the world. Leukemia is seen in Africa, but with a low frequency, unlike the experience in America and Europe where leukemia is more common and solid lymphoma is rare in children. Eventually, other cases in Africa were collected and a plot of the geographic distribution made. They were clustered along the equator in central Africa (extending more northerly to the west and southerly to the east in a plane angled about fifteen degrees to the equator) and did not follow racial or tribal (in Uganda thirteen tribes were affected) patterns. Nearly all cases were in children younger than eleven years old with a peak incidence at age five. The geographical distribution followed the "tsetse fly belt" of Africa and the suggestion has been made that this insect vector, which transmits "sleeping sickness," could be involved.

Modern genetic studies have shown that, of the endemic (African) Burkitt's lymphoma cases, ninety percent contain Epstein-Barr virus genome. Non-endemic (American) Burkitt's lymphoma cases do not (at least eighty-five percent do not) contain Epstein-Barr virus genome. This, the first recognition of a possible infectious etiology for cancer in humans came from epidemiological studies by a missionary doctor in Africa. The same virus has since been identified in the nasopharyngeal cancer seen in Asians. Both these malignancies grow rapidly and have high mortality rates.

Dennis Burkitt was not finished with his contributions to modern medicine. During his twenty-year service in Africa, he noticed that certain diseases, common in England and America, were almost unknown in the African villagers he treated. Among them were appendicitis, diverticulitis, and colon cancer. He surveyed hospitals in Africa and, of fifty-two which returned a questionnaire, forty-four had never seen a case of diverticular disease (bleeding, perforation, or inflammation), diverticulitis, or other complication of the presence of colon diverticula. He observed that the diseases did occur in Africans who had moved from villages to towns and cities and who had adopted a "European diet."[306] Appendicitis was similarly rare in African villagers; he reported that twenty-five African hospitals surveyed saw fewer than three cases per year.[307] In 1971, he published an analysis of colon cancer that noted a similar disparity between the incidence of this tumor in African villagers (3.5 cases per 100,000 men age thirty-five to sixty-four) versus Americans (51.8 cases per 100,000 men age thirty-five to sixty-four in Connecticut) in which the disease is fifteen times more likely in American men.

Burkitt had also noticed that his African patients, those who were villagers, ate a high bulk diet with unrefined flour used in its preparation and had voluminous bowel movements. A study of intestinal transit times, using radiopaque markers[308], shows that African villagers passed eighty percent of the markers (eaten in food containing barium pellets) in thirty-five hours while English schoolboys took eighty-nine hours to pass eighty percent of the barium pellets. The common theme in his work was the effect of low residue diets and transit time in the colon. The result of this research was increased interest in dietary fiber and a change in the diets of Americans and Europeans who became more health conscious. The association between colon cancer and dietary fiber presumed that bacterial fermentation of colon contents might produce carcinogenic derivatives of non-absorbed compounds plus the effect of prolonged exposure of colonic mucosa to these compounds because of slow transit time. Recently, attention has focused on the role of animal fat in the diet, and colon cancer has not been found to be associated with diverticulosis, so Burkitt's theory, at least with respect to cancer, has to be ruled unproven as yet.

With diverticulosis, his theory of etiology remains on better ground and studies using pressure gauges inserted into the sigmoid colon through the anus have confirmed spikes of high intracolonic pressure. The diverticula are located adjacent to small vessels, which penetrate the muscular wall of the colon to supply the mucosa. High intraluminal pressure may produce herniation of mucosa through the weak area adjacent to the blood vessels producing the pouch-like diverticulum. Bleeding, caused by erosion of diverticula through the adjacent vessels, is a common complication of diverticulosis and occurs in the absence of inflammation. High intraluminal pressure is probably the result of small volume stools (producing an effect predicted by the Law of LaPlace[309]) combined with excessive fermentation. No better explanation has appeared since Burkitt and the evidence from epidemiology seems unchallenged.[310] Appendicitis may be related to a similar phenomenon, although a hereditary factor, involving the anatomy of the appendix itself, is probably important as well.

CHOLESTEROL

In the 1950s, a study of Korean War casualties showed a startling seventy-seven percent of young soldiers had significant coronary artery disease at autopsy.[311]   In 1950, Gofman had shown that elevated cholesterol damaged arteries in laboratory animals.[312] With the use of a high-speed centrifuge, they were able to fractionate the cholesterol into two levels, "low density lipoprotein" cholesterol (LDL) and "high density lipoprotein" cholesterol (HDL). The rabbits, in which he had produced disease with a high cholesterol diet, had elevated levels of this low density fraction (LDL). Gofman then produced a clinical correlation in men recovering from heart attacks when low density lipoprotein cholesterol was found to be elevated compared to normal control subjects. A randomized controlled trial was carried out, stimulated by the shocking incidence of atherosclerosis in young battle casualties. This was poorly controlled but suggested that elevation of cholesterol was associated with increased risk of heart attack.

In 1952, Kinsell demonstrated that substitution of vegetable fat for animal fat led to a reduction in cholesterol levels.[313] It was soon discovered that the beneficial effect of vegetable fat was due to the unsaturated molecule.[314] The result was a reduction in consumption of red meat, heavily marbled with saturated animal fat, and the substitution of vegetable fats for cooking plus increasing consumption of low fat foods. A similar autopsy study conducted in the Vietnam War showed that the incidence of atherosclerosis in battle casualties' coronary arteries had declined to forty-four percent, still high but declining. Since that time, enormous efforts have been expended in the study of the metabolism of cholesterol.

The matter was complicated somewhat in 1972 when New York cardiologist Robert Atkins published a book describing a new diet.[315] The Atkins diet advocated a high-fat, low carbohydrate diet for weight loss. This, of course, was the exact opposite of what other cardiologists were now saying. The book became a bestseller and is still in print. Other cardiologists were furious and treated Atkins as a quack. The problem was that the diet worked and people using it lost weight. Atkins' theory is that man is a meat eater and carbohydrates do not suppress hunger as well as fat does. Thus, the low-fat diets, which tend to substitute pasta and other carbohydrates for fat, produce an increase in the consumption of calories and this results in obesity. The Atkins diet was a phenomenon but the trend in American and European medicine continued to be an emphasis on low fat diets, unsaturated fat in the diet and ultimately a series of expensive drugs that affect cholesterol metabolism. There was one problem; in spite of all the emphasis on low fat diets, obesity, including childhood obesity, has grown in the past thirty years. The proportion of the population described as obese increased from eight to thirteen percent, in 1950, to as high as twenty-five percent.

Other factors may be at work such as decreased exercise in both TV-addicted children and automobile driving adults. Childhood obesity has so increased the incidence of type II diabetes (at least both have increased-- no link is proven) that the name was changed from "adult onset diabetes" to type II. Research in recent years has suggested that insulin resistance is responsible for type II diabetes. Atkins and some of his supporters now suggest that high carbohydrate diets stimulate chronic high levels of insulin secretion and result in tissue insulin resistance. The Atkins diet, and its theoretical underpinnings, has been banished from serious research for thirty years. That may be changing, although a review of Medline still shows few supporters of Atkins.

SMOKING AND CANCER

Lung cancer was a rare disease early in the twentieth century. In 1922, the number of deaths recorded by the Registrar-General in Britain was 612. The death rate from lung cancer in 1901-1920 was 1.1 per 100,000 males and 0.7 per 100,000 females. In 1936-39 the death rate from lung cancer had increased to 10.6 in males and 2.5 in females, a ten-fold increase in males and about 3.5 times in females. Clearly, the increase in deaths was not related to population increase. From 1940-44 the death rate from lung cancer continued to increase by six fold. Similar increases were seen in the US and Canada. Reasons for this change were discussed and two possibilities seemed most likely: atmospheric pollution and tobacco smoking.

After World War II physicians continued to see increasing numbers of lung cancer cases and in 1950 American researchers Wynder and Graham (Evarts Graham who had performed the first pneumonectomy) reported that cancer risk increased with amount and duration of smoking and was rare in non-smokers.[316] Their study included 684 patients. Graham, a smoker himself, was to die of lung cancer in 1957. That same year Richard Doll and A. Bradford Hill published a case-control study, which is now considered a classic in epidemiological research, showing that cigarette smoking was clearly associated with lung cancer. Patients were interviewed and their smoking history was recorded in detail. Of 649 men and sixty women with lung cancer, 0.3 percent of the men and 31.7 percent of the women were non-smokers. The control group of patients (this is how a case-control study is designed) were of the same age, sex and social class of the cancer cases. The control group had other diagnoses, such as cancer of other organs or non-cancer illness, and 4.2 percent of the men and 53.3 percent of the women were non-smokers. The amount of smoking and the duration were both significant factors in the incidence of cancer. All of this is common knowledge now but this study was the first to clearly implicate smoking in lung cancer.[317]

The fact that this was not established fact could be judged from the letters to the editor in the October issue of the same journal questioning the association and blaming everything from arsenic in the smoke to saltpeter used to make manufactured cigarettes easier to light.

Within a few years, other respiratory diseases began to be associated with cigarette smoking.[318] Emphysema, in particular, reached near epidemic proportions among the World War II generation. In 1955, Doctor Doll published an extremely controversial report on asbestos and lung disease.

Gloyne and Wood had first described the effect of inhalation of asbestos in 1934.[319] They showed the direct effect on the lung, called "asbestosis." Doll began to study the incidence of lung cancer in asbestos workers in England and, against intense opposition by the largest asbestos mining company, published a study showing that these workers had a high risk of cancer, including a rare tumor called "mesothelioma."[320] The pressure from the asbestos industry was so powerful that the doctor who had originally drawn Doll's attention to the problem, asked to have his name removed from the paper before publication.[321]

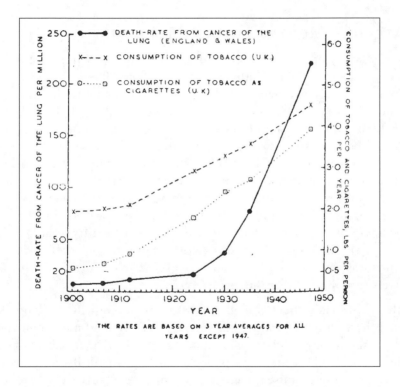

Figure 11 – Chart of tobacco consumption and lung cancer incidence from Doll and Bradford-Hill paper (1950)

Sir Richard Doll had one more contribution to make to epidemiology when he was asked by the World Health Organization to investigate a catastrophic poisoning episode in 1981 involving rapeseed oil in Spain. Spain, to protect its olive oil industry, does not allow the use of cheaper rapeseed oil for human consumption. To insure that the cheaper vegetable oil is not used in cooking, it is treated with aniline, a poisonous additive. In 1981, 30,000 poor Spanish residents became ill, and 1,000 died, after using rapeseed oil for cooking. The Spanish government insisted that the oil was not to blame; it must be an epidemic of some sort. Sir Richard Doll investigated and, resisting the government efforts at obstruction, published a WHO report in 1985. The entire incident is called "the Spanish Toxic Oil Syndrome" and, again, Doll showed his integrity in confirming the facts of the catastrophe.

MATERNAL MORTALITY AND MORBIDITY

The advent of antisepsis had reduced maternal mortality from twenty-six percent in some of the old filthy hospitals to about 200 deaths per 10,000 deliveries. Total maternal mortality, including home births, hovered around fifty per 10,000 in England after antisepsis was adopted, but, from 1880 until 1937, did not decline further. The Scandinavian countries had better results, with a decline from sixty-five in 1880 to about thirty per 10,000 births in 1900. The US, which did not collect uniform data prior to 1850, had worse mortality rates, largely a result of racial practices in the South. After 1936, the maternal mortality rate declined from about sixty-five deaths per 10,000 births to about thirty in 1950, the same mortality rates that Scandanavia experienced fifty years earlier. Why did the benefits of antisepsis and asepsis fail all these women? Poverty was the most probable answer except that a few experimental projects complicated that theory.

In the 1920s Mary Breckinridge, a frontier nurse-midwife in Kentucky, started the Kentucky Frontier Nursing Service. Trained nurse-midwives rode horses through isolated mountain terrain to deliver babies. Their patients, black and white, were poor and malnourished. By good obstetric practice, these nurses achieved astonishing resuls. The Frontier Nursing Service had one-tenth the maternal mortality of private obstetrics patients in the hospital of nearby Lexington.[322] A similar experience, called the "Rochdale Experiment," in England in 1929 reduced maternal morbidity from ninety per 10,000 births to one of the lowest in England. Much of the improvement has been attributed to antibiotics, blood transfusion and better obstetric education. The two experiments described above suggest that the last factor may be the most significant.

THE COMING OF AIDS

In 1981, several big-city medical centers described a new syndrome. Young homosexual men were seen with Kaposi sarcoma, a low-level malignancy usually seen in elderly Jewish or Italian patients, or *Pneumocystis carinii* pneumonia, an opportunistic pulmonary infection seen in immuno-suppressed patients with organ transplantation (on immunosuppressant drugs) or leukemia. *The Morbidity and Mortality Weekly Report* of the Center for Disease Control reported the first series in July of 1981.[323] Four weeks later a group from New York reported on a series of homosexual men with Kaposi Sarcoma.[324] In September, the *Lancet* published a report on the first eight patients and speculated that the cause might be exposure to sexually transmitted diseases. Initially there was suspicion that frequent exposure to sexually transmitted diseases (STD) might "exhaust" the immune system. The new sexual freedom enjoyed by homosexuals in the 1970s had led to an epidemic of STDs including hepatitis B (fifty percent of gay men tested in San Francisco had hepatitis B antibodies) and enteric parasites like *Giardia lamblia* and amebiasis. In New York, at the Gay Men's Health Project, thirty percent of patients seen had gastrointestinal parasites. Epidemiologists unfamiliar with gay life worried about the water supply until gay colleagues explained some of the sexual practices of the community. Gay bathhouses, especially in New York and San Francisco, and promiscuity provided the setting for the spread of the new plague. At first, it was called "Gay Related Immune Deficiency" or GRID.

Within a year, the new syndrome was named "Acquired Immune Deficiency Syndrome" to distinguish it from congenital disorders, with similar clinical manifestations, in children. Hematologists and immunologists noticed that the patients had an absence of T-helper lymphocytes, a phenomenon never seen before. By July of 1982, the Center for Disease Control had reports of 471 cases of the new syndrome. As of December 1983, the cause was still unknown, although a transmissible agent passed through sexual contact, blood transfusion or blood product injection (it had already appeared in hemophiliacs receiving AHG from pooled plasma) was probably responsible.[325,326] Within a year, it was apparent that recipients of blood transfusions were being infected[327] and mothers had infected their in-whom infants during pregnancy.[328] In 1981, French researchers at the Pasteur Institute saw a similar syndrome of persistent lymph node enlargement in homosexual men. They read the first American publication and realized that the two conditions were probably related. In January of 1983, a lymph node biopsy specimen was taken from a male fashion designer with a persistent cough and enlarged lymph nodes. The lymph node and a blood specimen were cultured and examined for evidence of a retrovirus.

In 1907, Peyton Rous had discovered that a virus caused a sarcoma (a form of cancer) in chickens.[329] Viruses were very difficult to study prior to the 1940s and the development of tissue culture techniques, but Rous was able to transmit the sarcoma to other chickens by injecting a cell-free extract of the original tumor. His discovery was received with considerable skepticism but he was eventually awarded the 1966 Nobel Prize for the discovery. A number of other animal cancer viruses were discovered as the years went by and, once analysis of genetic material was possible, they were found to be unusual. They did not have DNA as their genetic material. Instead, their genes were encoded in RNA, a violation of the rules of molecular biology, as it was understood at the time. After the discovery of the structure of DNA in 1953, the RNA viruses remained a problem. How did they replicate?

In 1955, Howard Temin, a graduate student in biology at Caltech, became interested in the RNA viruses. Temin eventually discovered that Actinomycin D, one of the Actinomycin family of antibiotics and anticancer drugs, which blocks the replication of DNA, would also block the replication of the Rous Sarcoma virus. He concluded that RNA viruses must transcribe their genes into DNA first, before replication.[330] His conclusion led him to postulate the existence of an enzyme, which must be present and must synthesize DNA from RNA. He called it "reverse transcriptase" and, once he thought to look for it, found it easily in infected cells. He decided to report his discovery at the Tenth International Cancer Conference in May of 1970. His report caused a sensation. Then he received a call from virologist David Baltimore who informed him that he, Baltimore, had also discovered reverse transcriptase and already had a paper submitted to the journal *Nature*. The journal published both papers in the same issue.[331] The RNA viruses quickly became known as "retroviruses" and reverse transcriptase became a sensitive test for their presence. Baltimore and Temin shared the 1975 Nobel Prize for this discovery.

Francoise Barré, the assistant to Jean-Claude Chermann in the retrovirus section of the Pasteur Institute (the two of them comprised the entire department), cultured the cells for a week before she detected reverse transcriptase, but it was there. It took twenty-three days before a high titer, conclusive evidence, was present. Soon trouble arrived because the T-cell culture was dying. The significance of this observation was not recognized for some time. The French researchers succeeded in keeping the culture alive by adding fresh T-cell lymphocytes acquired from placentas and umbilical cord blood. Eventually the connection became apparent;

AIDS was an immune deficiency disease because the virus was destroying the patients' T-cells. In the lab, this new retrovirus was killing T-cells.

In America, Robert Gallo was a famous virologist at the National Cancer Institute, part of the National Institutes of Health. He had discovered reverse transcriptase in human leukemia cells in 1970, setting off a sensation although no viral role in human leukemia was ever proven.[332] The reverse transcriptase was from a mouse leukemia virus contaminating the culture. Gallo had been studying a virus he named Human T-cell Lymphoma Virus (HTLV) for ten years although most oncologists regarded his results with skepticism. When the AIDS epidemic began, he proposed that the cause of the new disease was another of the family of HTLV viruses, known to be retroviruses. The French, after suggesting collaboration and believing that Gallo had agreed, sent a sample of the material from their patient for comparison with Gallo's virus. They were calling the virus they had discovered LAV, "Lymphadenopathy Associated Virus." The French had requested material from Gallo to perform their own comparisons but he did not provide the material they asked for, antibodies and DNA probes to test the new virus' genetic makeup. His concept of collaboration differed from theirs, as they were to learn to their cost.

Considerable political maneuvering developed placing the little-known French lab at a disadvantage with the well-known American institution. In September 1983, Jean-Claude Montagnier, the French virologist from the Pasteur Institute, who thought he was collaborating with Gallo, presented his results at an AIDS meeting at Cold Spring Harbor. He found a hostile reception. After Gallo attacked the French results as unrelated to AIDS and possibly caused by a contaminant, he quietly asked Montagnier for more of the LAV material! His public and private reactions were quite different. Gallo was proposing a new virus he called HTLV-3 as the cause of AIDS, but the French had better results in isolating the LAV virus from case material provided by the Center for Disease Control as well as from their own French cases. There was more than professional prestige at stake, because a new blood test to detect the virus in bank blood, as well as suspected new cases, was being developed. A patent for the new test was at stake. By 1987, it had become apparent that the French virus was the cause of AIDS and their test for the virus, derived from their own material, had a much higher rate of true positive and true negative results than Gallo's test. A true positive test should identify all the cases in which the disease is present. A true negative should exclude all cases in which the disease is not present. No test is perfect, but a high false positive rate subjects patients to unnecessary follow-up studies (or in the case of AIDS, panic at the prospect of death) and a high false negative rate misses many cases of the disease, which should be picked up (critically important in blood banks). Both false positive and false negative results were common with the test based on the Gallo material.

In March of 1985, 9,000 cases of AIDS had been reported in the US and 4,300 of those patients had died. By 1998, 22 million cases had been identified worldwide of which 1 million were children. About 600,000 of these cases were reported in the US. The prevalence of infection with the HIV (as it was named in 1994) virus has declined in the US since 1993, no doubt due to behavior changes and other prophylactic methods. In 1982, anti-hemophiliac globulin was produced from pooled serum and many (about 4,000) hemophilia patients were infected by AHG injections. Heat treatment of the concentrate used for AHG therapy has eliminated this source of infection, although the French had a scandal in the late 1980s because the health minister permitted use of existing stocks of untreated AHG (to save money) before ordering the heat-treated product.

1987 brought preliminary testing of zidovudine (AZT), the first drug shown to be effective in inhibiting replication of the virus. It is a nucleotide analogue, which binds to reverse transcriptase interrupting polymerization of the virus DNA from RNA. Significant side effects occur because the DNA polymerase of mitochondria (unlike nuclear DNA polymerase) also takes up the false nucleotide and muscle weakness results. This phenomenon is one more bit of evidence that mitochondria were once independent organisms, captured in early evolution in a symbiotic relationship with eukaryotic cells (cells with a nucleus unlike bacteria which do not have mitochondria). The HIV virus (like most retroviruses) also mutates as it replicates (the DNA replication is fraught with errors) and resistance to AZT develops quickly. Other reverse transcriptase inhibitors, less subject to the virus mutations, were developed and then protease inhibitors appeared. The new drugs have resulted in prolonged remissions for HIV infected patients. No vaccine has been developed and the virus' distressing tendency to mutate suggests that a vaccine may be difficult to produce. In one very discouraging example a patient, who had shown remarkable resistance to the HIV, became infected with a different strain and quickly developed full-blown immunodeficiency.[333] This has implications for possible vaccine development if new strains, unaffected by existing immunity, are constantly appearing. The thirteen strains of the poliovirus, in contrast, have remained stable since their discovery.

In 1994, a settlement of the patent dispute between the American government (the NIH) and the Pasteur Institute made it clear that the French had discovered the AIDS virus. The settlement raised serious questions about whether Gallo's lab had, either accidentally or on purpose, mixed the French virus with the American specimens and confused the true discoverer of the virus beyond definite resolution. A 1993 study by the NIH Office of Research Integrity concluded that Gallo had lied, his claim was "knowingly false when written," but, during a subsequent appeal by Gallo, the NIH lost its nerve and retracted the findings of its own ORI. The virus was renamed "Human Immunodeficiency Virus" (HIV) in a compromise between the claims of both groups. It also became clear that Francoise Barré, the true discoverer of the AIDS virus, like Rosalind Franklin thirty years before in the discovery of DNA, would never get any credit for her work. No one got a Nobel Prize for this momentous discovery (probably because of the controversy) and Robert Gallo left the National Cancer Institute under a cloud of his own making. A recent book describes the entire controversy in meticulous detail and is a fascinating read.[334] Another book, *The River*, goes into meticulous detail about the origin of the virus and speculates that HIV was transferred to humans in a batch of poliovirus, grown in chimpanzee kidney tissue culture, and used in making a live poliovirus vaccine in the 1960s. The author has conducted an enormous amount of research, identifying a few AIDS cases dating back to as early as 1959, but recent articles in *Nature* have disputed his theory.[335]

CARDIOLOGY

Section V of Osler's textbook is "Diseases of the Circulatory System." The connection between sudden death, myocardial infarction and coronary thrombosis was recognized. He also notes the connection between angina pectoris and coronary disease although he groups the section on angina with arrhythmias, in "Neuroses of the Heart." He comments on the thickening of the left ventricular wall in cases of Bright's disease, chronic renal insufficiency, but measurement of the blood pressure was to be brought back from Italy by Harvey Cushing in 1901, nine years after publication. Treatment of angina was amyl nitrite or nitroglycerin but the use recommended was a daily one and not for the immediate relief of symptoms as we would use it. In 1847, Ascario Sobrero discovered nitroglycerin. In 1849, he reported on the phenomenon of violent headaches occurring when the compound was tasted or applied to the tongue. Constantin Hering tested nitroglycerin on normal volunteers, confirming the observation, and advocated it as a remedy for headache; this was another example of homeopathy in which "like cures like." In 1859, Alfred Nobel began to study the use of nitroglycerin in mining (as an alternative to gunpowder) but an explosion in 1864, which killed his brother Emil, prompted a search for a safer form of the explosive. In 1866, he learned to mix the explosive liquid with diatomaceous earth, a form of silica, and the mixture proved to be stable. He named it "dynamite" and his fortune was made. In the meantime, Lauder Brunton, a chemist and pioneering pharmacologist, was studying amyl nitrite, which had been shown to dilate arteries. A search for similar nitrate compounds, and the recollection of the headache effects of nitroglycerin, prompted further study. Nobel and some of his employees noticed that tasting nitroglycerin would relieve angina pain. By 1905, Osler was advocating both drugs for angina, but it would be another seventy-two years before the mechanism of action was described. In 1977, Ferid Murad discovered that nitroglycerin was converted to nitric oxide, a potent vasodilator.

Osler described cyanotic congenital heart disease and recommended bleeding in severe dyspnea. Actually, his understanding of heart disease was quite sophisticated considering the limitations in diagnostic techniques, but Osler was unmatched as a physician at the time.

William Harvey, in his masterpiece *Anatomica de Motu Cordis et Sanguinis*, described not only the pulmonary and the systemic circulation but the coronary circulation as well. He asked, "For what should the coronary arteries pulsate in the heart save to drive the blood on by that impulse? And why should there be coronary veins except to acquire blood from the heart?" The next great advance after Harvey was by Lower, who demonstrated the pulmonary circulation, showed that oxygen is absorbed by the blood in the lungs and corrected several of Harvey's errors. More was to come in the mid nineteenth century. Carl Ludwig was head of the Institute of Physiology in Leipzig from 1867 on. Study of the physiology of the heart began with his invention of the kymograph (a smoked drum which rotated and on which a stylus scratched a tracing), the first instrument to permit quantitative measurement of small volumes and flows. His student, Adolph Fick, devised the method to measure cardiac output, which continues in use today. Fick was a mathematician and physicist and his contributions to cardiology were the product of his physics knowledge. The basic "Fick principle" is used every day and consists of the simple relationship: cardiac output=oxygen consumption/arteriovenous oxygen difference, and was published in 1856. It was thirty years before his calculation, based purely on theory, could be tested in dogs. J. Plesch finally accomplished the first application of the measurement in humans, in Germany in 1909. Bauman and Grollman, who inserted a spinal tap needle into the right atrium, made the first direct measurement in 1930. Theirs was a daring procedure.[336]

In 1914, Starling published a series of papers explaining the function of the heart that have stood without contradiction for almost ninety years.[337] Starling was born in London in 1866 and educated at Guy's Hospital Medical School where he was trained in physiology by another product of Ludwig's lab, Charles Woolridge. Only two years after Starling's return to Guy's as an instructor, Woolridge died suddenly. Starling was appointed to take his mentor's place and a few years later married Woolridge's widow. In ten years, Starling was Jodrell Professor of Physiology at University College and had already described capillary function and lymph flow, a concept known as "Starling's hypothesis" which has also been proven largely true. He discovered secretin in 1902 (a hormone released by the duodenum when exposed to acid) and coined the term "hormone." Starling's Law of the Heart, the explanation of autoregulation of cardiac output, occupied an entire issue of the *Journal of Physiology* (London).[338] His work has stood the test of time.[339] The Law of the Heart was the first explanation of congestive heart failure and hinted at effective treatment: reduction of venous pressure when it exceeds the optimal level on the famous "Starling Curve," which shows cardiac output and filling pressure plotted against each other. Modern cardiology has shown that the Starling curve, atrial pressure plotted against ventricle stroke volume, can be shifted by drugs but the principle remains the same and forms the basis for treatment of heart failure and shock.

ELECTRICAL ACTIVITY OF THE HEART

In 1781, Leopoldo Caldani, a professor of anatomy at Bologna, was able to induce a frog leg muscle to contract with a spark from a Leyden jar. His student, Luigi Galvani, participated in the experiments and twenty-four years later continued Caldani's work with stimulation of the crural nerve in frog leg preparation. The nerve stimulation caused the entire leg, not just a single muscle, to contract. Galvani also experimented with dissimilar metals in contact with muscles. He concluded that the muscle was capable of storing energy and contracted when this energy was released by contact with the metal. His contemporary, Alessandro Volta, disagreed and believed that the reaction between the two metals generated the electrical energy; Volta was correct. Volta did not believe that animal electricity existed. In this he was wrong, but his work resulted in the voltaic pile and, eventually, in the storage battery. In 1820, Hans Oersted, a Danish physicist, discovered that electrical currents in conductors would influence the needle of a compass nearby. Soon after, Andre Ampere showed that parallel wires would be attracted to each other if current flowing through them was oriented in the same direction; if the current flowed in opposite directions, the wires repelled each other. These observations ultimately led to Maxwell, Faraday, and experimental physics.

Another pathway led to the galvanometer and electrophysiology. Eventually, Carlo Mateucci, in 1843, was able to measure the electrical current of muscle contraction using a galvanometer developed by others over twenty years. In 1856, Kölliker and Müller identified an electrical current generated by the frog heartbeat. In 1872, Gabriel Lippman developed a very sensitive instrument called the capillary electrometer, which could measure these very small bioelectric currents. In 1881, Marey devised a photographic technique to record the measurements. By 1887, Walter Gaskell had demonstrated the sinus node and the atrio-ventricular node in the turtle heart and observed a short delay in transmission of the electrical impulse from atrium to ventricle. He showed that cutting the muscular bridge between atrium and ventricle stopped the transmission of the impulse, leaving the ventricle to contract at its own rate, and that the impulse originates in muscle cells, not in nerve ganglia.

Purkinje had shown the modified muscle of the conduction system in 1839. The next few years allowed precise delineation of the anatomy of the conduction system. In 1893, Wilhelm His demonstrated the connecting bundle between atrium and ventricle using embryology of the chicken heart to study how the pathway develops. A number of others worked on the problem and disputed His's priority. Kent, Mahaim, and James discovered the accessory pathways, now so important in electrophysiology and therapy of arrhythmias.

In 1887, Augustus Waller succeeded in measuring cardiac electrical activity from the surface of the body, a necessity for clinical application. He called the record an "electrogram" but did not believe that it would be of any clinical use. In 1893, Willem Einthoven, professor of physiology at Utrecht, began to improve the capillary electrometer. Over the next seven years, he described the waves of the electrical recording and discovered that people with heart disease had different electrocardiogram tracings from those with normal hearts. He was not satisfied with the existing instruments and began to develop a new machine that was more practical for clinical use; a machine he called the "string galvanometer." The device included a strong electromagnet and a quartz thread suspended between its poles. The deflection of the thread (or its shadow) was recorded on a moving photographic plate. The first instrument weighed 600 pounds and occupied two rooms. The quality of the recordings obtained was far superior to those of modern instruments. His first report, in 1901, changed cardiology. By 1906, after connecting the string galvanometer in Einthoven's lab to the hospital with a 1500-meter cable, recordings had been made of a number of types of cardiac disease. Left ventricular hypertrophy, P mitrale, and rhythm disturbances were the first abnormalities recorded.

In 1908, he published his second classic study, which included electro-cardiograms from a wide variety of cardiac diseases and included the effects of changes in heart rate, respiration and anesthesia on the ECG. Visitors came from all over Europe to see for themselves and learn the new method of examination. Finally, in 1912, he presented his third classic paper to the Chelsea Clinical Society in which he analyzed the relation-ship of voltages in the three limb leads and constructed the equilateral tri-angle now standard in all ECG interpretations. The relationship became known as "Einthoven's Law."[340] The following year he presented the method of calculating the heart's electrical axis during the cardiac cycle. In 1924, he was awarded the Nobel Prize in physiology for his work.

In 1912, James B. Herrick of Chicago, one of the greatest cardiologists (and physicians) of all time, described the classic signs and symptoms of coronary artery occlusion.[341] His paper was ignored at first, he says in his memoirs, because coronary artery disease was considered an autopsy find-ing and not a clinical entity. In 1918, Bousfield published the first ECG taken on a patient during an attack of angina pectoris, improving clinical diagnosis.[342] The next year, after conducting dog experiments, Herrick described the abnormal T waves in leads I and III in myocardial infarction. Over the next decade, the ECG changes in cardiac ischemia and infarction were intensively studied and the diagnosis could now be made in life.

In 1924, Einthoven, during a visit to the US, was astonished to see an ECG technician make the diagnosis of acute myocardial infarction just by look-ing at the ECG. He was visiting Dr. Samuel Levine at the Peter Brent Brigham Hospital when the technician walked in with a wet ECG and asked if she should call the house officer right away. Einthoven was amazed at the progress in the use of his instrument.[343] In 1928, the Cambridge Scientific Instrument Company of London built the first portable string electrocardiograph, a thirty pound instrument in a suitcase. A few years later, less sensitive, but lighter and more rugged galvanometers were devel-oped and then the modern amplified, direct writing instruments appeared. In 1919, Frank Wilson, of the University of Michigan, began to investigate the ventricular complex of the electrocardiograph and soon described bun-dle branch block, ventricular hypertrophy and, in 1930, published a classic paper on the mathematics of the Einthoven Triangle.[344] In the 1930s the chest leads were introduced, including the multiple "V leads," and accura-cy improved considerably compared to the classical three limb leads.

WENCKEBACH AND RHYTHM DISTURBANCES

Frederick Wenckebach (1864-1940), a Dutch-born physician, graduated from Utrecht in 1888, was an early electro-cardiographer, and became chief of the first medical university clinic in 1915 in Vienna. He adopted Enthoven's new machine and began to study electrocardiography as early as 1898, in spite of considerable doubt and even ridicule on the part of other practitioners of the day. The machine was not portable and the patient must be taken to the machine rather than the other way around. Rather than changes of cardiac ischemia, described above, he became interested in changes of rhythm. He discovered atrial fibrillation, and flutter; he described atrial and ventricular tachycardia. In referring to his work on the treatment of atrial fibrillation, he said, "I owe my reputation to the fact that I use digitalis in doses the text books say are dangerous and in cases that the text book say are unsuitable."[345]

His name is chiefly remembered for the intermittant heart block in which one beat is dropped of every four or so.[346] The classification of heart block (interruption of transmission between atria and ventricles) is now known from the work of Mobitz, who expanded the classification to include all forms of transmission disorders. Woldemar Mobitz was a Russian, born in St. Petersburg in 1889, who became professor of medicine at Freiburg, Germany, in 1928. He described the relationship between the Wenckebach phenomenon, in which the PR interval increases with each heartbeat until one atrial beat is not transmitted to the ventricle (after which the AV node "resets"), and the fixed second degree block in which one-half or one-third of all atrial beats is transmitted. The fixed block was first described by Englishman John Hay.[347] The Wenckeback variable block is now called Mobitz type I and the second Mobitz type II.[348]

Complete heart block, the dissociation of ventricular rate from atrial rate, was first described by Morgagni, (1682-1771), who examined a Padua merchant. "When visiting by way of consultation, I found with such a rarity of the pulse that within the sixtieth part of an hour the pulsations were only twenty-two - and this rareness which was perpetual - was perceived to be even more considerable, as often as even two (epileptic) attacks were at hand - so that the physicians were never deceived from the increase of the rareness they foretold a paroxysm to be coming on."[349] His description includes the slow pulse and the loss of consciousness that would be described again by two Irish physicians, a century later. Robert Adams (1791-1875) was an Irish surgeon who wrote treatises on gout and diseases of the heart. In the latter he described a sixty-eight-year-old patient with symptoms similar to those of Morgagni's patient.[350] William Stokes (1804-

1878) was educated at home by his physician father, who was a member of a religious sect and had resigned his position as Regius professor of medicine at Dublin University because of religious concerns. Stokes enrolled in the College of Surgeons School in Ireland in 1821, in a course of anatomy where his father had succeeded John Cheyne as professor of medicine. Initially, he was interested in chemistry and went to Glasgow University to study this under the professor of chemistry there, Thomas Thompson. After two years, however, he decided to switch to medicine and went to Edinburg where he made friends with professor William Pulteney Alison (1790-1859) and Dominic John Corrigan (1802-1880). Stokes graduated M.D. in 1825 with the dissertation *De ascite*. In 1825, Stokes also became a Licentiate of the King and Queen's College of Physicians, and a clinical instructor. He introduced the stethoscope to the medical school and this innovation caused much comment, often sarcastic, rather than laudatory. His book, *An introduction to the use of the stethoscope*, was the first on this topic in English. His description of the Stokes-Adams attack and Cheyne-Stokes respiration, the agonal respiration that often precedes death, are contained in his textbook on diseases of the heart.[351] He also describes paroxysmal tachycardia in the same work. These descriptions preceded the development of the electrocardiogram and Wenckebach later demonstrated the rhythm disturbances associated with the symptoms.

Wenckebach was the beneficiary of an example of serendipidy in discovering the first drug effective for arrhythmia. He was examining a patient with atrial fibrillation, a condition of irregular pulse with many complications, when he began to warn the patient about the seriousness of the condition. The patient said, "Oh, it's nothing. It will be gone when I come back tomorrow." Wenckeback asked him what he did to make it go away. He replied, "Oh, I take the quinine I use for my malaria." Wenckebach, like all the great scientific physicians of the era of discovery, investigated the patient's claim and found that, while quinine worked, quinidine (another extract of the bark) was better. The first anti-arrhythmic drug was discovered.[352]

CARDIAC RESUSCITATION AND THE DEVELOPMENT OF CPR

In 1848, the first sudden death during general anesthesia occurred, in a fifteen-year-old girl named Hannah Greener, while she was anesthetized with chloroform for the removal of a toenail. In 1860, the Boston Society for Medical Improvement analyzed forty-one such cases. In 1911, Levy demonstrated that deaths under chloroform anesthesia were caused by ventricular fibrillation. Several attempts with open chest cardiac massage had been unsuccessful but in 1901, Kristian Igelsrud, in Norway, succeeded in reviving a forty-three-year-old woman who suffered cardiac arrest under chloroform anesthesia during a hysterectomy. She recovered and went home. Soon after this, other cases were reported, all with open chest massage of the heart, although Sir William Arbuthnot Lane, in 1902, reported a successful cardiac massage with the surgeon's hand introduced through an appendectomy incision, compressing the heart through the diaphragm. In 1895, Oliver and Schafer described the action of epinephrine in the body and, two years later, pure epinephrine was isolated. In 1905, George Crile successfully revived a child after a cardiac arrest, under ether anesthesia for a brain tumor operation, using infusion of an adrenaline solution through the brachial artery and mouth-to-mouth breathing. That patient recovered and Crile followed her until she was an adult. Finally, in 1906 epinephrine was used to treat cardiac arrest by intracardiac injection. In other instances, Crile used closed chest cardiac massage. He was fifty years ahead of everyone else.

Vesalius had originally described ventricular fibrillation. In 1883, Sidney Ringer described the effects of calcium and potassium on myocardial contraction. By 1904, Maurice d'Halluin published *Cardiac Resuscitation*, in which he described using potassium to stop fibrillation and calcium chloride to restart or strengthen the heartbeat afterward. In 1904, George Crile's interest in electrocution was aroused by an incident in which he and his wife, horseback riding with a friend, were nearly electrocuted by a broken electrical conduit in the ground. The three horses were electrocuted. He was asked by the president of the Cleveland Electrical Illuminating Company to study electrocution. He and professor of physiology, J.J. McLeod, published an analysis of the problem in the *American Journal of the Medical Sciences* in 1905. They found that atropine administered before electric shock would protect animals from cardiac standstill. This, of course, is not a practical therapy in accidental injuries and Crile's interests were more about the effect of cerebral anoxia. In 1926, Donald Hooker, at Johns Hopkins University, devised a regimen for stopping electrically induced fibrillation in dogs. The drug injections worked but were not practical for use in a clinical situation except in the operating room. In 1930, Dr. Hooker began to work with William Kouwenhoven, a professor of electrical engineering at Johns Hopkins, who had been studying electrocution. The Consolidated Edison Company was trying to find a way to revive electrocuted workers and sponsored this work for years. They began to study not only the electrical current needed to stop the heart (ventricular fibrillation) but how to stop the fibrillation, and restart the heart, with electric current as well. They found that electrical shock, applied to the surface of the heart with two small paddles, could restore the heart rhythm. They had proven that dog hearts could be restarted with electrical current. Would it work in man? They obtained permission to experiment on an ape in the Philadelphia Zoo that was about to die from other causes. They found that ape hearts (and later found the same in monkey hearts) will not remain in ventricular fibrillation: they resume normal rhythm spontaneously. Back to the lab.

Carl Wiggers, a highly respected physiologist at Western Reserve, had been losing lab animals to ventricular fibrillation during his experiments and became interested in Hooker and Kouwenhoven's work. He came to Baltimore, observed their methods and returned to Cleveland where he repeated their experiments. By 1940, he had revived over 1,000 animal hearts from ventricular fibrillation. In particular, he learned that a short period of cardiac massage before defibrillation markedly improved the result. He also found that the use of a series of shocks worked better than a single shock. Claude Beck, in his work on coronary artery disease, to be described next, learned to defibrillate hearts in the dog lab. In 1937, he equipped the operating room with a defibrillator.[353] Beck developed a whole regimen for cardiac arrest in the operating room, which included open chest massage, endotrachial intubation and the use of procaine to improve defibrillation. After defibrillation, he used epinephrine and calcium chloride to restore normal cardiac function. In spite of his efforts, Beck was unsuccessful in reviving cardiac arrest in a patient until 1947.

The first successful use of his program was by Hubert Adams and Leo Hand at the Lahey Clinic in Boston. They were removing the lobe of a lung and were just closing the incision when the patient had a cardiac arrest. After twenty minutes of cardiac massage, endotrachial ventilation and administration of drugs, the heartbeat was restored and the patient recovered. In 1949, Beck and his associates in Cleveland began a training program to teach resuscitation to physicians and defibrillators became commonplace in operating rooms. In 1960, Kouwenhoven, Jude, and Knickerbocker described closed chest cardiac massage, mouth-to-mouth breathing and external defibrillation.[354] They had been working on these three techniques since 1951 when the Edison Electric Institute asked Kouwenhoven to develop a portable defibrillator. By 1957, he had an AC defibrillator that could be used in humans and he and his colleagues spent hours in the morgue perfecting the closed chest cardiac compression. Peter Safar, at the Baltimore City Hospital, had developed the concept of mouth-to-mouth breathing after studies showed that residual oxygen in expired air was sufficient to revive cardiac arrest victims. They incorporated Safar's method into the CPR program. After their initial report, many others studied the technique and compared its effectiveness to open chest massage. By 1967, closed-chest massage was standard and, in 1969, Johns Hopkins awarded Kouwenhoven an honorary MD degree. He had already received an Edison Medal in 1962.

THE PACEMAKER

Aldini, Galvani's nephew, first described electrical pacing of the heart in 1774, but his experience was with corpses and it would take more than a century before any practical application would exist. In 1872, Duchenne reported the successful stimulation of a child's heart during treatment of diphtheria. The first artificial cardiac pacemaker was constructed by Albert Hyman who, in 1932, reported successful pacing of human hearts using a transthoracic needle to pace the right atrium.[355] His device included a magneto and a hand crank. In 1950, Wilfred Bigelow, and his associates at the Banting Institute in Toronto, developed a pacemaker to use in cardiac surgery. Eventually a device was made using their design and became the first commercially built pacemaker. Their work, reported to the American College of Surgeons in 1950, created a stir, including a front-page article in the New York Times. Unfortunately, their device was designed to pace the atrium, not the ventricle, and so was of limited usefulness. Paul Zoll, who would design his own AC defibrillator in 1956, attended the meeting and met with Callaghan, one of Bigelow's associates, afterwards to discuss the pacemaker device. In 1952, Zoll reported a successful use of a transesophageal pacemaker for complete heart block in a patient. This was a monumental step, but the US Public Health Service did not think so, turning down his request for a $5,000 research grant. He then developed the external pacemaker, but it was limited by discomfort (from chest muscle contractions) and skin injury to short-term use. The implantable pacemaker had to wait for the invention of the transistor and, finally, in 1958, Ake Senning and Rune Elmqvist, in Sweden, implanted a pulse generator with rechargeable batteries and electrodes sutured to the myocardium. The device only functioned for three hours, and a replacement failed after eight days. The patient, an engineer, finally got a better pacemaker three years later. He actually collaborated with Senning and Elmqvist on the new version and lived twenty years with his improved model (which required twenty-four replacements).

Technological progress was rapid once the first prototypes had been built. In 1964, Chardack reported on the first sixty patients treated with an implantable pacemaker for complete heart block.[356] The pacemaker lead was sutured to the surface of the heart requiring a thoracotomy. Battery failure was a problem not solved for another twenty years. Eventually, lithium batteries were developed that lasted for years. The fixed rate determined by the pacemaker circuitry did not allow for increased cardiac output with exercise, a potential problem in children, many of whom developed complete heart block during repair of congenital heart defects. A synchronous pacemaker was developed that used an atrial lead to pick up the P wave and ventricular leads to stimulate the ventricle after a delay equal to the normal P-R interval.[357] This allowed a variable heart rate and approximated the normal atrial systole for ventricular filling but the battery life of these pacemakers was a drawback. They were usually replaced with fixed rate units after the child was fifteen years old, or so. This reduced the frequency of replacement from every six months to every eighteen months (at best). Eventually transvenous pacemakers were developed that did not require the heart be exposed to attach the lead and better batteries were available by the 1970s.

HYPERTENSION

The measurement of blood pressure began with Stephen Hales. In 1733, he published his observations on dogs and horses. He measured the arterial pressure in the horse by inserting a brass pipe into a vessel and attaching a glass tube nine feet in length. His first measurement was eight feet three inches above the horse's left ventricle and he noted the rise and fall of the column with the heartbeat. Poiseuille used a mercury manometer in 1828 and connected it to a needle inserted into the artery. Carl Ludwig's kymograph permitted recording of a continuous tracing of the pressure after 1847. Finally, Riva-Rocci invented the sphygmomanometer that allowed clinical measurement of blood pressure. In 1905, N.E. Korotkoff introduced the auscultatory method used today. Korotkoff was a young Russian surgeon interested in vascular surgery who began to use auscultation for better accuracy in determining arterial occlusion and stenosis.[358] The origin of the sounds heard over the artery, when partially compressed by the Riva-Rocci device, has been the source of speculation since his brief report.[359]

The regulation of blood pressure was not understood until endocrinology progressed enough to understand the humeral influences of adrenaline and other hormones. Harvey Cushing discovered the brain's autoregulatory system, in which an increase in intracranial pressure produced a corresponding increase in arterial pressure. William Bayliss, a physiologist, spent years studying the vasomotor system and his 1923 textbook of physiology summarized the state of knowledge at the time. Walter Cannon, Harvard physiologist and remembered for his study of the sympathetic nervous system, described the "fight or flight" phenomenon.[360] All these scientists tried to understand what changed blood pressure and why some people had pressure that was too high. Fredrick Mahomed, an English physician of Indian parentage, measured blood pressure in 1874 and recognized the association of kidney disease and hypertension. Richard Bright had described the pathology in the heart and kidneys in 1836[361] but the measurement of blood pressure, itself, would take another forty years. In 1879, Mahomed published his observations and made the connection between high blood pressure, the early stage, and renal disease, the late stage of Bright's disease.[362] Unfortunately, Mahomed died at the age of thirty-five from typhoid fever and what might have been a glorious career was cut short. Others have been given priority, but an earlier paper by Mahomed clearly points out the presence of high blood pressure before the onset of the albuminuria that heralded Bright's disease.

In 1913, Janeway discussed the association between high blood pressure and cardiac hypertrophy. He proposed a causal relationship between renal disease and hypertension and called the disease "nephritic hypertension." He speculated on the cause and described experiments in which the renal artery was partially occluded with paraffin emboli and others in which a portion of the kidney was removed. In both cases, the dogs did not become hypertensive. He discusses renin, discovered in 1898 by Robert Tigerstedt,[363] but rejects it as a factor. He is enthusiastic about epinephrine as a cause, but acknowledges the problems demonstrated by other's research showing no increase in circulating epinephrine in hypertension. Finally, he is reduced to speculating about "unknown, probably extra-renal causes" producing a vasoconstricting mechanism.

The improved understanding of etiology did not provide any useful therapy until Goldblatt discovered the effect of renal artery stenosis in the 1940s. His group produced hypertension in animals by constricting the renal arteries. This fit with the Bright's disease model but then they found that constricting only one renal artery also made the animal hypertensive. Why? And did this mean that all hypertension was renal in origin?[364] Did all hypertensive patients have renal artery stenosis? If so, maybe this was a discovery that would finally lead to a cure. Unfortunately, only a small fraction of hypertension is due to renal artery stenosis but those cases that are, can be cured with arterial reconstruction (or nephrectomy). Goldblatt's work did point to the kidney as the possible source of hypertension.

Blalock and Levy, in 1937, were able to produce hypertension by transplanting a kidney to a heterotopic location (to ensure that any nerves were cut) and constricting the artery. Releasing the constriction relieved the hypertension. Clearly, a hormone was at work and it was not epinephrine. Using Blalock's model Pickering's group discovered the role of renin.[365] Renin had been discovered, and named, in 1894 by Robert Tigerstedt of Stockholm, but its existence, or at least its role, was doubted (and rejected by Janeway in 1913) until Pickering's report. In 1939 Irwin Page, famous for his work in brain chemistry (he discovered serotonin), reported that renin was an enzyme whose substrate was a plasma protein he called angiotonin (later changed to angiotensin). A few years later his discovery led to the recognition of angiotensin converting enzyme after several groups realized that angiotensin had two forms, I and II, and that II was the active form. Angiotensin converting enzyme inhibitors (ACE Inhibitors) are widely used today. Gradually, the realization formed that there were several causes of hypertension and everybody was half-right: the kidneys, the adrenals, and the neuroendocrine system all contributed.

THE ANTI-HYPERTENSIVE DRUGS

Prior to 1950, there were only two effective means of lowering blood pressure, both surgical and of doubtful efficacy. Goldblatt's theory that all or most hypertension resulted from renal artery stenosis resulted in too many nephrectomies for what were called "Goldblatt kidneys." Renal artery repair awaited better techniques in vascular surgery and angiography to study the renal arteries. Even then, laboratory determination of blood renin levels eventually narrowed the application of this approach to a very small number of cases. Sympathectomy, advocated by Smithwick in the 1920s, was effective in lowering blood pressure but the effect was unpredictable, complicated by severe postural hypotension (blood pressure would drop when the patient stood up.) and tended to diminish with time. The observation by Langley and Dickinson, in 1889,[366] that nicotine blocks autonomic ganglia, prompted a search for drugs that would perform a "medical sympathectomy." Ganglionic blocking agents were developed to mimic the sympathectomy effect but they had frightening side effects. In 1949, hexamethonium, the first of the alpha-blockers, was introduced. To give an idea of how serious the side effects could be. This drug was recently used in an experiment at Johns Hopkins University. The purpose was to reduce pulmonary artery pressure in pulmonary hypertension by causing vasodilatation in the lung. A healthy young woman lab technician volunteered for the study and, after inhaling hexamethonium in a gas form, developed respiratory failure and died. Johns Hopkins was severely criticized for lax standards in human subject research, lost several large federal grants, and its human subject research program was suspended for several months.[367] Those early drugs were dangerous but, fortunately, safer ones were coming.

Another side effect of sulfanilamide resulted in the first drug to combine efficacy and safety. Patients receiving sulfanilamide in 1940 were found to develop metabolic acidosis with alkaline urine. Investigation of this phenomenon showed that the drug inhibited a renal carbonic anhydrase enzyme. The enzyme hydrates CO_2 in the kidney to form carbonic acid, which then dissociates into hydrogen ion and bicarbonate. The hydrogen ion enters the urine and is excreted, contributing to the body's acid-base balance. The bicarbonate is reabsorbed from the renal tubule. If the enzyme is inactive, too much hydrogen ion (a metabolic waste product) is retained in the body and acidosis results. The patient is acidotic with alkaline urine. Another effect of blocking the enzyme is increased excretion of potassium, which is exchanged for sodium when not enough hydrogen ion is available (sodium preservation takes precedence). The drug's effect leads to an increase in sodium and potassium in the urine, and a corresponding increase in urine volume.

THE MERCURIAL DIURETICS

Sulfanilamide is a weak diuretic, the first to be discovered since the organic mercury compounds (which poison the kidney) came into use in the 1920s. Frederick Wenckebach was professor of medicine in Vienna from 1915 to his retirement in 1929. The first effective diuretics were discovered by accident during his tenure. Mercury was still in use in the treatment of syphilis. Some syphilitic patients, who had developed syphilitic aneurysms of the ascending aorta, suffered congestive heart failure as a consequence. In October, 1919, a young girl with congenital syphilis was admitted to professor Wenckebach's clinic in Vienna. Dr. Paul Saxl was the attending physician and he prescribed intravenous salicylate of mercury, to be administered by the third year medical student. The student, Alfred Vogl, discovered to his dismay, that the salicylate was insoluble in water and could not be given as ordered from the pharmacy. Another physician suggested the use of a new anti-syphilitic called "Novasurol." Vogel administered the drug and discovered a dramatic increase in the patient's urine output. The nurses in the syphilitic ward left jugs at the foot of the bed to collect the patients' urine, not for tests but to discard it. They did, however, make accurate records of the volume, a sign of the new emphasis on scientific nursing. Vogl decided to try the same drug on a man in obvious heart failure. The patient passed ten liters of urine in the next twelve hours! Eventually they tried it on a boy with congenital heart disease who had no sign of syphilis. The medical student and the nurses finally convinced the professor that the mercury injection was doing something other than the effect on syphilis. It was eventually realized that organic mercury, in addition to its effect on syphilis,[368] was causing the kidney to release the inappropriate fluid conservation typical of heart failure.[369] These mercury compounds were toxic, had to be given by injection and stimulated allergic reactions that were sometimes fatal. They were of no use in treating hypertension.

THE NEW DRUGS

Analysis of the sulfanilamide side effect led to modification of the molecule to increase the diuretic effect and reduce the toxicity. Acetazolamide (Diamox), a chemical alteration of the molecule, was found to be 300 times as potent as a carbonic anhydrase inhibitor but it was not a very effective diuretic since the diuresis was limited by the limited amount of hydrogen ion normally excreted and by the harmful effect of acidosis and potassium loss. Another derivative, with a chlorobenzene side chain added, was a better diuretic but only half as effective in inhibiting carbonic anhydrase. Apparently, the two properties were not related after all. This set off a search for more effective molecules and chlorothiazide was discovered in 1958. Eventually, a family of synthetic compounds resulted including hydrochlorothiazide, the most effective diuretic with very little carbonic anhydrase activity. In addition to their diuretic properties, or perhaps because of them, they were found to be effective in reducing blood pressure and became the first drugs used, even after stronger and more effective compounds became available. In the 1960s the "loop diuretics," furosemide (Lasix) and ethacrynic acid were discovered. These were potent diuretics but not very useful in hypertension.

Rauwolfia serpentina is a root from which, in the sixteenth century, Garcia de Orta, a Portuguese physician, extracted a drug useful in insomnia. The Portugese called it "premium et laudatissimum remedium."[370] The same drug was known in ancient India where it was called *pagel-kadawa* and was used to put children to sleep.[371] Another compound, used in India for sedation, was called *Sarpagandha* and it contained *Rauwolfia serpentina benth*, another preparation of the root which varied somewhat in activity with the region where it was growing.[372] An effect on blood pressure was described in the Indian medical literature in 1931.[373] In 1949, Rustom Jal Vakil published a scientific study of the drug. Apparently, folk medicine was far ahead of traditional pharmacology in this case. He found that the dried root was being used in India for the treatment of high blood pressure and resolved to study the effects using a scientific approach. He surveyed other physicians in India and found that it was in common use. This was not the first vegetable extract to be advocated for hypertension but it was the first to be subjected to careful analysis. He found that seventy-seven percent of his study group of fifty patients had a significant drop in systolic blood pressure and seventy-three percent had a decrease in diastolic pressure. With longer periods of treatment, the results improved. He reported no toxic effects although depression was later found to be a significant side effect of the drug. The first effective drug for severe hypertension had been discovered.[374] In 1952, reserpine was isolated from *Rauwolfia* and, in 1958, it was synthesized. Eventually, reserpine was found to deplete nerve endings of norepinephrine and dopamine, effects that cause the psychiatric side effects. Chlorpromazine (Thorazine) has somewhat similar effects (by a different mechanism). It has been impossible to separate the anti-hypertensive effect from the depression side effect since both are caused by the same action of the drug.

A drug discovered in 1949 was another example of serendipity, similar to that in the case of sulfanilamide. Hydralazine-related anti-parasite drugs were being tested in the late 1940s when some animals exhibited a drop in blood pressure. Further investigations resulted in the clinical introduction of hydralazine as a drug for high blood pressure in 1953. Investigation of the mechanism of activity found that it was a vasodilator and acted on smooth muscle cells in small artery walls. A reflex increase in heart rate was a problem until it was combined with hexamethonium or reserpine, both of which block this effect. Another drug based on anti-parasite chemical structures was guanethidine, introduced in 1960 as a more potent anti-hypertensive. The mechanism of action of guanethidine, the subject of pharmacology lab experiments when I was a medical student in 1963, is an inhibition of reuptake of norepinephrine by the sympathetic nerve ending. This is similar to the mechanism of action of drugs that are used to treat depression but guanethidine does not enter the central nervous system, avoiding the side effects of reserpine. Tricyclic antidepressant drugs (to be discussed in another chapter) drastically inhibit the effects of guanethidine, however.[375] Severe postural hypotension has limited the usefulness of guanethidine and newer drugs have replaced it.

In 1948, Ahlquist postulated the existence of alpha and beta-receptors for adrenergic drugs. This would explain the contradictory actions of some drugs, especially epinephrine which relaxes some smooth muscle and contracts it in other areas. In 1958, Powell and Slater discovered an agent with beta blocking ability, confirming Ahlquist's hypothesis. The first beta-blocker was dichloro-isoproterenol, but it was not clinically useful. Finally, Black and Stephenson introduced propanolol, which became the first of the beta-blocker agents and a new chapter in the treatment of hypertension opened.[376] In 1968, the Bayer Company developed another family of drugs. This story began in 1963 when the chief pharmacologist was asked to study two newly synthesized coronary vasodilators. They had undesirable cardio-depressant side effects, and this observation would provide another example of serendipity. They mimicked the effects of calcium withdrawal. Additional calcium neutralized the drug's effect on cardiac muscle. They were also neutralized by beta-adrenergic drugs or digitalis glycosides, both of which increase calcium availability. Eventually, calcium antagonism became a new pharmacological principle and muscle cell biology was better understood. These drugs had no natural analog; they were purely synthetic. Most of their effects are cardiac but they were found in the search for vasodilators. The family is called "calcium channel blockers."

Finally, pharmacology research began to use the information about drug mechanism of action to search for new approaches to the problem.[377] Since reserpine lowered blood pressure by reducing the availability of norepinephrine at nerve endings, maybe interference with the body's synthesis of the chemical would be useful. The synthesis of norepinephrine follows three steps beginning with the amino acid tyrosine. Tyrosine is acted upon by the enzyme tyrosine hydroxylase to become dopa (dihydroxy phenylalanine). In the next step, dopa becomes dopamine under the influence of another enzyme, dopa decarboxylase. Finally, dopamine, acted upon by another enzyme, dopamine beta-hydrolase, becomes norepinephrine. It was found that alpha-methyl-dopa, a synthetic analogue of dopa, would block the step in which dopa becomes dopamine by inhibiting dopa decarboxylase.[378] The drug alpha-methyl-dopa became "Aldomet" a very effective antihypertensive drug still in use. Pharmacology research had progressed until hypertension was finally treatable and new drugs continue to appear.

DIRECT ATTACK ON CORONARY ARTERY DISEASE

Atherosclerosis has been found in the arteries of Egyptian mummies, including that of Menenphtah, the Pharoah supposedly drowned in the Red Sea during the Hebrew exodus.[379] The ancients did not mention the disease and medical history is silent regarding the coronary arteries until Lower demonstrated intercoronary anastomoses in 1669. He showed that injection of one coronary artery would fill the other by what we now call collateral branches. In 1850, Sir Richard Quain finally correlated cardiac muscle damage with coronary artery calcifications. The muscle changes Quain saw in his microscope were not "fatty changes," as he described them, but ischemic areas or infarction.[380] In 1882, William T. Porter conducted a series of fruitful experiments that showed ligation of the left coronary artery in dogs resulted in ventricular fibrillation and death. In later work, he showed that ligation resulted in infarction of muscle in the distribution of the ligated artery. The intercoronary anastomoses were not sufficient to prevent muscle death; the intramuscular branches of coronary arteries are end arteries. Osler was familiar with the role of coronary thrombosis in chest pain, infarction and sudden death. He was the first to refer to the anterior descending branch of the left coronary as "the artery of sudden death." J.B. Herrick presented a paper describing the diagnosis of coronary thrombosis in the living patient in 1912 but was disappointed by the response.[381] His later work on electrocardiography has been described already.

The first diagnostic test to use cardiac physiology was the exercise electrocardiogram, which Einthoven first performed in 1908. His case did not show any abnormalities and the only difference between the resting and exercise tracing was an increase in heart rate. In the 1930s interest in ECG before and after exercise resumed, although there were warnings that it could be dangerous. Master and Oppenheimer, a physiologist, tried to standardize the various approaches to the exercise ECG and Master began to record the tracing during, as well as after, the exercise.[382] In 1958, Paul Wood of London described the ischemic depression of the ST segment during the exercise test and further clarified the interpretation.[383]

CARDIAC CATHETERIZATION

Claude Bernard performed cardiac catheterization on animals and gave the procedure its name in 1844. He measured the temperature of the blood in the heart with a very long thermometer. Combustion was assumed to occur in the lungs and it was this process that warmed the blood. If this were true, the pulmonary venous blood should be warmer than that in the pulmonary artery. Bernard succeeded in measuring the temperature in the right ventricle by passing his long thermometer down the jugular vein of a horse. He then passed the instrument down the carotid artery into the left ventricle. The blood in the right ventricle was warmer than that in the left, disproving the theory. Body heat comes from the peripheral tissues (and the liver, which has the highest temperature) where oxidation takes place and Bernard took the first step toward this understanding of metabolism with his long thermometer. He also showed that the ancients, with their concept of a "cooling" function in the lungs, were not that far from the truth. Bernard also measured pressures in the cardiac chambers.

The definitive research on this subject was performed by Chauveau and Marey, French physiologists (Chauveau was a professor of veterinary medicine), who, in the 1860s, measured pressures in the left ventricle and aorta simultaneously and identified the isometric phase of ventricular contraction, recording their observations on a kymograph drum.[384] The isometric phase is prior to opening of the aortic valve when the ventricular pressure, while rising, is still less than diastolic pressure in the aorta. During this part of the cardiac cycle, the volume in the ventricle does not change; no blood is yet pumped into the aorta. (Charles Atlas, the bodybuilder, built muscles with isometric contraction that he called "dynamic tension") Fick's experiments are described earlier and no further progress in the application of this method to human disease occurred until Werner Forssmann, a surgical resident in Germany, performed the insertion of a ureteral catheter (a thin catheter used for treatment of kidney disease), through an arm vein, into the heart. At first, he experimented on cadavers. Next, he inserted a catheter into the atrium of a patient dying of peritonitis to instill a solution of glucose, epinephrine and strophanthin. With no antibiotics available for another fifteen years, the drugs were ineffective and the patient died. At autopsy, the catheter could be seen entering the right atrium. Next, he inserted a catheter into his own arm vein, advanced it into what he thought was the atrium and walked downstairs to the x-ray department to document the position with a chest x-ray. He later described the details of his first self-catheterization. First, being a junior resident physician, he had to convince the clinic surgical supervisor to give him the ureteral catheter. He was so successful in convincing her of the importance of his work that she insisted she be the first subject for cardiac catheterization. Unable to dissuade her, he convinced her to allow him to strap her down to the operating table so she "would not fall off." When she was strapped down he inserted the catheter into his own vein, then released her and she assisted him in walking down to the x-ray department. His report, which appeared in 1929,[385] stimulated several others, one of whom used the Fick principle to measure cardiac output. Forssmann experimented with injection of x-ray dye into the catheter but the primitive contrast agents of the time were not capable of visualizing the heart because of dilution. He was unable to continue his research and eventually became a urologist in private practice in the Schwarzwald.

In 1936, Andre Cournand learned the technique of right heart catheterization, now well established for pulmonary angiography, and developed the method as a diagnostic procedure in cardiac disease. In 1941, Cournand and Ranges published their seminal paper.[386] Between 1941 and 1945, they improved catheters, including the construction of a double lumen catheter, and trained a large number of students who then carried the method all over the world. Richards, Cournand, Darling and Gillespie used right heart catheterization to study congestive heart failure and the effect of venous pressure on cardiac output. In doing so, they proved that Starling's work on dogs was applicable to man and his Law of the Heart was correct.[387] They performed critical work on shock and blood loss for the military during the War. By 1947, intensive study of congenital heart disease had reached a point where left heart catheterization was going to be the next step. In 1950, Zimmerman succeeded in reaching the left ventricle through the ulnar artery and in 1967; Judkins developed the technique used today, via the femoral artery. All used methods developed by Cournand and his group. Judkins was an Army general medical officer assigned to a post with no urologist. He learned about catheters and spent years developing new types, many of which are still in use. In 1956, Cournand, Forssmann (who had been rebuffed by Sauerbruch when he wanted to pursue his research in 1929), and Dickinson Richards shared the Nobel Prize in Medicine for cardiac catheterization. Cournand had sought out Forssmann to ensure that he received credit for his pioneering work.

CORONARY ANGIOGRAPHY

In the late 1950s, F. Mason Sones, a radiologist at the Cleveland Clinic, conducted experiments in coronary angiography using the new x-ray systems that allowed a rapid series of x-rays, known today as ciné angiography. The initial attempts to visualize the coronary arteries were disappointing. Injection of contrast material in the root of the aorta, above the aortic valve, had already been used to assess valve insufficiency. It did visualize the coronary arteries, but the contrast was poor and any stenosis of an artery rendered visualization of the distal runoff branches impossible. The next attempt involved a brief occlusion of the aorta (with a balloon) above the injection site to divert the maximum volume of contrast into the coronary vessels. This worked well in dogs but was unsatisfactory in humans because of the larger size of the human aorta. Cardiac arrest, to improve visualization, was produced by injection of acetylcholine, but the early attempts were complicated by a death in one of the first cases.[388] Direct cannulation of the coronary orifice was avoided because of fear of cardiac arrest and the primitive state of the defibrillation equipment. Sones avoided this problem largely with a catheter of new design and reported his first experience in 1959.[389] By 1962, he had performed coronary angiograms by direct cannulation of the coronary orifice in 1,020 patients. The fear of ventricular fibrillation, which had inhibited others prior to the development of the AC defibrillator by Kouwenhoven, proved unfounded. In 954 of the 1,020 patients, both coronary artery orifices were entered. Four years later a successful method of treating the lesions Sones identified was finally developed.

270   Frederick M. Allen, *Studies Concerning Glycosuria and Diabetes* (1913).

271   FG Banting, and CH Best, JB Collip, WR Campbell and AA Fletcher, "Pancreatic Extracts in the Treatment of Diabetes Mellitus," *Canadian Medical Association Journal,* 2:141-146 (1921).

272   Seale Harris, *Banting's Miracle* p 98, J.B. Lippincott Co. (1946).

273   Seale Harris, pages 99-103.

274   Michael Bliss, *The Discovery of Insulin*, MacMillan Press (1982).

275   EP Joslin, LI Dublin and HH Marks, "Studies on diabetes mellitus: I Characteristics and trends of diabetes mortality throughout the world," *American Journal of the Medical Sciences*186:753-73 (1933).

276   GB Gruber, "Zur Frage der Periarteritis Nodosa, mit besonderer Berücksichtigung der Gallenblasen- uncd Nieren-Beteiligung," *Virch-Arch.,* 247:441 (1925).

277   Arnold Rich, "Hypersensitivity in Disease with Especial Reference to Periarteritis Nodosa, Rheumatic Fever, Disseminated Lupus Erythematosis and Rheumatoid Arthritis." *The Harvey Lectures XII,* 106-147 (1946).

278   Thomas Addison, *On the Constitutional and Local Effects of Disease of the Suprarenal Capsules,* S. Highley, London (1855).

279   William Osler, "On Six Cases of Addison's Disease with the report of a case greatly benefited by the use of the suprarenal cortical extract," *Proceedings of the Johns Hopkins Medical Society, Hopkins Hospital Bulletin,* 7:208-209 (1896).

280   F.A. Hartman and K.A. Brownell, "The hormone of the adrenal cortex," *Proceedings of the Society for Experimental Biology and Medicine* 27:938 (1930).

281   GW Thorn, HR Garbut, FA Hitchcock, FA Hartman, "The effect of cortin upon the renal excretion of sodium, potassium, chloride, inorganic phosphorus and total nitrogen in normal subjects and in patients with Addison's disease," *Endocrinology,* 21:202-212 (1937)

282   T Reichstein, J von Euw, "Euber Bestandteile der Nebennierenrinde: Isolierung der Substanzen Q (desoxycorticosterone) und R sowie weitere Stoffe," *Helvetius Chim Acta* 21:1197-1210 (1938).

283   George W. Thorn, "The Adrenal Cortex," The 1967 Thayer Lectures, *The Johns Hopkins Medical Journal* 123:49-77 (1968).

284   M. Vialli and V. Erpsamer, "Cellule enterocromoffine e cellule basogranulose acidofile nei vertebrati Zischr," *Zellforsch U. Mikr. Anat.* 19:743 (1933).

285   M. Rapport, A. Green and I.H. Page , "Purification of the Substance Which is Responsible for Vasoconstrictor Activity of Serum," *Federation Proceedings* 6:184 (1949).

286   Harvey Cushing, "The hypophysis cerebri: clinical aspects of hyperpituitarism and hypopituitarism." (Oration on Surgery, given to the Section on Surgery of the American Medical Association held in Atlantic City in June, 1909) , *JAMA* 53:249-55 (1909).

287   JE Collip, E Anderson, DL Thompson, "The adrenotropic hormone of the anterior pituitary," *Lancet* II, 347-50 (1933).

288   George W. Thorn, F.T.G. Prunty and P.H. Forsham, "Clinical studies on the effects of pituitary adrenocorticotrophic hormone," *Transactions of the Association of American Physicians* 60:143 (1946).

289   Jules Bauer, "The so-called Cushing's syndrome, its history, terminology and differential diagnosis," *Acta Medica Scandanavia*, 137:412-416 (1950).

290   JM Charcot and A Joffroy, "Cas de paralysie infantile spinale avec lesions des cornes anteriores de la substance grise de la moelle epiniere," *Archive of Physiologie and Normal Pathology,* Paris 3:134 (1870).

291   AG Gilliam, "Epidemiological study of an epidemic diagnosed as poliomyelitis occurring among the personnel of the Los Angeles County General Hospital during the summer 1934," *Public Health Bulletin* (Washington) no. 240, pp 1-90 (1938).

292   M Brodie and WH park, "Active immunization against poliomyelitis," *New York State Journal of Medicine,* 35:815 (1935) and *JAMA* 105:10 (1935).

293   JA Kohlmer, "Susceptibility and immunity in relation to vaccination in acute anterior poliomyelitis," *JAMA* 105:1956-62 (1935).

294   JP Leake, "Poliomyelitis following vaccination against this disease," *JAMA* 105:2152 (1935).

295   AB Sabin and PK Olitsky, "Cultivation of poliovirus in vitro in human embryonic nervous tissue," *Proceedings of the Society for Experimental Biology and Medicine,*(N.Y.), 34:357-59 (1936).

296   Farbu E, Gilhus NE., "Former poliomyelitis as a health and socioeconomic factor. A paired sibling study," *Journal of Neurology.* Apr;249(4):404-9 (2002).

297   Tam SL, Archibald V, Tyreman N, Gordon T., "Effect of exercise on stability of chronically enlarged motor units," *Muscle Nerve.* Mar;25(3):359-69(2002).

298   JF Enders, TH Weller,and FC Robbins, "Cultivation of the Lansing strain of poliomyelitis virus in cultures of various human embryonic tissue," *Science* 109:85 (1949).

299   *New York Times*, page 1, (January 19, 2003).

300   Charles Huggins and Philip Johnson Clark, "Quantitative Studies of Prostatic Secretion. The effect of castration and of estrogen injection on the normal and on the hyperplastic prostate glands of dogs," *Journal of Experimental Medicine* 72:747-762 (1940).

301   A.T. White, "The Question of Castration for Enlarged Prostate," *Annals of Surgery* 24:265 (1893).

302   Charles Huggins, R.L. Stevens Jr. and Clarence V. Hodges, "Studies on Prostate Cancer. II The Effects of Castration on Advanced Carcinoma of the Prostate Gland," *Archives of Surgery* 43:209-223 (1941).

303   Charles Huggins, "Effect of Orchiectomy and Irradiation on Cancer of the Prostate," *Annals of Surgery* 115: 1192-1200 (1942).

304   Myron Karon MD, "A Strategy for Further Advances in Treatment for Childhood Leukemia," *Cancer Chemotherapy* , pp 191- 201 (1975).

305   Denis P Burkitt, "Sarcoma involving jaws in African Children," *British Journal of Surgery* 46:218-223 (1958-59).

306   Denis P Burkitt, "Related Disease- Related Cause?" *Lancet* ii:1229-1231 (1969).

307   Denis P Burkitt, "The Aetiology of Appendicitis," *British Journal of Surgery*

58:695-699 (1971).

308 JM Hinton, JE Lennard-Jones and AC Young, "A new method for studying gut transit times using radiopaque markers," *Gut* 10:842-847 (1969).

309 The Law of LaPlace reads, Tension in the wall = Pressure X Radius of the wall. This is the law that governs the behavior of soap bubbles, balloons, aneurysms and other hollow structures that contain gas or fluid under pressure. The higher the pressure, the greater the radius and the structure tends to expand as it increases in size. In a small colon, with small volume contents, the pressure can rise quite high.

310 J Simpson, JH Scholefield, RC Spiller, "Pathogenesis of colonic diverticula," *British Journal of Surgery* 89(5):546-54 (2002).

311 Joseph A, Ackerman D, Talley JD, Johnstone J, Kupersmith J, "Manifestations of coronary atherosclerosis in young trauma victims--an autopsy study," *Journal of the American College of Cardiology* 22(2):459-67 (1993).

312 JW Gofman, et al. "The role of Lipids and Lipoproteins in Atherosclerosis," *Science* 3:167 (1950).

313 LW Kinsell, et al. "Dietary Modification of Serum Cholesterol and Phospholipid Levels," *Journal of Clinical Endocriniology,* 12:909 (1952).

314 EH Ahrens Jr, David H Blankenhorn and TT Tsaltes, "Effect on Serum Lipids of Substituting Plant for Animal Fat in Diet," *Proceedings of the Society for Experimental Biology and Medicine* 86:872 (1952).

315 Robert C Atkins, *Dr. Atkins Diet Revolution,* David McKay (1972).

316 E.L. Wynder and Evarts Graham,"Tobacco smoking as a possible etiologic factor in bronchogenic carcinoma," *Journal of the American Medical Association*, 143:329 (1950).

317 Richard Doll and A. Bradford Hill, "Smoking and Carcinoma of the Lung," *British Medical Journal,* p 739-748 (Sept 30,1950).

318 Anderson AE Jr, Hernandez JA, Holmes WL, Foraker AG., "Pulmonary emphysema. Prevalence, severity, and anatomical patterns in macrosections, with respect to smoking habits," *Archives of Environmental Health.* May;12(5):569-77. (1966).

319 Stephan Gloyne and W. Burton Wood, "Pulmonary Asbestosis," *Lancet* ii 1383-5 (1934).

320 Richard Doll, "Mortality from lung cancer among asbestos workers," *British Journal of Industrial Medicine* 12:81-86 (1955).

321 Chris Beckett, "An epidemiologist at work:The personal papers of Sir Richard Doll," *Medical History* 46:403-421 (2002).

322 Mary Breckinridge, *Wide Neighborhoods: A story of the Frontier Nursing Service,* New York (1952).

323 Michael Gottlieb, et al., "Pneumocystis pneumonia – Los Angeles," *Morbidity Mortality Weekly Report*, July 3:30 (25) (1981).

324 A. Friedman-Kien, et al. "Kaposi's Sarcoma and Pneumocystis Pneumonia among homosexual men: New York City and California," *MMWR*, 30:305 308 (1981).

325 NJ Ehrenkranz, et al. "Pneumocystis carinii Pneumonia among Persons with Hemophilia A," *MMWR* 31:365-367 (1982).

326 SH Landesman and J Vieira, "Acquired Immune Deficiency Syndrome (AIDS), A Review," *Archives of Internal Medicine*, 143:2307-9 (1983).

327 A Ammann, et al. "Possible Transfusion-associated Acquired Immune Deficiency Syndrome (AIDS)- California," *MMWR* 31:652-654 (1982).

328   R O'Reilly, et al., "Unexplained Immunodeficiency and Opportunistic Infections in Infants – New York, New Jersey, California," *MMWR* 31:665-667 (1982).

329   Peyton Rous, "A transmissible avian neoplasm: sarcoma of the common fowl," *Journal of Experimental Medicine* 12:696 (1910).

330   Howard M Temin, "The effects of Actinomycin D on growth of the Rous Sarcoma Virus in vitro," *Virology* 20:577 (1963).

331   David Baltimore, "Viral-RNA dependent DNA polymerase," *Nature* 226:1209 (June 27, 1970).

       Howard M Temin and Satoshi Mizutani, "RNA-dependent DNA polymerase in virions of the Rous Sarcoma Virus," *Nature* 226:1211 (June 27, 1970).

332   Robert C Gallo, et al, "RNA dependent DNA polymerase of human acute leukemia cells," *Nature* 229:927 (1970).

333   Ramos A, Hu DJ, Nguyen L, Phan KO, Vanichseni S, Promadej N, Choopanya K, Callahan M, Young NL, McNicholl J, Mastro TD, Folks TM, Subbarao S., "Intersubtype human immunodeficiency virus type 1 superinfection following seroconversion to primary infection in two injection drug users," *Journal of Virology* 76(15):7444-52 (2002).

334   John Crewdson, *Science Fictions*, Little, Brown and Company (2002).

335   Berry, N. et al. "Analysis of oral polio vaccine CHAT stocks," Nature 410, 1046-1047 (2001). Blancou, P. et al. "Polio vaccine samples not linked to AIDS," *Nature* 410, 1045-1046 (2001).

336   A. Grollman, *The Cardiac Output in Man in Health and Disease*, Charles C. Thomas (1932).

337   Carleton B Chapman and Jere H Mitchell, *Starling on the Heart*, published by Dawsons of Pall Mall (1965).

338   SW Patterson, H Piper, EH Starling, "The Regulation of the Heart Beat," *Journal of Physiology* (London) 48: 465 (1914).

339   MF O'Rourke, "Starling's law of the Heart: an appraisal 70 years on," *Australian New Zealand Journal of Medicine* , 14:879-87 (1984).

340   W. Einthoven, "The Different Forms of the Human Electrocardiogram and Their Significance," *Lancet* i:853 (1912).

341   James B Herrick, "Clinical Features of Sudden Obstruction of the Coronary Arteries,", *JAMA* 59: 2015 (1912).

342   G. Bousfield, "Angina Pectoris," *Lancet* ii:457 (1918).

343   Samuel A. Levine, "Willem Einthoven: Some historical Notes on the Occasion of the Centenery Celebration of His Birth," *American Heart Journal*, 61:422 (1961).

344   FN Wilson, "The Distributions of the Potential Differences Produced by the Heart Beat within the Body and at Its Surface," *American Heart Journal* , 5:599 (1930).

345   Frederick Wenckebach, *Lancet*, ii: 633. (1937).

346   K.F. Wenckebach, "Zur Quoted in Analyse des unregelmässigen Pulses," *Zeitschrift für klinische Medizin* 36:181-199 (1899).

347   John Hay, "Bradycardia and cardiac arrhythmia produced by depression of certain functions of the heart," *Lancet* i:139-143 (1906).

348   Woldemar Mobitz, "Über die unvollständige Störung der Erregung-süberleitung zweischen Vorhof und Kammer des menschlichen Herzens," *Zeitschrift für die Gesamte Experimentelle Medizin,* Berlin 41:180-237 (1924).

349   Giovanni Morgagni, *De sedibus et causis morborum per anatomen indagatis(On the Seats and Causes of Diseases, Investigated by Anatomy)* (1769).

350 Robert Adams, *Cases of Diseases of the Heart, Accompanied with Pathological Observations*. (1827).

351 William Stokes, *The Diseases of the Heart and Aorta*, Dublin, Hodges & Smith, Philadelphia (1854).

352 Allen B.Weisse, *Heart to Heart*, Rutgers University Press, page 8. (2003).

353 Claude Beck and Fredrick Mautz, "The Control of the Heart Beat by the Surgeon," *Annals of Surgery*, 106:532-33 (1937).

354 WB Kouwenhoven, JR Jude, GG Knickerbocker, "Closed chest cardiac massage," *JAMA* 173: 1064 (1960).

355 S Hyman, "Resuscitation of the stopped heart by intracardiac therapy," *Archives of Internal Medicine*, 50:283 (1932).

356 William Chardack, "Heart Block Treated with an Implantable Pacemaker," *Progress in Cardiovascular Diseases*, 6:507-537 (1964).

357 DA Nathan, S Center, Wu Chang-You and W Keller, "An implantable synchronous cardiac pacemaker," *Circulation* 27:682 (1963).

358 Translation by TH Lewis, "Clinical Sphygmomanometry," *Bulletin of the New York Academy of Medicine,* 17:871 (1941).

359 William Dock, "Korotkoff's Sounds," *NEJM* 302:1264-1267 (1980).

360 Walter Cannon and D de la Paz, "Emotional Stimulation of Adrenal Secretion," *American Journal of Physiology* 28:64 (1911).

361 Richard Bright "Cases and Observations Illustrative of Renal Disease Accompanied with the Secretion of Albuminous Urine," *Guy's Hospital Report*, London I:338 (1836).

362 FA Mahomed, "On Chronic Bright's Disease, and its essential symptoms," *Lancet* i:46 (1879).

363 R Tigerstedt and Bergman, "Niere und Kreislauf," *Skandinavia. Archiv fur. Physiologie*, 8:223 (1898).

364 H. Goldblatt "The renal origin of hypertension," *Physiology Review*, 27:120 (1947).

365 EM Landis, H Montgomery, D Sparkman, "The effects of pressor drugs and of saline kidney extracts on blood pressure and skin temperature," *Journal of Clinical Investigation,* 17:189 (1938).

366 JN Langley and WL Dickenson, *Proceedings of the Royal Society*, Series B, 46:423 (1889).

367 G. Kolata, "Johns Hopkins death brings halt to U.S.-financed human studies," *NY Times (Print)*. Jul 20:A1, A18. (2001).

368 P. Saxl and R. Heilig, "Über die diuretische Wirkung von Novasurol und anderen Quecksilberpraparaten, *Wien klinik Wchnschr* 33:943 (1920).

369 Allan B. Weisse, *Heart to Heart*, Oral history of William Dock who was present at Wenckeback's clinic in Vienna when the mercurial diuretics were discovered, pages 7 to 9, Rutgers University Press (2003).

370 H.J. Doin, "Biological Research in the Pharmaceutical Industry with Reserpine," in F.J. Ayd and B. Blackwell, ed., *Discoveries in Biological Psychiatry*, Lipincott pages 142-152 (1970).

371 R.N. Chopra, *Indigenous drugs of India*, Art Press, Calcutta (1933).

372 N.S. Kline, "Use of *Rawolfia serpentina benth* in neuropsychiatric conditions," *Annals of the New York Academy of Sciences* 59:107-114 (1954).

373 G. Sen and K.C. Bose, "*Rawolfia serpentine*, a new Indian drug for insanity and

high blood pressure," *Indian Medical World* 2:194 (1931).

374   R.J. Vail, "A clinical trial of *Rawolfia serpentine* in essential hypertension," *British Heart Journal* 11:350-355 (1949).

375   Robert Maxwell, "Guanethidine after twenty years: a pharmacologist's perspective," *British Journal of Pharmacology,* 13:35-44 (1982).

376   JW Black and JS Stephenson, "Pharmacology of a new beta-adrenergic receptor blocking compound," Lancet ii:311-14 (1962).

377   Max Wilhelm and George DeStevens, *"Antihypertensive Agents,"* *Drug Research,* 20:197-259 (1976).

378   TL Sourkes, "Inhibition of Dihydroxyphenylalanine Decarboxylase by Derivatives of Phenylalanine," *Archives of Biochemistry and Biophysics,* 51:444 (1954).

379   ER Long, "Development of our knowledge of arteriosclerosis," in *Cowdry's Arteriosclerosis,* Ed. Blumenthal (1967).

380   R. Quain, "On fatty diseases of the heart," *Medical Chirurgical Transactions,* 33:120 (1850).

381   JB Herrick, "Certain clinical features of sudden obstruction of the coronary arteries," *Transactions of the Association of American Physicians,* 27:100 (1912).

382   AM Master ,R Freidman, S Dack, "The electrocardiogram after standard exercise as a functional test of the heart," *American Heart Journal,* 24: 777-93 (1942).

383   P Wood, M McGregor, O Magidson, W Whittaker, "Effort test in angina pectoris," *British Heart Journal,* 12:363 (1958).

384   Described by Andre Cournand in "Cardiac Catheterization," *Acta Medica Scandinavia Supplement* p 579 (1975).

385   W Forssmann, "Die Sondierung des Rechten Herzens," *Klinica Wochnschraft,* 8:2085 (1929).

386   A Cournand and HA Ranges, "Catheterization of the right auricle in man," *Proceedings of the Society for Experimental Biology,* 46:462 (1941).

387   Dickenson W Richards, Andre Cournand Robert C Darling, and William Gillespie, "Pressure in the Right Auricle of Man, in Normal Subjects and in Patients With Congestive Heart Failure," *Transactions of the Association of American Physiologists,* 56:218-21 (1941).

388   JS Lehman, RA Boyer, and FS Winter, "Coronary Arteriography," *American Journal of Roentgenology,* 81:749 (1959).

389   Sones, "Cinecardioangiography," *Clinical Cardio-pulmonary Physiology,* Second Edition, New York, Grune and Stratton, (1960).

19

Cardiac Surgery

THE FIRST OPERATIONS ON THE HEART, AS MIGHT BE EXPECTED, WERE TO repair injuries and the first success was by Rehn, of Frankfurt, in 1896.[390] More cases followed and, ten years later, a forty percent success rate was reported. The First World War provided the opportunity for many surgeons to gain experience in the treatment of cardiac injuries. A few reported successful removal of intracardiac missiles but infection was a major barrier to patient survival in those cases. Bullet emboli from cardiac wounds were also observed. An embolus, is an object (usually a blood clot) which is carried along in the flow of blood much as a stick is carried along by flowing water in a stream. The embolus moves with the flow of blood so long as the vessel diameter is larger than the diameter of the object. Arteries, however, grow progressively smaller as branches are given off. Eventually the artery is smaller than the embolus and it lodges like a cork in a bottle. The obstruction of the artery by the embolus may cause severe consequences, such as a stroke if the affected artery is in the brain.

Osler recognized constrictive pericarditis and described the typical findings. The pericardium surrounding the heart is diseased and compresses it, interfering with filling between heartbeats. He recommended aspiration of large pericardial effusions (fluid collections in the pericardial sac) that were compromising cardiac function, but he had no recommendation for the constrictive version where the membrane itself is doing the compressing. An effusion is usually sterile and caused by diseases like lupus erythematosus (The "red wolf," an autoimmune disease) or cancer. The constrictive version does not involve fluid, but the membrane, itself, shrinks and compresses the heart. The cause may be tuberculosis, common in 1900, cancer or autoimmune disease. In 1907, Henle attempted to treat the condition surgically, but failed. Ludwig Rehn, who had successfully repaired a cardiac wound, attacked the problem of constrictive pericarditis in 1913. In 1920, he set down the basic principles of surgical therapy (removal of enough of the pericardium to release the heart from its restriction) and described his own series of four cases treated successfully. In

1929, Edward D Churchill performed the first pericardial resection for constriction in the United States.

RHEUMATIC FEVER

Rheumatic fever was a feared disease of children until modern times brought the introduction of penicillin. Group A streptococcus infection, usually pharyngitis, is the cause through an immune reaction affecting the heart valves. There has been considerable research on the reason for the heart valve damage and there seems to be a cross reaction between the bacterial wall carbohydrates and glycoproteins (proteins with a carbohydrate molecule attached) of the valve. The most severe cardiac injury is mitral stenosis, where the mitral valve leaflets fuse at the commissures (the cleft between the valve leaflets) leaving a small slit opening between atrium and ventricle. In 1902, Sir Lauder Brunton wrote, "Mitral stenosis is not only one of the most distressing forms of cardiac disease, but in its severe forms it resists all treatment by medicine. On looking at the contracted mitral orifice in a severe case of this disease one is impressed by the hopelessness of ever finding a remedy which will enable the auricle to drive the blood in sufficient stream through the small mitral orifice, and the wish unconsciously arises that one could divide the constriction as easily in life as one can after death." He spent some time in the laboratory practicing a procedure to open the fused commissures and, in February 1902, proposed the operation in the *Lancet*.[391]

A controversy ensued and an editorial condemned his proposal. Some of the criticism was due to a misunderstanding of the defect in mitral stenosis; it was thought to be due to a weak heart, not mechanical obstruction. It would be another twenty-five years before anyone dared to approach the mitral valve.

Lockwood reported on the history of cardiac and pericardial surgery to date in the 1929 *Archives of Surgery*.[392] In the same issue of Archives, Cutler and Beck reported their attempts, and those of others, at correction of valvular stenosis.[393] In the first reported case, by Doyen in 1913, an attempt to relieve pulmonary valve stenosis by use of a valvutome (a cutting device inserted into the valve opening) was unsuccessful and the patient died.

Tuffier, also in 1913, reported a finger dilatation of a stenotic aortic valve performed by invaginating the aortic wall to dilate the valve. This was successful, and the patient was reported to be alive four years later in a subsequent report.

Cutler and Beck attempted seven operations for mitral stenosis, all of which proved fatal. They did describe one success, by Souttar in 1925, in which the procedure was insertion of the finger through the atrial appendage (an ear shaped flap of atrium) and dilatation of the valve with the finger only.[394] The patient was a young girl and Souttar had planned to use a valvutome but, because the valve was soft, he used only his finger. She recovered and reported only slight breathlessness with exertion three months later. Sadly, his lead was not followed up and mitral valve surgery waited another twenty years after Beck and Cutler to resume progress. Beck and Cutler, in planning their approach to the mitral valve, had studied hearts fixed in formaldehyde. The fixed (embalmed) mitral valve was stiff and the leaflets could not be pried apart with finger pressure in these specimens. Beck and Cutler, therefore, devised a valvutome to cut these leathery leaflets and that addition to the procedure brought the failure of their attempts. Cutting the leaflet blindly, as they did, resulted in mitral insufficiency and the patients succumbed to pneumonia and heart failure. The cardiac valves resemble small half parachutes; tearing the parachute canopy results in failure and a massive leak back through the valve. In one of their cases they could not locate the valve and closed without any relief of the stenosis; she also died. They did report one temporary success, in 1923. An eleven-year-old girl had resection of part of the mitral valve using the cardiovalvutome. She recovered from the operation and their report a month later stirred worldwide hope that a treatment of severe mitral stenosis was at hand. She did not have complete relief of the stenosis, however, and died of the disease four years later. Souttar had the only successful result before 1948, and he had not used the valvutome. His patient subsequently died (five years later) of a cerebral embolus, for which there was no treatment at the time. Patients with abnormal mitral valves had dilated left atrial chambers, frequently resulting in spontaneous clotting in the atrium. These clots could break loose at any time with disastrous consequences. Anticoagulant drugs, when they came along, reduced this risk.

CONGENITAL HEART DISEASE

The discovery of anticoagulant drugs made the next developments possible. Heparin, in particular, allowed direct surgical approaches to cardiac and vascular disease (See chapter 15). Congenital heart defects were the first to yield to the progress in cardiac surgery and the first successes were with extra-cardiac lesions that did not require stopping the heart or opening a cardiac chamber. The ductus arteriosus connects the left pulmonary artery with the aorta and is open in fetal life as a bypass, carrying oxygenated blood from the placenta around the non-functional lungs.

It closes soon after birth when arterial oxygen saturation rises and pulmonary artery flow resistance drops. In 1907, John Munro, chief surgeon at the Boston City Hospital proposed correction for those cases in which the ductus remains open after birth. In fetal life the flow is from pulmonary artery to aorta because the pulmonary resistance is higher than systemic resistance (the lungs are not inflated yet). If the ductus does not close at birth, the flow reverses and constitutes a short circuit flooding the pulmonary circulation, now a low resistance, low-pressure system, with a high volume of blood from the aorta. Simply ligating the ductus stops the short circuit and corrects the defect.

Munro practiced a technique for ligation on cadavers and presented his work to the Philadelphia Academy of Surgery but never succeeded in making the diagnosis on a live patient.[395] In 1936, Maude Abbot published an atlas of congenital heart defects and described ninety-two patients who had died of patent ductus arteriosus. Some of the patients had died of bacterial endocarditis, secondary to local injury to the aortic or pulmonary artery lining by the "jet effect" of a small ductus acting like a nozzle on blood flow through the abnormal channel. The flow jet damaged the lining of the pulmonary artery resulting in infection at the site of injury. The first attempt at correction was by John Strieder who divided a patent ductus in a young woman with bacterial endocarditis on March 6, 1937. She survived the operation but died on the fourth postop day. At autopsy, bacterial vegetations were found, filling the pulmonary artery from the ductus to the pulmonary valve, and Strieder gave up the procedure.

At Children's Hospital in Boston Robert Gross, unaware of Strieder's work in the same city, was developing a technique for closure of the ductus in children. Closing the defect early would avoid the problem of bacterial endocarditis (actually, endarteritis but the other term is usually used). On August 17, 1938, Gross performed the first successful correction of a congenital heart defect.[396] Children were less likely to have developed bacterial endocarditis and it has been a principle ever since Gross' operation to close the ductus in childhood, even in the absence of symptoms, to avoid that devastating complication. Willis Potts, a pediatric surgeon in Chicago, improved the procedure by developing the first vascular clamp.[397] This allowed complete division of the ductus, a very short structure, with almost no risk of a clamp slipping off the stump before the sutures were tied. The clamp had teeth to prevent slipping and yet did not crush the tissue avoiding the risk of sloughing of the stump and delayed hemorrhage.

Coarctation of the aorta, a narrowing of the vessel just distal to (below) the location of the ductus was the next lesion to be corrected. Coarctation severely narrows the aorta, resulting in hypertension above the constriction and poor circulation below. Endocarditis is also a complication of this lesion and the cause is the same, a jet effect damaging the lining of the aorta below the narrow segment. The problem with the repair was, and still is, the fact that the blood supply to the spinal cord comes off the aorta below the constriction. Clamping the aorta, while the narrow segment is repaired, risks paraplegia. Clagett, at the Mayo Clinic performed the first successful correction in the U.S., in 1947. Clarence Crafoord, a famous Swedish surgeon, had successfully repaired coarctation in two patients in 1944.[398]

BLUE BABIES AND THE BLALOCK-TAUSSIG OPERATION

Fallot described the most common "blue baby" heart defect, tetralogy of Fallot, in 1888. A patient with the tetralogy has a ventricular septal defect, plus stenosis of the pulmonary artery so that flow is from right to left, instead of left to right, as in a simple ventricular septal defect. The normal right ventricular pressure is much lower than that in the left but the pulmonary stenosis causes right ventricular hypertrophy (the third component of the four). The fourth defect is an overriding aorta which is more to the right (displacing and narrowing the pulmonary artery origin) than normal and which overrides the ventricular septal defect. The children are blue from birth and have poor pulmonary flow causing very poor exercise tolerance. The blue color is produced by mixing venous blood, which is darker because of non-oxygenated hemoglobin (a darker red than when oxygenated), with arterial blood. Cyanosis, the blue color, can be produced by other diseases associated with low oxygen concentrations in arterial blood. Few blue babies reach adulthood without at least partial correction.

In 1930 Helen Taussig, a Johns Hopkins cardiologist, was placed in charge of the children's cardiac clinic. By 1935, she had become interested in surgical correction of congenital heart disease. She saw children with tetralogy and noticed that, on fluoroscopy of the chest, the pulmonary arteries were small. She sought ways to prevent the closing of the ductus in these cases but was unsuccessful. Next, she began to discuss the possibility of creating an artificial ductus to augment pulmonary blood flow. She spoke to Robert Gross about it, but he was not interested. He is reported to have told her, "Madame, I close off patent ductuses, not create them."[399] Alfred Blalock became chief of surgery at Johns Hopkins in 1940 and, unlike his immediate predecessors, he was already interested in cardiac surgery. He had experimented with connecting the left subclavian artery to the pulmonary artery in an attempt to produce pulmonary hypertension in dogs.

In 1930, while at Vanderbilt University Medical School, Blalock hired a young black man as his laboratory technician. Vivien Thomas had been forced to drop out of college for financial reasons and took the Vanderbilt job in January 1930, as the Depression deepened. Blalock began to teach Thomas how to perform surgical procedures on dogs as the professor became too busy to do all the work himself. Thomas also learned to perform laboratory tests and became Blalock's assistant in all his research work. When Blalock moved to Baltimore in 1940, Thomas came with him and became the supervisor of the Johns Hopkins surgical research laboratories. Thomas and resident William Longmire (later to be chief of surgery at UCLA) worked on the operation that was to be used in 1944 on "blue babies." They devised the clamp, known as the "Blalock clamp," that became one of the first vascular clamps. The dogs tolerated the procedure well and did not develop pulmonary hypertension. When Helen Taussig came to Blalock, the idea was already there.

Blalock performed the first operation for tetralogy of Fallot on November 29, 1944. Vivien Thomas stood directly behind him and pointed out technical details from his own experience in the research lab. The patient was a fifteen-month-old girl who was severely cyanotic and weighed only ten pounds. The operation connected the left subclavian artery to the left pulmonary artery. The child had a difficult postop course but recovered, gained weight and was discharged two months later. Her improvement was temporary and another shunt six months later was unsuccessful. The second patient was an eleven-year-old girl who could not walk more than thirty feet. Her operation was more complex because she had a right sided aortic arch, not unusual in tetralogy, and the shunt was performed with the right subclavian artery. She recovered well and her exercise tolerance was much improved three weeks later. The third case had the best result and that child, six years old and bedridden preop, had an excellent recovery. In May 1945, Blalock and Taussig presented their landmark paper to an immense response.[400] The operation did not cure the defect but these children had been condemned to a short and miserable life before this advance. Ten years later, total correction became possible with cross circulation, then total bypass. The barrier had been broken.

Vivien Thomas continued as supervisor of the surgical research laboratories at Johns Hopkins even after the retirement of Dr. Blalock in 1964. In 1976, Thomas was appointed Instructor in Surgery at Johns Hopkins School of Medicine and at his retirement in 1979 he was named emeritus Instructor in Surgery. In 1976, Thomas was honored by the university with a degree as Doctor of Laws by Johns Hopkins University.

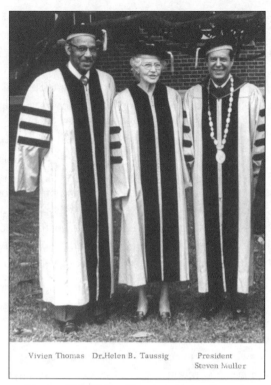

Vivien Thomas Dr.Helen B. Taussig President
Steven Muller

*Figure 12 – Vivien Thomas, Helen Taussig
and University President.*

MITRAL STENOSIS

After World War Two, progress on mitral stenosis resumed. It had been nearly twenty years since Beck and Cutler presented their grim report on attempts to relieve this fatal consequence of rheumatic fever. When I was a child, a family friend (the daughter of an orthopedic surgeon) developed rheumatic fever at the age of six (about 1943) and spent two years at bed rest in La Rabida Sanitarium in Chicago. The treatment, the only one available at the time, was successful and she did not develop the heart disease. In the intervening years, attempts had been made to relieve the pulmonary venous hypertension of mitral stenosis indirectly, by connecting the pulmonary veins to the azygous vein (which drains to the right atrium), but this worsened the low cardiac output by reducing flow through the stenotic mitral valve.

In 1948, Charles P Bailey reported the first successful surgery for mitral stenosis since Souttar.[401] He had studied fresh hearts with mitral stenosis and concluded that it would be possible to either stretch or cut the fusion of the cusps at the commissures to avoid mitral insufficiency afterward. He had proven in the dog lab that mitral insufficiency was not tolerated and, had the Brigham group anticipated his experiments in 1920, a different approach might have been tried. His first attempt in humans, in 1945, was unsuccessful and the patient died on the operating table. His next attempt, in 1946, was on a woman in very poor condition. He could not find the mitral orifice with the valvutome and was obliged to insert his finger to find and dilate the valve. This seemed to be successful and he did not use the cutting instrument. She improved, but died after two days. At autopsy, the valve commissures were torn open but not far enough and the stenosis was only partially relieved. He concluded that thrombus formation at the site of tearing had restricted the opening and decided to use heparin with the next case. The next case, however, died because of postop bleeding (heparin had been used to avoid clotting postop) and excessive fluid administration. The mitral valve at autopsy was still not completely opened.

The next case, on June 10, 1948, also died although the patient's heart had stopped before valvotomy was attempted. During attempts at resuscitation, he dilated the valve with a finger but the heart could not be restarted. Later the same day the first successful commissurotomy was performed on a twenty-four-year-old housewife. A small knife, retracted into a sheath along the surgeon's index finger, was advanced into the left atrial appendage and used to cut the commissure. The patient recovered and had an excellent result. There is a story, which Dr. Bailey confirms, that he had been told no more mitral valve surgeries would be permitted in Philadelphia hospitals because of the series of intra- and postoperative deaths.[402] He scheduled the last two cases on the same day and, after the first patient died on the table at Philadelphia General Hospital, took a taxicab to Episcopal Hospital and, without mentioning the earlier case, performed his second mitral valve surgery of the day. That case was successful and the operation was judged acceptable after all.

Ten days later, he presented the results of his last case to the American College of Chest Physicians in Chicago. His patient was present at the meeting, having traveled to Chicago with Bailey. By early 1949, he had performed another five mitral commissurotomies with two survivors and a third, who survived for two months postop. One patient had a successful mitral commissurotomy but died on the sixth postop day of a cerebral embolus, a hazard of left heart surgery. Dwight Harken, in Boston, performed a partial excision of a mitral leaflet and released the commissures in a successful operation four days before Bailey presented his results. The same year, Lord Brock performed a finger dilatation of a stenotic mitral valve with a good result. All three of them had been working on parallel paths. Soon the operation was being performed in most countries but the problem of mitral regurgitation could not be addressed until a heart-lung machine had been developed.

The surgeon who discussed Dr. Bailey's report at the College of Chest Physicians meeting was Horace Smithy. Dr. Smithy was a thoracic surgeon in Charleston, South Carolina who had actually performed eight mitral valve surgeries himself with five survivors. He used the method of Cutler and Beck but immediately adopted the Bailey finger-fracture technique. Dr. Smithy was driven to develop cardiac surgery because he, himself, suffered from aortic stenosis. After the meeting he had Dr. Bailey listen to his chest, and they agreed that, without a heart-lung machine, there was nothing that could be done. Dr. Smithy had already asked Alfred Blalock to attempt a repair but Blalock was not willing to attempt what he considered a hopeless task on a colleague. Subsequently, Dr. Smithy brought an aortic stenosis patient to Johns Hopkins, where he and Dr. Blalock attempted to perform a closed aortic valvotomy using the Cutler instrument. The patient died on the table. Blalock did not make any further attempts and Dr. Smithy died of his aortic stenosis on October 28, 1948, four months after discussing Bailey's case. He was thirty-four years old.[403] His family endowed a chair in cardiac surgery at Medical University of South Carolina.

THE HEART-LUNG MACHINE

Preservation of life while the heart is stopped has taken two paths in medical research. It was known very early that the brain will die when deprived of circulation for a few minutes. George Crile's work eventually determined how long the brain could survive without circulation. One path in research was to find a mechanical means of continuing the circulation while the heart is stopped. In 1885, Frey and Gruber devised a crude system to accomplish this. They oxygenated blood by having it flow over a rotating cylinder in an atmosphere of oxygen gas. A ten c.c. syringe with two one-way valves pumped the blood and the apparatus was driven by an electric motor. In 1920 the aviator, Charles Lindberg, working with Alexis Carrel, devised a system for oxygenating perfusion fluid (not yet blood) to keep organs alive.[404] In 1995, Jacobi used an excised animal lung to oxygenate blood in an *in-vitro* system. Professor S.S. Brukhonenko, a Russian scientist, used Jacobi's approach in 1926 when he and S. Tchetchuline designed a similar machine that used diaphragm pumps to circulate the oxygenated blood. They used their device to perfuse isolated organs, then an entire animal.[405]

In 1931, the eventual developer of the heart-lung machine, John Gibbon, spent a night at the bedside of a patient with massive pulmonary embolism. He was a surgical research fellow and his job was to watch this young woman, who was fifteen days postop from a routine cholecystectomy when she had her embolus, to determine if she was going to die without the desperate attempt to directly remove the embolism. The procedure, known as the "Trendelenberg operation," had never been performed successfully in the United States. Trendelenberg had described his operation in 1908, but most patients died from infection or blood loss prior to 1924 when Professor Kirschner of Koenigsberg, Germany performed the first successful pulmonary embolectomy in which the patient recovered. The operation was reported in the June 7, 1924 issue of *JAMA* Four years later Kirschner's patient was alive and well.

Gibbon sat there for seventeen hours with his young patient, in the operating room (they had moved her bed into the operating room to be ready in an instant if the operation was needed), until her blood pressure became unobtainable and Dr. Churchill began the operation in her bed. The procedure, opening the pulmonary artery and removing the clots, took only six minutes, but she died. I have assisted with a Trendelenberg procedure in a patient's bed with the same outcome. After his fellowship Gibbon moved back to Philadelphia but continued (with almost no encouragement from others) to work on the concept of heart lung bypass. In the fall of 1934, he returned to Boston and was given space in the Massachusetts General Hospital, in the old Bullfinch Building where the Ether Dome is, to work on the idea. The most difficult problem was the oxygenator. It must oxygenate a sufficient volume of blood per minute yet be gentle enough to avoid hemolysis of the red blood cells. Gibbon lacked funds and was forced to improvise. No one thought that he would accomplish anything and the country was in the depths of the Depression. He made his own valves from rubber lab flask corks. The initial machine could oxygenate 500 c.c. of blood per minute, far below human requirements but more than anyone else had accomplished. His wife (a trained lab assistant before they were married) helped him in the lab, and sometimes with his search for stray cats, the subjects of his experiments. His pump was based on the design of Dale and Schuster.[406] Finally, he succeeded in maintaining cats with complete occlusion of the pulmonary artery, the equivalent of the fatal pulmonary embolism suffered by his patient in 1931.

An improved blood pump was designed by Dr Michael DeBakey in 1934, and became the standard pump for heart-lung bypass thereafter.[407] By 1941, Gibbon had developed a machine large enough for dogs, and possibly for man, but his work was interrupted by the war.[408]

When Gibbon returned from the war, the Dean of the medical school, Jefferson Medical College, advised him to contact IBM for engineering help in building a larger and more efficient heart-lung machine.[409] The Endicott Research Laboratory, an IBM facility, had assisted others in basic research projects. Thomas Watson, chairman of the board of IBM, was impressed with Gibbon's ideas and promised help. Subsequently, Gibbon provided the medical concepts and IBM did the engineering work. By 1950, Gibbon had a reliable machine that permitted open-heart surgery in dogs, but the oxygenator was still too small for man.[410] About this time Thomas Stokes and John Flick, surgical residents working with Gibbon improved efficiency of the oxygenator by using a wire screen, instead of a smooth surface, to exposed the blood to oxygen. Next, the solid steel cylinder was replaced by a series of wire mesh screens that exposed both sides to oxygen. They learned to avoid air embolism and their mortality in dogs improved from an early eighty percent to ten percent, still too high for human use. Others were working on the problem, as well, and other designs were being tested in other countries. The oxygenator continued to be an obstacle and some tried to avoid the problem with other approaches.

In December 1950, Clarence Dennis, at the University of Minnesota, used a heart-lung machine in development there to repair a huge atrial septal defect in a young girl. She did not survive the operation. Finally, Gibbon attempted his first case, a fifteen-month-old girl with severe congestive heart failure who was thought to have an atrial septal defect. They opened

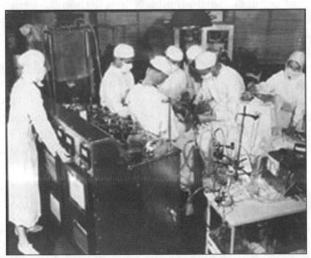

Figure 13 – Gibbon performing open-heart surgery with his heart-lung machine in 1953. His machine is behind him.

her atrium while on heart bypass, but found that there was no atrial defect; the preoperative diagnosis was wrong. She died soon after surgery and a patent ductus arteriosus, a correctable lesion not reachable from their incision, was found at autopsy.

On May 6 1953, Gibbon was ready for another attempt. This was an eighteen-year-old girl with an atrial septal defect. They placed her on bypass and repaired the defect without difficulty. She recovered and, several months later, repeat cardiac catheterization showed the defect closed. Hers was the first successful open heart surgery with total heart bypass. Gibbon performed two more open-heart surgeries in July 1953, but both patients died and Gibbon became discouraged. He had spent nineteen years working on this problem and was tired. He declared a one year moratorium on further efforts.

OPEN HEART SURGERY

C. Walton Lillehei next took up the task in Minnesota. Clarence Dennis had left and taken his heart-lung machine with him. Lillehei was not a cardiac surgeon but he decided to reexamine the fundamental questions of cardiac surgery and heart-lung bypass. He had finished his surgical residency in 1950, only to discover a lump in his neck. A biopsy was positive for cancer and he had radical surgery plus radiation therapy during the next year. Once he recovered, Dr. Wangensteen, the chairman of the department, asked him to take over research on heart-lung bypass. In 1953, Lillehei and several collaborators worked on cross-circulation, a technique to connect two individuals' circulation and the other major path of this research. Others had tried it and eventually they perfected their method in the dog lab.

They decided to use the technique to attempt repair of fatal heart defects in children and infants. The first patient was a one-year-old boy in congestive heart failure from a large ventricular septal defect. The boy's father was the circulation donor for the operation. The operation, on March 26, 1954, went well, but the boy died of pneumonia eleven days later. A month later, they tried again with a four-year-old boy who also had a VSD. They were successful. By August, they had performed open-heart surgeries with six survivors and follow-up cardiac catheter studies confirmed success. On August 31 1954, they performed the first correction of tetralogy of Fallot, again using cross circulation. During the first year, they performed forty-five open-heart operations on severely ill children with two thirds of the patients surviving the surgery; these were incredible results. One donor had severe hypotension and received open chest cardiac massage but recovered.[411] A critic of the technique had commented that it was the only operation he knew with a possible 200% mortality rate. In 1955, Lillehei and the Minnesota team received the Lasker Award; the Nobel Committee was no longer interested in clinical research.

PULMONARY BANDING

There was another approach for small children with ventricular septal defects. These patients go into congestive heart failure because of the volume of flow passing through a large VSD from the left ventricle to the right. In tetralogy of Fallot, the pulmonary stenosis limits the volume passing from left to right because the right ventricular pressure is as high, or higher, than that on the left. In fact, flow reverses because the pulmonary stenosis is so tight. The tetralogy patient has too little pulmonary blood flow and improves with the Blalock-Taussig operation, which increases it. The VSD patient has too much pulmonary flow, because of the low resistance of the pulmonary circuit and goes into heart failure as the short circuit overloads the heart's ability to pump enough volume. In 1951, Muller and Dammann at UCLA, decided to produce an artificial pulmonary stenosis by placing a band around the pulmonary artery just above the valve. Emile Holman and Claude Beck, pioneers in so much of cardiac surgery, had produced artificial stenosis in the animal lab in 1928.[412] In 1951 Hufnagel produced pulmonic stenosis by removing a segment of vessel wall.[413] On July 11, 1951 Muller and Dammann operated on a five-month-old child who was in congestive heart failure with what appeared to be a single ventricle without pulmonary stenosis. They constricted the large pulmonary artery to one-third its size by excising a wedge of the artery using the technique of Hufnagel. The child recovered from the surgery and, six months post-op, was free of heart failure.[414] By 1972, when I was a cardiac surgery resident banding of the pulmonary artery was standard treatment of the small child in heart failure with a VSD. The children did well, although one, operated on at the age of four days, was hospitalized for eighteen months after banding. He survived, returned for repair of the septal defect at the age of five years, and is today a successful businessman.

THE BUBBLE OXYGENATOR

John Kirklin, at Mayo Clinic, resumed work with a mechanical heart-lung machine using Gibbon's model as the starting point. By October 1955, they had sixteen survivors from thirty-six operations, all severely ill patients with end-stage heart defects. At Minnesota Richard DeWall began working on a bubble oxygenator, a concept that had been experimented with for years but one with a major problem of gas embolism. Bubbling oxygen gas through the blood was efficient if the problems with gas embolism could be overcome. By 1955, they had solved the problems and the machine was used in seven children with congenital heart disease. All the surgeries were successful and the device quickly became the standard, especially after a disposable version was developed.

ARTIFICIAL VALVES

In the years before heart-lung bypass became possible, mitral commissurotomy was the only procedure available for cardiac valve disease. When I was a third year medical student one of my first patients was a young girl admitted to the hospital with rheumatic heart disease. She was about twenty-three and had been through two mitral valve surgeries since the age of fifteen. The first had been a commissurotomy that left her with severe mitral regurgitation from a tear in a valve leaflet. The second operation, after the development of open-heart surgery in the late 1950s, was an attempt at repair of the mitral valve, which failed. She had wide-open mitral regurgitation with an enormous heart and poorly compensated congestive heart failure. My mother's brother Joe had died of the same condition in 1926, at a time when surgery was not an option. This was the fall of 1964 and, one year later, Albert Starr reported his first series of mitral valve replacements with a new artificial valve. Unfortunately, my patient had traveled from her home in the Midwest to California to visit relatives. The relatives, out of ignorance or carelessness, had not maintained her salt-free diet. Her heart failure decompensated and she was admitted to the hospital where an allergic reaction to a mercurial diuretic, all we had in those days, killed her.

The first attempt at valve replacement actually preceded the development of the heart-lung machine. In the 1940s, Charles Hufnagel, then a surgical resident at the Peter Bent Brigham Hospital in Boston, began to study the problem of transplantation of kidneys. The kidneys were rejected, a story to be told in another chapter, but the blood vessel anastomoses were not damaged by the rejection. Because of this observation, Hufnagel began to study homografts, preserved segments of artery, as possible arterial grafts. In another branch of his research program, he discovered a new material that was to be used in surgery for the next sixty years, methyl methacrylate, also known as Plexiglas. Hufnagel constructed methyl methacrylate tubes to use as arterial prostheses. Eventually, he turned his attention to aortic valve disease, especially aortic insufficiency. He built a series of ball valve prostheses and his research laid the foundation for all that would come after. Eventually he built a prosthetic valve with a hollow Plexiglas sphere inside a cage that was designed to be placed in the descending aorta.

The concept was to assist cardiac output by preventing the reverse flow associated with severe aortic regurgitation. He placed the valve in hundreds of dogs, some of which lived for five years with the valve in place. On September 11, 1952, almost a year before Gibbon's first successful open-heart surgery, Hufnagel implanted the first prosthesis in a patient. She was a young woman with severe aortic regurgitation, congestive heart failure and angina pectoris.

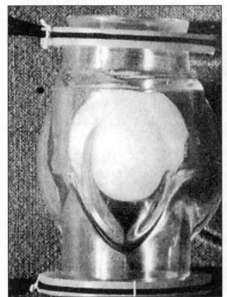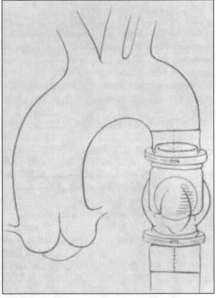

Figure 14 & 15 – The Hufnagel valve with its plastic ball and Plexiglas cage. On the right it is shown in position in the descending aorta.

At surgery, he found that she also had a coarctation of the aorta, which made the operation very difficult. She survived the procedure and lived another several years, dying of the uncorrected aortic regurgitation. He went on to implant many valves that were relatively free of complications. The patients' chief complaint was about the noise of the clicking ball and Hufnagel finally developed a noiseless nylon ball. It was said that the clicking of the valve with the plastic ball could be heard by others standing nearby if the patient opened his or her mouth. The prosthesis did not correct the basic problem with the aortic valve but it did provide palliation until better valves and open-heart surgery came along. The procedure did not, however, have anything to offer the mitral insufficiency patient.

STARR AND EDWARDS

In 1958, a retired engineer named Lowell Edwards met University of Oregon surgeon Albert Starr and told him that he wanted to build an artificial heart. Edwards was convinced that the heart could be duplicated as a hydraulic system. Starr suggested that they try to build a valve first, and then worry about a whole heart. Two years later, they had a usable artificial valve that could replace the human mitral valve. Their first patient was a young woman who, like my patient in 1964, had already been through a commissurotomy and an attempted repair of her incompetent mitral valve. She survived the operation but died eleven hours postop from an air embolus to her brain after being turned in bed. The second patient, a man named Philip Admundson, lived fifteen years with his artificial valve and died from a fall off a ladder. In May of 1963, a patient named Virgil Roberts received three Starr-Edwards valves, in the same operation, in the aortic, mitral and tricuspid locations. The following fall Dr. Starr began a talk on artificial valves at a national meeting by projecting a photograph of Virgil

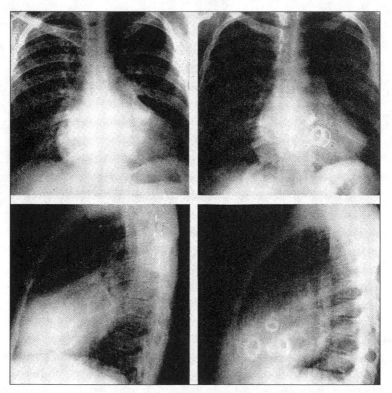

Figure 16 – The first triple valve replacement case.
The postop x-rays, with the valves in place, are on the right.

Robert's chest x-ray.[415] It brought the audience, all thoracic surgeons, to their feet. By March of 1965, the design had been modified several times based on the early experience in patients and the version called Model 6120 became the standard for twenty years. Edwards had financed much of the research himself and, in 1961, he established a new company, Edwards Laboratories, to make the valves commercially. By 1965, the new operation was becoming the standard for treatment of mitral insufficiency, but it was too late for my patient.

The Starr-Edwards valve used a metal cage and a silicone rubber ball. The Hufnagel valve used a plastic cylinder and ball which would not be suitable for placement in the root of the aorta, even after open heart surgery became available, because the plastic cylinder would obstruct the coronary artery orgins just above the normal valve location. In 1957, Hufnagel dealt with this objection by designing a plastic cage that had openings for coronary flow. These valves were implanted in dogs for periods of up to six months but were never used in humans.[416]

CORONARY ARTERY BYPASS

When I was a fourth year medical student in 1965, I reviewed the world literature on the state of surgery for coronary artery disease as a student project. It was a dismal task. Claude Beck (who had worked with Elliot Cutler on mitral valve surgery in the 1920s) spent years trying to develop a successful surgical approach to the coronary arteries. His first attempt was based on the observation of tiny connections between the coronary arteries and small vessels in the pericardium. Later, similar connections were identified between the branches of coronary arteries.[417] He stripped the pericardium and grafted various structures including omentum (the fatty apron in the abdomen that hangs down from the colon) and even pectoral muscle to establish connections between the blood supply of these other structures and the small branches of coronary arteries in the heart muscle. In 1935, Beck operated on his first patient, a forty-eight-year-old coal miner. Beck abraded the heart surface with a burr and then attached a graft of the left pectoral (chest) muscle in hopes that communication between the arterial circulations would develop. The patient recovered and was free of chest pain seven months later. By 1937, he had performed ninteen of these "Beck I" procedures and, in spite of fifty percent mortality, he persevered. Eventually, he tried another approach. Physiologists had demonstrated, as far back as 1895, that the heart could be perfused with blood through the coronary sinus (into which flow the coronary veins), reversing the flow in the coronary system. Beck tried placing a vascular graft into the coronary sinus to augment flow when the coronary arteries were diseased. This was called the "Beck II" procedure, but his results were poor and few procedures were attempted.[418]

Another procedure produced an interesting clinical research study. The ideal way to assess the value of a proposed treatment is to conduct what is called a "randomized controlled trial," often abbreviated "RCT." This involves the use of a placebo, a "sugar pill" that has no effect, and comparing the result to the drug or treatment under study. To avoid bias from enthusiasm by the participants, doctor or patient, neither knows which is the sugar pill. A third party keeps track of the results and, when the study period is over, breaks the code and tells everyone whether the treatment worked or it was all a result of the "placebo effect," the power of suggestion that can result in improvement in symptoms and sometimes even in objective tests. For example, thirty percent of ulcers will heal with sugar pills and any antacid must show a better result to be considered effective.

It is difficult to use randomized controlled trials in the evaluation of surgical procedures since it is obvious who got the surgery and who did not. A sham operation is needed and this is rarely possible for ethical reasons. In 1955, the principle of the Beck operation, collateral circulation from small arteries around the heart, prompted a new treatment that was ultimately subjected to a randomized trial. Italian surgeons reported improvement in angina after ligation of the internal mammary arteries.[419] The internal mammary arteries run just beneath the sternum, the breastbone, and connect with tiny vessels that supply the pericardium, the membrane that covers the heart. These surgeons proposed ligating the internal mammary arteries below the heart to increase the pressure in the small branches, the pericardiacophrenic arteries. Suddenly blocking an artery will raise the pressure above the block because the kinetic energy of flowing blood is converted to additional pressure. They reported improvement in the angina pain of patients subjected to the operation, a very simple procedure that could be performed under local anesthesia. In 1957, *Reader's Digest* printed an optimistic article about this procedure[420] and several other surgical groups had reported positive results. Surgeons at the University of Washington, among others, suggested that this procedure could be studied in a randomized trial since the operation was such a small procedure, an incision on each side of the sternum about an inch long.

A series of patients was divided into two study groups, half had the internal mammary artery ligated, and the other half had a sham operation in which the two small incisions were made but no deeper procedure was carried out. A number of patients reported excellent results including one who had reversion of an abnormal electrocardiogram to normal. In a "double blind" study, which this was, neither the patients nor the physicians know who got the real drug, or operation in this case. The records are kept in code until it is time to see the results. When the code was broken, the operation had produced no benefit.[421] The patient whose electrocardiogram improved had had a sham operation![422] The development of coronary arteriography, described earlier, reduced the reliance on relief of symptoms as a criterion of success of treatment. These studies showed that symptomatic relief was unreliable as a measure of results, even in severe cardiac disease.

In the past several years, a similar randomized control trial was performed on another surgical procedure that involved a small skin incision. Arthroscopy, described in the section on modern orthopedics, has been applied to osteoarthritis of the knee. The procedure, arthroscopy and lavage, or debridement, of the knee joint, was reported to show about a fifty percent rate of improvement. This is a different procedure from the repair or removal of injured cartilage in younger patients. A recent study included a randomized series of VA patients to study the effectiveness of this procedure in osteoarthritis of the knee.[423] The result was similar to that of the internal mammary artery ligation subjects. Half of the patients received a sham operation (a small skin incision only) and their results were equal to those with either lavage or debridement. All the patients, regardless of the study group they were placed in, had about a fifty-five percent improvement on the knee pain scale at two years. These results confirm the earlier studies' warnings about the hazards of using symptomatic improvement to assess surgical intervention.

THE VINEBERG OPERATION

The next development in coronary artery disease was another unlikely procedure. A Canadian surgeon named Arthur Vineberg reported that implanting (by simply tunneling the bleeding artery into the heart muscle) the internal mammary artery into the heart muscle resulted in collateral connections developing between the coronary arteries and the graft vessel.[424] The first report was an animal study and few were impressed. This time, Vineberg had angiography that showed the development of collaterals but the size of the vessels was too small to explain the improvement in symptoms. In 1962, Vineberg reported a human experience with thirty-six cases of whom thirty-one survived the operation. He reported sixty-six percent symptomatic improvement although less than fifty percent had long-term good results.[425] A 1965 report, of a series of

Vineberg operations, by Effler (at the Cleveland Clinic), with angiography by Mason Sones, got immediate attention.[426]   The angiographic results lent some credibility to his claims and, indeed, some patients continue to show collateral connections twenty-five years after the procedure.

CORONARY ARTERY BYPASS GRAFTS

Everything changed in 1968 with the publication, by Rene Favaloro, of a new technique.[427] Favaloro reported fifteen patients in which he divided the right coronary artery beyond a point of severe narrowing and performed an end-to-end bypass graft using saphenous vein. The other end of the saphenous graft was attached to the aorta. All patients survived and postoperative angiography confirmed that the grafts were open and functioning. Why it should have taken so long, after Robert Linton began using saphenous vein to bypass leg artery obstructions, to adopt the procedure to coronary disease is one of those "Why didn't I think of that?" mysteries.[428] Claude Beck was so close to the right idea with his coronary sinus grafts if he had only thought of putting them into the artery! Part of the problem was poor visualization of the disease before Sones developed the angiography technique. Still, it took nearly ten years after good angiography before Favaloro, at the Cleveland Clinic, came up with the idea. By 1970, Effler and Favaloro were attacking the left coronary artery although others, through fear of the risk, would delay left coronary surgery until 1972. Their report[429] described the new method, which did not divide the artery, and included 188 patients with only four deaths, a mortality rate of 2.1 percent. The modern era of coronary artery surgery had arrived. By 2000 over 500,000 such operations were being performed in the United States each year.

ANGIOPLASTY

In 1978, Andreas Gruntzig reported a new technique of dilating coronary artery stenosis with a balloon catheter. He developed a new, non-elastic balloon in 1974 and began study of the technique in the femoral artery. In 1976, he began dilatation of coronary artery lesions and in 1978; he reported his results in the first fifty patients.[430] They were able to dilate sixty-six percent of the vessels and only two patients died, at two and six months post-procedure. Follow-up angiograms in sixteen patients showed restenosis in two. They were unable to dilate vessels in eighteen patients, seventeen of whom underwent bypass grafting-seven emergently. They were unable to dilate main stem left coronary disease and stressed that complications required a cardiac surgery team standing by for emergency bypass, if problems arose. Both of these concerns remained as significant problems in the future, but the technique, aided in a few years by stent technology that reduced restenosis, has replaced a large proportion of surgical coronary bypass since 1979.

390   Rehn "ueber penetrierende Herzwundin und Herznaht," *Archive fur Klinich Chirurgerie* 55:315 (1897).

391   Lauder Brunton, "Mitral Stenosis," *Lancet* I (1902).

392   Ambrose L Lockwood, "Surgery of the Pericardium and Heart," *Archives of Surgery*, 18:417-474 (1929).

393   Elliot Cutler and Claude S Beck, "The Present Status of the Surgical Procedures in Chronic Valvular Disease of the Heart," *Archives of Surgery* , 18:403-416 (1929).

394   HS Souttar , "The Surgical Treatment of Mitral Stenosis," *British Medical Journal* 2:603 (1925).

395   John C Munro, "Ligation of the Ductus Arteriosus," *Annals of Surgery* 46: 335-38 (1907).

396   Robert E Gross , J.P. Hubbard, "Landmark article Feb 25, 1939: Surgical ligation of a patent ductus arteriosus. Report of first successful case," *JAMA* 251:1201-2 (1984).

397   T.G. Baffes. "Willis J. Potts: his contributions to cardiovascular surgery," *Annals of Thoracic Surgery* 44:92-6. (1987).

398   Clarence Crafoord and G. Nylin, "Congenital Coarctation of the Aorta and Its Surgical Treatment," *Journal of Thoracic Surgery* 14:347-361 (1945).

399   Allen Weisse, *Heart to Heart*, page 43.

400   A Blalock and HB Taussig, "The surgical treatment of malformations of the heart in which there is pulmonary stenosis or pulmonary atresia," *JAMA* 128:189 (1945).

401   Charles P Bailey, "The Surgical Treatment of Mitral Stenosis (Mitral Commissurotomy)", *Diseases of the Chest*, 15:377-397 (1949).

402   Allen Weisse, pages 77-78.

403   Allen Weisse, pages 79-80.

404   Alexis Carrel and Charles Lindberg, "The culture of whole organs," *Science* 81:621-623 (1935).

405   Described in WR Probert and DG Melrose, "An early Russian Heart Lung Machine," *British Medical Journal* 1:1017 (1960).

406   HH Dale and EA Schuster, "A Double Perfusion Pump," *Journal of Physiology* (London), 64:356-64 (1928).

407   Michael DeBakey, "A Simple Continuous-flow Blood Transfusion Instrument," *New Orleans Medical Surgical Journal*, 87:386 (1934).

408   JH Gibbon Jr. and CW Kraul, "An Efficient Oxygenator for Blood," *Journal of Laboratory and Clinical Medicine*, 26:1803 (1941).

409   Ada Romaine-Davis, in her exhaustive history of Gibbon's work, *John Gibbon and His Heart-Lung Machine*, credits a medical student named E.L. Clark with suggesting IBM.

410   TL Stokes and J H Gibbon Jr., "Experimental   Maintenance of Life by a Mechanical Heart and Lung During   Occlusion of the Vena Cavae Followed by Survival," *Surgery, Gynecology and Obstetrics*, 91:138 (1950).

411   C. Walton Lillehei, "Controlled cross ciculation for direct-visiobn intracardiac surgery:correction of ventricular septal defects, atrio-ventricular communis and tetralogy of Fallot," *Postgraduate Medicine*, 17: 388-396 (1955).

412   Emile Holman and Claude Beck, "The physiologic response of the circulatory system to experimental alterations; effect of aortic and and pulmonic stenosis," *Journal of Clinical Investigation* 3:283 (1926).

413   C.A. Hufnagel, B.B. Roe and A.C. Barger, "A technique for producing pulmonary artery stenosis," *Surgery* 29:77 (1951).

414   William H. Muller and J. Francis Dammann, Jr, "The treatment of certain congenital malformations of the heart by the creation of pulmonic stenosis to reduce pulmonary hypertension and excessive pulmonary blood flow," *Surgery, Gynecology and Obstetrics* 95:213-219 (1952).

415   Albert Starr "Surgery for Multiple Valve Disease," *Annals of Surgery* 160:596-613 (1964) This article includes the famous x-ray of the first patient to receive three artificial valves.

416   Charles A. Hufnagel, Paulo Diaz Villegas, Hector Nahas, "Experiences with New Types of Aortic Valvular Prostheses," *Annals of Surgery* 147:636-645 (1958).

417   PM Zoll,S Wssler and MJ Schlessinger, "Interarterial Coronary Anastomosis in the Human Heart, with Particular Reference to Anemia and Relative Cardiac Anoxia," *Circulation*, 4:797 (1951).

418   Claude S Beck, "Coronary Artery Disease – Physiologic Concepts – Surgical Operation," *Annals of Surgery*, 145:439-60 (1957).

419   M Battezzati, A Taglioferro, G DeMarchi, "La ligature delle due artere mammare interne nei disturbi di vasculorizzione del miocardio: nata preventive relatives di prinii dati spermentoli e clinica," *Minerva Medicina* 46:1178-1188 (1955).

420   Ratcliff, "New Surgery for Ailing Hearts," *Reader's Digest* 71:70-73 (1957).

421   EG Dimond, CF Kittle, JE Crockett, "Comparison of internal mammary artery ligation and sham operation for angina pectoris," *American Journal of Cardiology* 5:483-486 (1960).

422   LA Cobb, GI Thomas, GH Dillard, KA Merendino, RA Bruce, "An evaluation of internal mammary artery ligation by a double blind technic," *New England Journal of Medicine* 260:1115-1118 (1959).

423   J. Bruce Moseley, Kimberly O'Malley, et all. "A controlled trial of arthroscopic surgery for osteoarthritis of the knee," *New England Journal of Medicine* 347:81-88 (2002).

424   AM Vineberg, "The development of an anastomosis between the coronary vessels and a transplanted internal mammary artery," *Canadian Medical Association Journal*, 55:117-19 (1946).

425   Arthur Vineberg, "Surgery of Coronary Artery Disease," *Progress in Cardiovascular Diseases*, 4:391-418 (1962).

426   DB Effler, FM Sones, Jr, LK Groves, E Suarez, "Myocardial revascularization by Vineberg's internal mammary artery implant," *Journal of Thoracic and Cardiovascular Surgery,* 50: 527-31 (1965).

427   Rene G Favaloro, "Saphenous Vein Autograft Replacement of Severe Segmental Coronary Artery Occlusion," *Annals of Thoracic Surgery* 5:334-339 (1968).

428   Robert R Linton, "Some Practical Considerations in the Surgery of Blood Vessel Grafts," *Surgery* 38:817 (1955).

429   Rene Favaloro, Donald B Effler, et al. "Severe segmental obstruction of the left main coronary artery and its divisions," *Journal of Thoracic and Cardiovascular Surgery,* 60:469 (1970).

430   AR Gruntzig, A Senning and W Siegenthaler, "Nonoperative dilatation of coronary artery stenosis," *New England Journal of Medicine,* 301:61 (1979).

20
Critical Care Medicine and Anesthesia

IN 1896, GEORGE CRILE BEGAN TO STUDY SHOCK, PARTICULARLY "SURGICAL shock," the postoperative instability that Cushing was prepared, that first day of his residency, to administer strychnine to counteract. Crile tried all the drugs favored by surgeons in Europe and America. None seemed to produce any improvement. He resolved to study the blood pressure and pulse to see what the relationship was between them and the familiar manifestations of shock: cool skin, confusion, air hunger, and death. He found that saline infusion, in spite of maintaining blood pressure, did not improve survival of dogs. The Spanish-American War interrupted his studies in 1898, but offered practical experience. He operated on a young trooper who had been kicked by a horse. At surgery, he repaired a ruptured spleen and administered postoperative saline infusion (given subcutaneously in those days except in the laboratory). The patient did not survive. In 1903, Crile published *Blood Pressure and Surgery*, summarizing his six years of research. He devised a pressurized pneumatic suit that was effective in restoring blood pressure.

In my resident days we used such a device, called a "G-suit," and paramedics, until recently used a similar device called a "MAST" suit (Medical Anti-Shock Trousers). Crile had his suit manufactured by the Goodyear Rubber Company. He tried adrenalin infusions and found those effective, as well. He concluded that low blood pressure is the basic defect in surgical shock (Remember that routine blood pressure measurement would only come in 1902 after Cushing brought back the Riva-Rocci apparatus from Europe). He referred to closed chest cardiac massage in patients who had suffered cardiac arrest. He used his own blood pressure measuring apparatus (made from laboratory glassware), until his associate, Myron Metzenbaum called his attention to the Riva-Rocci apparatus. In 1903, he gave a talk to the Boston medical community, at the invitation of Dr. Councilman, which created a sensation. He told the group that all the stimulants used by other surgeons to treat shock were worthless.

That year he turned to the study of blood transfusion, already summarized in the chapter on blood. (See Chapter 15). Starling's work over the next twenty years provided the theoretical basis for understanding the relationship between blood volume, cardiac output and blood pressure. World War I provided extensive experience to young surgeons, as every war does, but progress was slow afterward. In the 1920s, Walter Dandy, who succeeded Harvey Cushing as chief of neurosurgery at Johns Hopkins (after Cushing returned to Boston), set up a small room adjacent to his operating room to provide "around the clock" care of his postoperative patients.[431] The Los Angeles County General Hospital, which opened in 1933, had a Postoperative Anesthesia Recovery (the PAR) area on the same floor as the main operating rooms. This was the first such facility to be designed in a hospital.

RESPIRATORS

THE IRON LUNG

Another major addition to the therapeutic armamentarium of the critical care physician was the invention of the respirator. Initially, the stimulus for this new device was not surgical at all but the increasing incidence of paralytic polio. Bulbar polio (involving the lower portion of the brain that controls breathing and other primitive functions) is a particularly devastating form of the disease in which the respiratory muscles are paralyzed and the patient asphyxiates. Dr. Philip Drinker, at the Harvard School of Public Health, and Louis A. Shaw, a physiologist, devised the first apparatus that would provide artificial ventilation in 1929.[432] Initially they worked on animals and built a small tank powered by air pressure. Inevitably, it became known as "the iron lung."[433] The first use in humans was in premature infants, to help them to breath. The results were dubious. The first patient with polio to be treated with the iron lung was a little girl. The air pump was a household vacuum cleaner. The doctors sat with her until she died. The second patient was an adult man and the nursing care was much more difficult. Still, he did survive and, rewarding their efforts, he recovered from the respiratory paralysis and a year later was walking with leg braces. After his recovery, he returned to the Massachusetts General Hospital to address the staff that had cared for him.

Early in their experience they built a "room respirator," similar to the Sauerbruch chamber, which held four patients, each with his or her head sticking out a hole in the wall. Amazingly, they could care for adults and children (even one only a year old) in the same room. Initially they had trouble with clearing airway secretions and some other hospitals became discouraged with the device because of misuse, especially with patients who did not require ventilation. Eventually they used tracheostomy in many cases to improve tracheal toilet (suctioning secretions). The Drinker Respirator continued in use into the 1960s when better positive pressure ventilators came along.

POSITIVE PRESSURE VENTILATION

Chevalier Jackson described the technique of endotrachial intubation in 1913[434] but its use was limited until better systems of delivering the anesthetic gas were devised. Elsberg first described the use of Meltzer's endotrachial tube (See Chapter 14) in a patient in 1910.[435] Continuous insufflation was used at a pressure of ten millimeters of mercury and a mixture of air and ether was given. The patient had a lung abscess and the operation was successful. After World War I, Magill and Rowbotham, British Army anesthetists, adopted the semi-open system of ventilation in anesthesia, which duplicated respiration. MaGill advocated the use of endotrachial anesthesia and invented a type of curved foreceps that could be used to assist in directing the tube into the trachea. He also described a technique of passing an endotrachial tube through the nose and directing the tip into the trachea, using the laryngoscope to aid visualization.[436] Both Magill and Rowbotham, by a fortuitous circumstance, had been assigned to the Queen's Hospital for Facial & Jaw Injuries at Sidcup, in 1919. Both had served in the Royal Army Medical Corps but had no experience as anesthetists. They were forced to learn how to admininister anesthesia to war veterans undergoing reconstruction of facial injuries which would not allow the usual open drop ether technique or the use of face masks. Their enthusiasm and inventiveness was to change the entire field of anesthesia.

THE EVOLUTION OF THE ANESTHESIA MACHINE

The invention of the bubble feed bottle, by Cotton and Boothby at the Boston City Hospital in 1910, allowed the anesthetist to measure the rate of oxygen administration. The gas was bubbled through water and the bubbling rate was proportional to the flow rate.[437] The same system was used to measure ether flow in machines built for the British Army in World War I.[438] In 1920, Rowbotham invented the large diameter endotrachial tube we are familiar with, and the insufflation catheter, which sent a continuous stream of air into the trachea but which did not control the airway, was gradually abandoned.[439] The cuffed endotrachial tube was invented by two Americans, Henry Janeway—who also invented the

L-shaped laryngoscope (Jackson's instrument was U-shaped) and G.M. Dorrance. The improved tube would wait until advances in anesthesia made a closed system useful. Ralph Waters, head of one of the first academic anesthesia departments in the world, and Arthur Guedel reintroduced the cuffed endotrachial tube to improve the efficiency of the closed circle anesthesia machine, invented by Waters. Guedel demonstrated the effectiveness of the cuffed tube by submerging his pet dog, anesthetized and intubated, in a tank of water. He then removed the dog from the water, extubated it and watched it shake the water from its fur coat to the amusement of the spectators.[440] The dog's name was "Airway."

In 1915, Dennis Jackson, a pharmacologist at Washington University in St. Louis, invented the sodium hydroxide canister to absorb the CO_2 in the expired air. This was useful even in early "to-and-fro" anesthesia machines like those used in World War I. Oxygen and ether were added to the exhaled air and, with the removal of the CO_2, the same moist warm air could be recirculated in a closed system. Waters introduced just such a system in 1924, using Jackson's principle.[441] The introduction of cyclopropane for anesthesia by Waters in 1930 popularized the closed system machines. Initially, the CO_2 cannister was close to the face, but Brian Sword produced the modern system, with the canister mounted on the machine, in 1930.[442] Cyclopropane was much easier to use for induction; ether takes forever to put the patient to sleep, but it was explosive. The Dräger company in Germany built CO_2 absorption devices for mine rescue operations and, in 1925, built their Model A anesthesia machine for use with nitrous oxide/oxygen combinations or ether. Nitrous oxide was so expensive in Germany that the device did not become popular until after World War II. Now, the endotracheal tube came into its own, but open drop ether would be common until the 1960s. In 1931, Waters discovered another application of the endotrachial tube as a result of an accident. The tube was too long for the patient and the tip passed down the right main-stem bronchus, ventilating only one lung. This is not an unusual complication and every surgeon and anesthesiologist is alert for this problem. Waters immediately recognized the possible application of this development to lung surgery. He applied the technique to thoracic surgery in which one lung may be inflated without the other.[443] This allowed safer lung surgery, which then rapidly advanced to pneumonectomy as described in Chapter 11.

HENRY K. BEECHER

Critical care medicine and anesthesia developed concurrently in the post-war era. In the 1930s, interns still administered ether anesthesia with a mortality rate that is frightening to those of us accustomed to modern medicine. In 1936, Henry K. Beecher completed his surgical training at the Massachusetts General Hospital under Edward D. Churchill, who then appointed him Chief of Anesthesia for the hospital. It did not matter to Churchill that Beecher had never spent any time in a formal anesthesia training program. Following Beecher's appointment, Churchill reported that the mortality rate of lung lobectomy performed for bronchiectasis declined from fifty percent in 1932 to five percent in 1938-39. The decline in mortality for this operation was so spectacular that other surgeons doubted Dr. Churchill's results when presented. It is likely that the technical improvements advocated by Ralph Waters contributed.

Beecher viewed his role as one of learning and teaching the physiology of the anesthetized patient, rather than developing technical skill in the handling of apparatus. In 1936, shortly after assuming the role of chairman he established the Anesthesia Laboratory of the Harvard Medical School at the Massachusetts General Hospital. This was the first research facility established to study the problems of anesthesia, described by Dr. Beecher as the bridge between pharmacology and surgery. In 1938, he published the *Physiology of Anesthesia,* a title that captures his emphasis. When the US entered World War II, he joined the army and, after service in North Africa, landed at the Anzio Beachhead with a military medical unit. Here he observed that wounded soldiers seem to require less pain medication than civilian patients suffering from similar injuries. He concluded that the wound had produced euphoria by removing the casualty from battle. The prospect of imminent death in combat had been removed by a wound the soldier was likely to survive and which might even result in returning him to home. The term "Million Dollar Wound" became popular. These observations would eventually lead him to his discovery of the placebo effect after return to civilian life. He studied the effects of narcotics and his research eventually led to concerns about the ethics of human experimentation and informed consent.

In 1954, Beecher and Todd published the first outcome study of anesthesia and found that the use of curare, a long acting muscle relaxant derived from arrow poison, resulted in a much higher mortality rate than similar surgical procedures performed without its use.[444] Curare had been introduced in 1940 as a muscle relaxant for electroconvulsant (shock) treatment in psychiatry. The paralysis prevented fractures (See the chapter on psychiatry). The drug had been discovered by European explorers in South America, where it was used by natives as arrow poison. Claude Bernard had shown that it acted on the nerve junction with muscle and prevented the effect of nerve stimulation, but did not prevent direct stimulation of the muscle electrically. Its first use in anesthesia came in 1942, but endotracheal intubation was required to prevent asphyxia. Because cyclopropane frequently required intubation anyway, the combination quickly came into common use.[445] Harold Randall Griffith, who introduced the use of curare in Canada in 1942, was honored with a commemorative stamp by that country in 1991. During the Second World War, the technique evolved into a combination of narcosis, analgesia and muscle relaxation, now called "balanced anesthesia," which is still in use.[446]

Beecher became concerned when the records suggested that paralyzed patients under anesthesia were at risk for reasons that his research would later explain. Ether potentiates the paralysis effect of curare and, without the ability to measure oxygen concentration in blood (still ten years away), patients did not get adequate oxygen while recovering from anesthesia. The study, and the fact that they published it in a surgical journal rather than an anesthesia journal, produced a furor. The very large series of patients studied and the rigor of the statistical methods forced critics to conduct their own serious analysis of the safety of muscle relaxants and prompted improvement in anesthesia care. One practical effect was the adoption of short acting muscle relaxants, like succinylcholine, whose effect lasted only a few minutes. The long acting agents are still in wide use but better monitoring of oxygen and CO_2 levels, plus the use of drugs to reverse the paralysis, have markedly reduced the risk.

In 1959 Dr. Henrik Bendixen, a member of the department at the MGH, began to study ventilation standards after finding that alveolar collapse developed in animals maintained on the usual volume settings for ventilation. In 1960, the Clark oxygen electrode was perfected and was used to determine arterial oxygen concentrations in anesthetized patients. Oxygen levels were found to be unexpectedly low during anesthesia and in the postoperative period. Here was the explanation of the outcomes study of 1954. In 1963, a four bed Respiratory Unit was opened at MGH under Dr. Henning Pontoppidan and Henrik Bendixen, after which anesthesiologists began to move out of the operating room into critical care. Respiratory therapists, blood gas technicians and the advent of the volume-controlled ventilator followed.[447] Anesthesia and critical care medicine advanced hand in hand after Beecher opened his experimental laboratory.

In 1956 a new synthetic gas, a fluorinated hydrocarbon related to aerosol propellants, like those used in spray cans, was introduced. Fluorinated compounds are very stable and hundreds were tested in mice for potential use as anesthetic agents. The chemical structure was modified during the research so these compounds are early examples of "designer drugs."[448] Ether is inflammable and cyclopropane, a superior anesthetic agent, is explosive. Neither drug can be used safely with electrocautery unless extraordinary precautions are taken. Even with great care occasional disasters occurred. Halothane was a tremendous improvement and quickly became the most common anesthetic agent in use. In the mid-1960s, reports of postoperative liver failure began to appear. Halothane is metabolized to a trifluoroacetyl halide compound that is capable of binding to hepatic microsomal (protein synthesis cellular organelles) proteins. These hapten structures may function as antigens and autoimmunity results. There is a genetic susceptibility to the problem and repeated exposure (characteristic of immune conditions) seems to be necessary for the severe hepatic injury. Other fluorinated hydrocarbon anesthetic agents, developed since halothane was introduced, seem to avoid the problem.[449]

THE INTENSIVE CARE UNIT

During the Second World War, the knowledge of physiology, anesthesia, and bacteriology began to come together in a new discipline although no one realized it at first. In the First World War, the battle casualties in shock were at first assigned to the "moribund ward." With the realization of what was happening to these men, chiefly the contribution of Ernest Cowell who measured blood pressure and realized that the shock was due to hemorrhage, the military surgeons began to transfuse casualties and save them. The "moribund ward" became the "resuscitation ward," the first Intensive Care Unit. The Los Angeles County General Hospital Post-Anesthesia Recovery Room, called the PAR, was located on the same floor as the operating rooms and was equipped with the primitive apparatus used in resuscitating patients from anesthesia at the time. Here, nurses experienced in the care of patients emerging from anesthesia could watch them; in the case of ether, this could take hours. The concept of placing patients at increased risk in a special nursing unit was long in coming but it began here and in Walter Dandy's special nursing unit at Johns Hopkins.

For World War II, antibiotics (sulfa drugs at first and then finally penicillin) were available and medical training had improved in the previous twenty years, especially in surgery and anesthesia. In the Mediterranean Theater of Operations Edward D. Churchill set up a "Chest Center" to study casualties with heart and lung injuries. The surgeons learned a great deal about the care of these critical injuries and about trauma patients in general.[450] The Chest Center surgeons identified a new syndrome they called "Traumatic Wet Lung." This condition is now know as Adult

Respiratory Distress Syndrome, or ARDS, and is still one of the two or three greatest challenges in the care of the critically ill patient. Lyman Brewer, a young thoracic surgeon from Los Angeles, was one of those assigned the task of improving the care of these patients. Severely wounded men developed a wet cough, increasing bronchial secretions, and then, finally, pulmonary edema, a condition also seen in acute heart failure and severe mitral stenosis. Many of these patients had chest wounds but some did not. In 1937, Barach had described the use of positive pressure ventilation in acute pulmonary edema from heart failure.[451] In 1944 Lyman Brewer, and the other thoracic surgeons of the eleventh Field Hospital, began to use an anesthesia machine, fitted with a manometer to measure the airway pressure, and a tightly fitting facemask to treat traumatic wet lung with positive pressure ventilation. Having the patient breathe in an atmosphere of higher pressure seemed to push the excess fluid that was leaking from capillaries into the lung small air sacs, the alveoli, back into the vascular space and improved oxygen exchange. Over 167 patients were treated using this apparatus and most survived.[452]

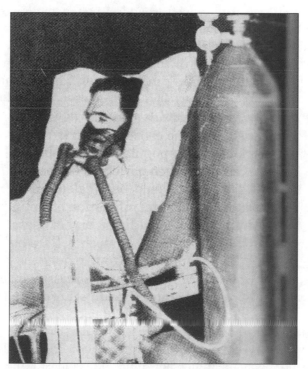

Figure 17 – Here is a traumatic wet lung patient receiving
an IPPB treatment in Italy, near Cassino, in 1943.
Photo from Brewer, et al, Surgery in World War II

The Draeger Company[453] had been making anesthesia machines since 1907(originally not intended for anesthesia-see above) but they were not suitable for long-term use and were not automatic. The anesthetist manually ventilated the patient under anesthesia by squeezing a rubber bag. By 1944, anesthesia machines made by this company were adapted to this new form of therapy until better machines for the purpose were available. The Drinker respirator (the "Iron Lung") is not suitable for the ventilation of patients with increased lung stiffness or resistance. During the Los Angeles polio epidemic in 1949 (already described – See Chapter 18), a bellows device was added to Drinker respirators which permitted positive pressure ventilation through the tracheostomy for some patients. This modification seems to have reduced the mortality of bulbar polio from eighty percent to seventeen percent in that group but the effect was not widely appreciated until later

In 1946, Dr. Brewer returned to Los Angeles and convinced an engineer named Ray Bennett to adapt a pressure sensitive valve, used for oxygen masks in high altitude flying during the war, to civilian use. Bennett had developed these valves to support wounded aircrew members, who were having trouble breathing, until they could get home to base. It was not too great a step to adapt the system to this use. The first Bennett respirator was the result. Bennett continued to manufacture respirators of improving efficiency and others, notably Forrest M. Bird, produced similar devices. The Bird respirator, a small green plastic box, was introduced in 1958 and was widely used in the 1960s and 70s. Bird's machine was air-driven and very portable. Until the 1960s, these devices all used pressure sensitive valves, which provide little control of the volume of gas delivered to a stiff lung. They are fine for administering Intermittent Positive Pressure Breathing (IPPB) to patients requiring treatments of fifteen minutes several times per day and were soon modified to deliver a fine spray of medication to the lungs as well. The use of central venous pressure monitoring became less cumbersome when a technique for percutaneous insertion of subclavian catheters was standardized in the 1970s.[454]

Blood gas measurements became possible in the 1960s and the limitations of the pressure sensitive respirators eventually prompted a change to volume-controlled ventilators by 1971. A volume controlled respirator will deliver a measured volume of air with each breath; the pressure controlled respirator will deliver a measured pressure for so many seconds each cycle but there is no way to determine how much air is inhaled (the amount can be measured by collecting the exhaled air but it cannot be controlled). The volume respirator usually has a release valve to avoid excessive airway pressure but it is much more effective with stiff lungs. Some of the concepts of volume-controlled ventilation were discovered during a disastrous polio epidemic in Denmark in 1952. In that incident 2,241 cases occurred in Copenhagen and, of these, 345 were bulbar polio requiring ventilation. Copenhagen had one Drinker respirator. The medical schools were closed and 250 medical students manually ventilated these patients using anesthesia machines and bag-valve systems. At times, the students, who worked in shifts around the clock, were ventilating seventy patients at once.[455] Lessons about humidification, care of endotrachial tubes and the use of blood gas measurements to control the respiratory assistance were learned.

In 1963, Engstrom described the first volume controlled respirator.[456] His machine delivered a fixed volume of gas per breath (driven by a piston) and a bag arrangement allowed the patient to breathe spontaneously at a rate higher than that set by the machine. A glass cylinder filled with water functioned as a safety valve to release any pressure higher than the limit set by the amount of water in the cylinder. It was crude by later standards but it was the first volume controlled respirator we had. The Mörch respirator was a low flat machine designed to fit under the patient's bed. It did not have a safety valve and was usually used with an uncuffed tracheostomy tube, in my own experience.[457] Bennett later designed a better device, called the "MA-1,"introduced in 1967. It could assist the patient, or take over breathing completely, and highly modified models are still in production. John H Emerson, who had improved the Drinker respirator, also built a volume respirator that competed with the Bennett machines.

Community hospitals began to construct intensive care units in the 1950s for a variety of reasons. In 1958, at Baltimore City Hospital, Dr. Peter Safar opened the first modern intensive care unit. He had done pioneering work in the development of mouth-to-mouth breathing which would be combined with the closed chest cardiac massage being studied nearby at Johns Hopkins. (See the section on CPR in Chapter 18.) The new technology demanded skilled nurses and inhalation therapy technicians to operate the new machines. Private rooms and private duty nurses, still the standard at the Massachusetts General Hospital surgical service in 1965, were isolated and expensive. Many private duty nurses did not want to care for critically ill patients and were not comfortable with new technology, primitive as it was. Physicians taught ICU nurses to read ECG tracings and to recognize arrhythmias on the new monitors that began to appear by 1960. It seemed that better and more economical care could be delivered by putting all the critically ill patients in one place.[458] Eventually the ICU would have hazards as well as benefits. Infection became the bane of these units with their concentration of patients with multiple problems. They were noisy, and cardiac patients, who also would benefit from more intensive monitoring, acquired their own facility, the "coronary care unit." The coronary care unit was quiet and most patients were monitored with electrocardiogram leads. Los Angeles County Hospital built a coronary care unit in 1966 with plans to have ECG tracings read by computer. Respirators and patents with non-cardiac problems, including postop cardiac surgery patients who often required respirators for a day or more, went to the ICU.

The Vietnam War changed trauma care enormously. The helicopter got the casualties to the hospital so quickly that the mortality rate was less than five percent of those admitted. Vascular surgery saved many limbs that would have been lost in Korea, let alone World War II. It did bring a severe lesson in resuscitation that everyone thought had already been learned in previous wars. In 1966 G. Tom Shires, a professor of surgery, published a series of studies suggesting that patients suffering from major blood loss and trauma had better outcomes if resuscitated with lactated Ringer's solution, a salt solution, than with blood.[459,460] The use of saline had been controversial in World War I but the matter was thought to be settled until these studies were published. The result was that young surgeons and anesthesiologists in Viet Nam used huge volumes of salt solution to treat casualties and only used blood for severe anemia. By 1968, a new entity called "Da Nang lung" was a major problem in Vietnam (Da Nang was a large base where the military hospital was the "in-country" referral center for the smaller military hospitals). Da Nang lung looked an awful lot like traumatic wet lung and an inquiry into this new disease prompted a review of Shires' original studies that had encouraged the aggressive saline administration. Francis D. Moore, author of the definitive book on postop care,[461] analyzed the study published by Shires and found a methodological error. The recommended volumes of salt solution were too high, due to an error in measuring the distribution of radioactive isotopes in Shires' studies. Military surgeons, following Shires' enthusiastic recommendations, were giving casualties too much fluid and producing acute respiratory insufficiency, a condition that was named Adult Respiratory Distress Syndrome (ARDS). *The Journal of Trauma*, in 1968, devoted an entire issue to the problems of respiratory insufficiency, Da Nang lung, its etiology and treatment.[462] A number of suggestions were made in the symposium that began the modern era of critical care. Moore and Shires published a joint article calling for moderation in the adoption of new methods[463] and care of the wounded was modified.

The syndrome continued to be a problem, and was not solely a trauma problem, as it became increasingly apparent that the pulmonary reaction was related to a variety of noxious stimuli associated with critical illness.[464] New methods of airway pressure control, including applying positive pressure during exhalation (called Positive End Expiratory Pressure or PEEP[465]), were effective in reducing the pulmonary edema and more of these patients survived. Bennett further developed the volume controlled respirator, the "MA-I," in the 1970s and it became the most popular machine for the next twenty years.[466]

Pediatric critical care required the development of a small respirator that could provide artificial respiration for infants. Finally, small respirators, suitable for infants, appeared about 1970. During my residency training in 1968, I operated on a premature infant weighing one pound ten ounces, smaller than any surviving premature infant to date, let alone one having abdominal surgery. We had no ability to provide artificial respiration but she survived without all the intensive care apparatus typical of the care of small premature infants today. Four years later all that had changed and another child I cared for in 1972 spent eighteen months on a respirator after surgery for a huge ventricular septal defect. He is alive and healthy today.

TOTAL PARENTERAL NUTRITION

Nutrition has always been a serious problem for critically ill patients, especially those on respirators or with GI tract injuries that prevent eating solid food. The usual intravenous fluids add fifty grams of glucose to each liter of solution. This provides an isotonic solution (the same concentration of electrolytes as plasma) of water for intravenous use, to avoid hemolysis of red blood cells. When added to other solutions to make them isotonic it provides some calories. If three liters of five percent (five grams of glucose per 100 ml of solution) solution are infused per day, the patient receives about 750 calories (150 grams times five calories per gram), not enough to maintain adequate nutrition but something. Using hypertonic solutions (ten percent glucose, for example), to increase caloric intake, causes phlebitis in peripheral veins. An attempt to increase caloric intake by the intravenous route using lipid solutions (nine calories per gram and less osmotic effect) ended in the early 1960s after several severe allergic reactions to Lipomul, the lipid suspension. In 1968 Stanley Dudrick published a study in which he maintained litters of beagle puppies on a total intravenous nutrient regimen from birth.[467] The puppies on the IV nutrition (a mixture of hypertonic glucose (often twenty-five percent glucose solutions), amino acids and electrolytes) developed normally and the era of "total parenteral nutrition" had arrived. His next report, the same year, described the first patients maintained on this program, 300 adults and twelve newborns, with one infant maintained for 400 days on total parenteral nutrition with normal growth and development. Critically ill patients could be given thousands of calories per day without using the GI tract. The central venous catheters that were now ubiquitous, provided the route for the highly concentrated solutions Dudrick used. A new lipid suspension called "Intralipid" came into use and the allergic problems seen in the earlier era did not appear. Tube feeding, which had been used for years but was troubled with hyperosmolar coma (from inadequate water in the solutions) and diarrhea complications, improved as nutrition research, much of it prompted by Dudrick's work, became a serious topic.

THE SWAN-GANZ CATHETER

In 1970, H.J.C. Swan and William Ganz described a new catheter which allowed the placement of the tip of this catheter into the pulmonary artery from an arm vein.[468] The catheter, afterwards called the "Swan-Ganz catheter," had a small balloon at the tip which, when inflated, caused the blood flow to pull the catheter along into the heart and then into the pulmonary artery. Fluoroscopy, required for traditional cardiac catheterization, was not necessary and the catheter could be inserted at the patient's bedside in the ICU. It was connected to a pressure transducer (a monitoring device) and the pressure tracing told us the location of the catheter tip. This new device allowed direct measurement of pulmonary blood flow, pressure and cardiac output. Fick's principle was now available at the bedside to monitor the effect of the new drugs coming along and to control cardiac physiology as had never previously been possible. Arterial catheters permitted continuous monitoring of arterial pressure and frequent determinations of arterial blood gas concentrations without the need for frequent arterial puncture. New drugs came along. In 1972 the standard of care in an ICU with a (non-cardiac) shock patient was a central venous pressure catheter, a volume controlled ventilator (although they were still primitive then), and isoproterenol, a beta adrenergic pressor agent that was an improvement over epinephrine and norepinephrine but was still subject to many problems. Soon new drugs became available and progress in the care of the critically ill steadily increased.

431 A. McGehee Harvey, "Neurosurgical Genius: Walter Dandy," *Hopkins Medicine* 135: 364-65 (1974).

432 Philip Drinker and Charles McKhann, "The Use of a New Apparatus for the Prolonged Administration of Artificial Respiration," *JAMA* 92:1658-1660 (1929).

433 P Drinker and LA Shaw, "Apparatus for prolonged administration of artificial respiration; design for children and adults," *Journal of Clinical Investigation*, 7:229 (1929).

434 Chevalier Jackson, "The Technique for Insertion of Intratracheal Insufflation Tubes," *Surgery, Gynecology and Obstetrics* 17:507-9 (1913).

435 Charles A. Elsberg, "Clinical Experiences With Intratracheal Insufflation (Meltzer), With Remarks Upon the Value of the Method for Thoracic Surgery," *Annals of Surgery* 52:23-33 (1910).

436 Ivan W. Magill, "Endotracheal Anaesthesia," *Proceedings of the Royal Society of Medicine,* xxii pages 83-87 (1929). Reprinted in *Anaesthesia* 33:1-4 (1978).

437 F.G. Cotton, W.M. Boothby and J.T. Gwathmey, *Anaesthesia* , Appleton & Co., New York , page 161 (1914).

438 G. Marshall, "Two types of portable gas-oxygen apparatus," *Proceedings of the Royal Society of Medicine* 13:16-19 (1920).

439 H.A. Condon and E. Gilchrist, "Stanley Rowbotham. Twentieth century pioneer anaesthetist," *Anaesthesia* 41: (1) 46-52 (1986).

440 A.E. Guedel and R.M. Waters, "A new intratracheal catheter," *Current Research in Anesthesia and Analgesia* 7:238-9 (1928).

441 Ralph M. Waters, "Clinical scope and utility of carbon dioxide filtration in inhalation anesthesia," *Anesthesia and Analgesia* 3:20-22 (1924).

442 Brian C. Sword, "The closed circle method of administration of gas anesthesia," *Anesthesia and Analgesia* 9:198 (1930).

443 J.W. Gale and Ralph M Waters, "Closed endobronchial anesthesia in thoracic surgery: preliminary report," *Current Research in Anesthesia and Analgesia* 11:283-7 (1934).

444 Henry K. Beecher and D.P. Todd, "A study of deaths associated with anesthesia and surgery," *Annals of Surgery*, 140:2-34 (1954).

445 E. Randall Griffith and G.E. Johnson, "The use of curare in general anesthesia," *Anesthesiology* 3:418-20 (1942).

446 Thandla Raghavendra, "Neuromuscular blocking drugs: discovery and development," *Journal of the Royal Society of Medicine* 95:363-367 (2002).

447 Henry K. Beecher and Mark D. Altschule, *Medicine at Harvard. The First Three Hundred Years,* University Press of New England (1977).

448 Richard S. Atkinson and Thomas B. Boulton Eds., *The History of Anaesthesia* , Parthenon Publishing Group, page 221-2 (1989).

449 J.P. Bunker, et al, Eds. *National Halothane Study: A Study of Possible Association Between Halothane Anesthesia and Post-operative Hepatic Necrosis.* U.S. Government Printing Office, Washington, D.C. (1969).

450 Lyman Brewer III, "Respiration and Respiratory Treatment. A Historical Overview," *American Journal of Surgery* 138:341-354 (1979).

451 AL Barach, J Martin and M Eckman, "Positive pressure respiration and its application to treatment of acute pulmonary edema," *Annals of Internal Medicine* 12:754-795 (1938).

452   L A Brewer III, PC Samson, B Burbank and C Schiff, "The wet lung in war casualties," *Annals of Surgery* 123:343 (1946).

453   L Rendell-Baker and JI Pettis, "The development of positive pressure ventilators," *In The History of Anesthesia*, Royal Society of Medicine (1987).

454   Cordell Bahn and Michael Kennedy, "Catheterization of the superior vena cava," *Surgery* Jan;73(1):115-7 (1973).

455   HCA Lassen, "The epidemic of poliomyelitis in Copenhagen, 1952," *Proceedings of the Royal Society of Medicine*, 47:67-71 (1952).

456   CG Engstrom, "The clinical application of prolonged controlled ventilation," *Acta Anesthesiology Scandanavia* (supplement) 13:1-52 (1963).

457   Block AJ, Ball WC Jr., "Acute respiratory failure. Observations on the use of the Morch piston respirator," *Annals of Internal Medicine*. 65:957-76 (1966).

458   Julie Fairman, "Economically Practical and Critically Necessary? The Development of Intensive Care at Chestnut Hill Hospital," *Bulletin of the History of Medicine* 74:80-106 (2000).

459   Charles J Carrico, C. Dale Coln and G. Tom Shires, "Salt administration during surgery," *Surgical Forum* 17:59-60 (1966).

460   G Tom Shires, "Shock and Metabolism," *Surgery, Gynecology and Obstetrics*, 124:284 (1967).

461   Francis D Moore, *Metabolic Care of the Surgical Patient*, Saunders (1959).

462   " Proceedings of the Conference on Pulmonary Effects of Nonthoracic Trauma," *Journal of Trauma* 8:623-983 (1968).

463   Francis D Moore and G Tom Shires, "Moderation," *Annals of Surgery,* 166:300-301 (1967).

464   David Ashbaugh, Boyd Bigelow, Thomas Petty and Bernard Levine, "Acute Respiratory Distress in Adults," *Lancet* ii, August 12, 319-323 (1967).

465   Ashbaugh DG, Petty TL, Bigelow DB & Harris TM: "Continuous positive pressure breathing in adult respiratory distress syndrome," *Journal of Thoracic and Cardiovascular Surgery* 57:31 (1969).

466   Thomas L Petty, "A Historical Perspective of Mechanical Ventilation," *Critical Care Clinics* 6:489-504 (July 1990).

467   Stanley J Dudrick, Douglas W Wilmore, Harry M Vars and Jonathan E Rhoads, "Long term total parenteral nutrition with growth, development and positive nitrogen balance," *Surgery* 64:134-147 (1968).

468   HJC Swan, W Ganz, et al, "Catheterization of balloon tipped catheter," *NEJM* 283:447-451 (1970).

21
Transplantation

AUTOTRANSPLANTATION OF TISSUE IS ANCIENT, GOING BACK TO THE REPAIR of amputated noses in India. Damion and Cosmas, the early saints and martyrs, were believed to have transplanted a leg from a black Moor to a white man and are often depicted in medieval paintings standing by the bed-side of a patient with one black and one white leg. In 1869, Jean Casimir Guyon reported the first modern example of transplantation, small skin grafts applied to a large open wound. Jacques Reverdin, in Geneva, got the same idea from watching burn wounds heal. Second degree burns heal, not just from the edges, but from islands of skin which arise in the center of the burn developing from skin appendages like sweat glands and hair follicles. Third degree burns are, by definition, deep enough to destroy these appendages and do not heal this way. A third degree burn will heal from the edges, but, beyond a limited area, they will never heal completely. The hair follicles and sweat glands that survive a "partial thickness burn" are skin-derived struc-tures and "de-differentiate" into skin again; this new skin spreads to fill the bare surface. Reverdin observed this phenomenon and, independent from Guyon, thought of skin grafts.

Eduard Zirm, in 1906, devised corneal transplants, removing corneas from cadavers and, benefiting from the cornea's avascularity, which pre-vents rejection, transplanting the cornea to patients blind from corneal opacity, usually scarring from injury. In 1890, William Halsted reported a series of successful skin grafts to close leg ulcers. In 1887, he performed the transplant of a dog's hind leg from one side to the other but did not report the experiment until many years later. Alexis Carrel, in 1906, reported transplanting a leg from one dog to another, then the trans-plantation of both kidneys from a male to a female dog.[469] His report stated that the animal was up and about, doing quite well on the eighth day. Two years later, he revealed that the dog in his earlier paper became ill on the ninth day and subsequently died. Following this experience (belatedly acknowledged) he switched his studies to the cat and per-formed *en masse* transplantation of the kidneys, together with the aorta

380 A Brief History of Disease, Science and Medicine

and vena cava. These functioned satisfactorily up to the sixteenth day, but all eventually failed. In 1910, Carrel summarized his experience and concluded that the technical challenge had been overcome, at least for the kidney. The long term failure of his efforts was, in his words: "due to the influence of the host, that is, the biological factors." There the matter would remain for another fifty years.

In 1923, two different surgeons were attempting to breach the barrier again. Dr. Williamson, at the Mayo Clinic, repeated Dr. Carrel's experiments with more modern equipment and methods. He was able to analyze the urine produced by the transplanted kidney and prepared excellent photomicrographs of the rejection process in the kidney. He reported that: "As yet we do not feel justified in attempting to explain definitely any of the observations that we have made in this preliminary report."[470] Dr. Williamson believed that blood groups, only recently discovered, had something to do with the rejection phenomenon and observed that some transplanted organs functioned much longer than others. The other surgeon working on the problem that year was Emile Holman, a surgical resident at Johns Hopkins and later professor of surgery at Stanford. Dr. Holman was treating a five year old child who had suffered a severe "degloving injury" (that is an injury that strips skin from the limb) of the leg. Dr. Holman recognized that the child was going to need skin grafts to close the wound and believed that the mother might be a suitable donor. He tested the child and mother for blood type and they were compatible. He then removed "151 small deep, pinched grafts" (tiny grafts snipped off, often by creating a series of bumps with local anesthetic and shaving the tops off with a scalpel) were removed from the mother's thigh and applied to the inner and anterior granulating(healing) surface of the child's denuded leg." Seven days later another 168 additional pinch grafts were removed from the mother's thigh and applied to the balance of the denuded surface of the child's leg." After three days the grafts were "taking," that is they were healing. Two weeks later, he noticed an extensive skin rash over the child's entire body. Thinking that this might be an allergic reaction to the mother's tissue, he removed the grafts and the rash subsided.

After digesting this experience he decided to try again with a twenty-eight-month-old child who had suffered severe burns. He applied grafts from three different donors and, after about a month, all the skin grafts were rejected. He noted that subsequent grafts from the same donor increased the rapidity of the rejection of the secondary grafts, but did not affect the rate of rejection of those from another donor. His conclusion was: "It seems plausible to suppose, therefore, that each group of grafts develops its own antibody, which is responsible for the subsequent disappearance of the new epidermis." He was very close to a major part of the answer.

THE BIOLOGY OF TRANSPLANTATION

In 1916, Lillie, demonstrated that cattle twins often share a placental circulation even though identical twins almost never occur in cattle. There are two placentas but the vessels often interconnect. When the twins are of opposite sex, the female is sterile and is called a "freemartin." In 1945, Dr. Owen, a teacher of veterinary science at the University of Wisconsin, observed that, when this occurs, each twin has circulating blood cells of two types, its own and the other twin's. Some of these cases of dual blood types persist, suggesting that each twin's bone marrow has been colonized by the other twin's marrow stem cells. This situation is called a "chimera" after the mythical animal with the head of a lion, body of a goat, and tail of a dragon. To survive, a chimera must be "tolerant" of the other twin's cells. A few years later, a woman in Sheffield, England donated blood and the blood bank lab had difficulty typing it. The pathologist, Dr. Dunsford, discovered that she had two sets of red cells, some type A, and the others type O. He called the blood donor and asked her if she was a twin. She reported, quite surprised, that she had had a twin brother who died at three months of age. She was obviously not a "freemartin," as she had several children; the cattle analogy did not extend to humans. With this case, and Owen's report, as stimulus, other similar cases were discovered.

In 1959, Woodruff, a transplant surgeon in Edinburgh, would confirm that chimerism in humans did confer tolerance when he exchanged skin grafts between a brother and sister, fraternal twins with two red cell types, and showed that they were not rejected.[471] In the 1950s, a group at Stanford experimented with chickens, performing skin grafts between varieties of chickens like Rhode Island Red and Plymouth Rock. The grafts took and the researchers concluded that the breeds must be close genetically. They were wrong; later investigators found that newly hatched chicks were "anergic," they accepted skin grafts that, when a few days older, they would reject. Drs. Cannon and Longmire, at UCLA, repeated the experiment, but also used older chicks and found that the age was the critical factor. The newborn chick had "natural tolerance" to grafts from other individuals. The task now was to figure out how to produce tolerance in an adult.

The Second World War was to give tremendous impetus to this work, as in so many other fields of research in medicine. The bombing of London produced a large number of burn injuries. The Cocoanut Grove Restaurant fire in Boston, in November, 1942, stimulated interest in resuscitation of major burn injuries. Nearly five hundred people died, many of inhalation injuries suffered due to burning upholstery in the closed space of the restaurant. One hundred fourteen were taken to the Massachusetts General Hospital in a two hour period, of whom thirty nine were alive at admission. Many of the dead showed the cherry red color of carbon monoxide poisoning and most had few or no burns. Of the living patients admitted, seven died during the first three days, all of pulmonary injury from inhalation of toxic gases. Many patients arrived at the hospital with minimal burn injury only to die of pulmonary insufficiency or carbon monoxide inhalation within a few minutes. All of the physicians involved in the care of these patients commented on the similarity of the Cocoanut Grove cases to the fatal cases in the Cleveland Clinic fire of 1929. In that instance, a fire in the x-ray department produced a cloud of toxic fumes from burning nitrocellulose x-ray film. There were 129 deaths, many of them physicians and nurses, in that fire, most of pulmonary injury. The film stock for x-ray film was changed to gelatin after that disaster. The burning upholstery in the night club produced a similar toxic gas and, in both instances, the pulmonary injury resembled that from phosgene gas, a war gas used in World War I.

The treatment of the surface burn, itself, was uniform, the occlusive method: covering the burn surface with a bland ointment and then sterile gauze or sheets (except on the face). After fluid administration to treat shock, sterile strips of gauze saturated with boric acid were applied. Intravenous sulfadiazine was given. The dressings were changed after five to ten days and the boric acid gauze was replaced. For third degree burns, wet dressings containing boric acid were used until skin grafts could be applied. They did not debride (remove dead tissue)or cleanse the burn surfaces even though some patients had come in covered with dirt or even feces. This approach had become popular after the experiences at Pearl Harbor, on December 7, 1941, where many burn cases were treated and the old methods of debridement and the use of tannic acid on burns were abandoned because of the volume of casualties. Topical administration of sulfa drugs was not used because systemic absorption had been observed and the blood levels could be better controlled by intravenous administration. Ironically, the treatment of burns would be revolutionized twenty-five years later by the use of another sulfa drug, sulfamylon, applied topically. Boric acid was used because it had been used successfully to treat *Bacillis pyocyaneus*, now commonly known as Pseudomonas, and these patients did not become infected with that organism.

Of the thirty-two patients surviving, only ten had third degree burns. Of those ten cases, nine required skin grafting. Severe burns occurred especially on the hands and fifteen hands required grafting. Backs and legs were also extensively burned in female cases, probably due to a lack of protection by clothing. Hands were treated with full-thickness grafts to preserve function. The results in these cases were excellent and an entire issue of *Annals of Surgery* was devoted to an extensive discussion of the care of these victims.[472] As a result of these experiences, and those at Pearl Harbor, survival of patients with major thermal burns improved. What happened when the burn wound was so extensive that skin graft donor areas on the victim were inadequate? In the usual burn case, skin was taken from one area, the "donor site," and transferred to the burn site. The skin graft is thin, called "split thickness" (because it leaves enough skin to heal the donor site), and is taken from the donor site using a dermatome. The method originated with Thiersch in Germany and is used today. If the burn is larger than the area available for donating skin, the second set of grafts must wait until the donor site heals, a period of weeks. The possibility of using skin from another individual to cover a major burn would be very helpful in the most serious cases.

In 1942 and 1943, Dr. Gibson and Mr. Peter Medawar, at the Glasgow Royal Infirmary, began a study of the use of skin grafts in burn cases. Dr. Gibson was a plastic surgeon and Mr. Medawar was a lecturer in zoology at Oxford. They studied the fate of pinch grafts used on burn cases, a study similar to that reported by Emile Holman in 1923. In their first case in Glasgow, two sets of pinch grafts had been used: some taken from the patients' own skin, autografts, and some from other people, allografts or homografts (these last two terms are synonyms). Their observations confirmed those of Dr. Holman, homografts were rejected. They also noted that a "second set" of homografts were rejected much more quickly than the first set from the same donor. Their final conclusions were: "The time relation of the process, the absence of a local cellular reaction, and the accelerated rejection of the second set of homografts suggest that the destruction of the foreign epidermis was brought about by a mechanism of active immunization." The rejection of homografts was an example of immunization, just like vaccination.

Following this introduction, Mr. Medawar returned to Oxford and continued the research, supported by the War Wounds Committee of the Medical Research Council. He conducted animal experiments and used a rabbit model to study graft rejection. By 1944, he had completed an extensive study of transplant immunology. He began to study younger animals, moving in the direction taken by Longmire and Cannon in their chicken study. In 1953, Medawar, Billingham and Brent published *Actively Acquired Tolerance of Foreign Cells* describing experiments in which allografts could be induced to take and survive on the recipient. In newborn or fetal animals, a transplant of foreign tissue caused the animal to become "tolerant" of the tissues from that donor. Subsequent transplants were accepted as if the donor were the same animal as the recipient. Mice were running around in Medawar's laboratory with patches of fur of different colors, from different strains, and they had no ill effects from these transplants. Actively acquired tolerance was not a practical approach to the problem of transplants in humans, but it identified the factors involved in rejection and how it might be prevented, at least in theory. In December of 1960, Medawar and Burnet, who had proposed the original theory of tolerance, were awarded the Nobel Prize.

THE ARTIFICIAL KIDNEY AND THE FIRST ATTEMPT

The first attempt at kidney transplant in man did not wait until the rejection problem was solved. It was a desperate situation. The British described a new kidney syndrome, based on war experience, called "acute tubular necrosis." It began as the "crush syndrome." This condition was seen in people who were trapped beneath the rubble in bombed out buildings in the Blitz. Often, the patients were alive and in only mild distress when they were found, but deteriorated after being removed from the rubble and taken to the hospital. In some of these cases the legs or other portions of the body were crushed and the circulation interrupted by pressure. When circulation was restored, the tissue seemed to produce toxic substances that caused shock, even when the patient was not in shock when found. Now these people could be kept alive with blood transfusion and intravenous fluids, but their kidneys shut down and they died of the toxic effects of kidney failure.

In Holland, a man named Willem Kolff was working on an alternative but it would be the 1950s before his work would offer a usable therapy. In 1947, a young woman was admitted to the Peter Brent Brigham Hospital after suffering a severe uterine infection that resulted in septic shock. She was successfully treated for the shock, but her kidneys stopped working and she went into acute renal failure with no urine output for ten days. Finally she became comatose and death was near. Dr. George Thorn, director of the medical service, asked Charles Hufnagel to try a kidney transplant. He had been performing animal kidney transplants for some time as part of his research on blood vessels. Dr. Ernest Landsteiner was the urology resident and Dr. Dave Hume was the surgical intern. Hume was sent out to find a potential cadaver donor and, when he found a donor, obtained permission, and they had removed the donor kidney under sterile conditions, they asked to use an operating room to perform the transplant. The administration disapproved of this irregular procedure and refused permission for the use of an operating room. The transplant was performed in a small procedure room at the end of the hall under the light of two gooseneck lamps. It was after midnight, since they had waited for the donor to die before removing the kidney. Hufnagel, Landsteiner, and Hume performed the operation, transplantation of a kidney, to the patient's antecubital fossa (the anterior surface of the elbow). They knew it would eventually be rejected, so they put it in a location easy to return to. The renal artery was connected to her brachial artery and the renal vein to the basilic vein. The kidney immediately began to make urine and the ureter was left to drain into a basin. The kidney was partly covered with skin and the rest with moist sterile saline-soaked gauze. By the next day, she was waking up as the kidney continued to work beautifully. After two days, she was alert and entirely clear mentally. After another day and a half, the urine output declined, rejection was beginning, and they removed the transplanted kidney. Two or three days later, her own kidneys resumed making urine and she recovered completely. The first kidney transplant in a human had been an unqualified (although temporary) success.

Chronic kidney disease was the ideal subject for the first attempts at transplantation. Kidneys are paired, act as simple filters, although they also have some more complicated endocrine functions, and are tolerant of the ischemia time between removing the donor kidney and connecting it to the new recipient's blood supply. Kidneys can survive for hours, if kept cool, and are often flown across the country to suitable donors. The first task was to find a way to treat chronic kidney failure so that patients could be kept alive while the problems of transplantation were solved. Patients with kidney failure are unable to control their internal environment. Fluid volume and plasma chemistry become deranged and the nitrogen wastes of protein metabolism cannot be excreted. The patient develops edema, called "dropsy" by the ancients, and the accumulation of wastes produces coma after a week or so. Most of these derangements could be corrected by simple filtering of the blood.

In 1914, physicians at Johns Hopkins University demonstrated that "dialysis" through a semi-permeable membrane could remove waste products. A semi-permeable membrane is one which will allow the passage of small molecules like sodium and potassium, but retains large molecules like plasma proteins. The blood was on one side of the membrane and a salt water solution approximating the normal composition of plasma on the other. The small molecules (plus water of course) could diffuse through the membrane and excess concentrations, mostly waste products, would equalize on both sides. The normal kidney does this at a microscopic level in the glomerulus, the basic structure of the kidney. In the 1930s, Dr McEwen, in Chicago, resumed work on the concept using a membrane made from a plastic material called "celloidin." The blood clotted and the celloidin didn't make a very good semi-permeable membrane.

Heparin solved the blood clotting problem. Cellophane tubing was being made for sausage casings and this proved to be usable as a dialysis system. Heparinized blood was pumped through cellophane tubing immersed in a bath of salt solution. Willem Kolff, in wartime Holland, first constructed a working dialysis machine, under the noses of the occupying Nazis. His first report in English was published in 1944, but went unnoticed during the War.[473] In 1946, he published a lengthy description of his work in Dutch, then English.[474] Kolff had learned about cellophane in 1938 from professor Brinkman, a biochemist. Brinkman had used cellophane to measure osmotic pressure, the force exerted by a salt solution confined in a semi-permeable membrane. It will absorb water until the molecular concentration is the same on both sides of the membrane or pressure is applied to the solution. Kolff constructed a crude dialysis device and found that urea, the principle waste product accumulating in renal failure, could be removed easily from blood. Then the Germans invaded Holland. He moved to a smaller town where he could work without German interference and, on March 17, 1943, he treated his first renal failure patient. Over the next fifteen months, prior to the Allied invasion, he treated fifteen patients with one long term survivor.

In 1947, Kolff visited the US, but he had given away all of his machines to hospitals for further research. In Boston he met Dr. Thorn, whose experience with Hufnagel's temporary kidney transplant had convinced him that acute renal failure patients would recover if kept alive with an artificial kidney until their own kidneys recovered. The Peter Brent Brigham Hospital built another machine from Kolff's plans and added additional engineering work to overcome problems with febrile reactions during dialysis. Dr. John Merrill had just finished his residency training and assumed a major role in the study of renal failure. A team of five men was assembled to work on kidney dialysis. By 1950, the Kolff-Brigham kidney was in use and they reported thirty-three dialysis treatments in twenty-five patients. The device was used on Korean War casualties and many acute renal failure patients survived as a result. Chronic renal failure patients were another matter. Dialysis machines were in very short supply when I was a medical student in 1965; the Los Angeles County Hospital had two machines. Kidney transplantation needed another look. In March of 1951, a transplant was performed in Springfield Massachusetts. The recipient was a thirty-seven-year-old man with chronic renal failure who had received several dialysis treatments on the machine at the Brigham Hospital. The donor was a man with cancer of the ureter. The kidney was normal and the decision was made to try to transplant it. There was, of course, no way to prevent rejection. The recipient survived for five weeks until the kidney was rejected.

David Hume, who had participated in the first human kidney transplant, now took over a renewed study of transplantation in humans with the first operation on April 23, 1951. Rejection still occurred although it seemed to be delayed in these chronically ill patients. They were placing the new kidney in the thigh to facilitate removal after rejection. Results were poor long-term until Dr. W, a twenty-six-year-old physician with chronic renal failure. His transplant was enclosed in a polyethylene bag in an attempt to reduce rejection but his postop course was complicated by bleeding, poor function of the transplant, and swelling and hematoma around the transplanted kidney. Three weeks postop, things changed. The kidney started to produce urine, his wounds healed, and he recovered his appetite and energy. He was the first patient to be discharged home with the transplanted kidney.

Renal function remained good, but his blood pressure began to rise until, nearly six months postop, he died of complications of the hypertension with a functioning transplant. His own kidneys had not been removed and they had functioned as a Goldblatt kidney, producing severe hypertension that could not be controlled. Thereafter, the recipient's own diseased kidneys would be removed. The autopsy confirmed the absence of rejection in the transplant. The reason why his transplant was not rejected is a mystery; the polyethylene bag may have helped, but it was found to be torn. Tissue typing was still in the future and perhaps the donor (a young woman dying during heart surgery) and recipient were an accidental match. That first series included nine patients, then Dr. Hume was called up by the Navy Reserve to active duty in the Korean War. Dr. Joseph Murray succeeded him at Brigham on the transplant team. When Dr. Hume returned from military service, he found there was no room for him at the Brigham and, in 1956, he moved to Virginia, where he became chairman of the department of surgery at Medical College of Virginia. There he continued his work on transplantation as he and his associate, Dr. Richard Lower, performed both kidney and heart transplantation.

Dr. Murray would eventually share the 1990 Nobel Prize for the success of transplantation. In his Nobel Address he mentions Dr. Hume briefly twice. Dr. Hume was killed in a plane crash in 1973. He had given a seminar at USC and, because of engine trouble, left his personal plane in California returning to Virginia on a commercial flight. He came back to Los Angeles to pick up his plane, but found that the weather was heavily overcast. He did not have an instrument rating and an instructor pilot warned him to wait for better weather or leave the plane. Impatient to get home and reluctant to make another round-trip, he took off into the overcast...and crashed in the mountains north of Los Angeles. The great pioneer of transplant surgery, who should have shared the Nobel Prize, died too soon. He has been forgotten like many others in the history of medicine. I had the pleasure of spending time with him during my training.

IDENTICAL TWINS

On October 26, 1954 Mr. R.H. was admitted to the Peter Bent Brigham Hospital with chronic renal failure. The unique situation with Mr. R.H. was that he had an identical twin. In 1950, a paternity dispute in England had been solved by demonstrating that skin grafts could be exchanged between identical twins. This work was prompted by Medawar's research on immunology and skin grafting. The staff in Boston first performed studies to prove that the brothers were, in deed, identical. Small skin grafts were exchanged between the brothers and were not rejected. The next issue was an ethical one: should a healthy person be asked to donate one kidney to rescue another? Also, was there any hereditary tendency for the second twin to develop kidney failure himself? On December 23, 1954 the transplant was performed, the first from a live related donor. The kidney was placed in the lower abdomen and the ureter implanted in the bladder. The patient's diseased kidneys were not removed. He recovered but his blood pressure, high preop, did not come down. Keeping the case of Dr W. in mind, the patient's own kidneys were later removed. The transplant team waited a year before reporting the success of this procedure. In the meantime, the patient married one of his nurses. The public, especially other physicians, considered the case a medical freak. By 1970, however, forty-nine such cases had been reported throughout the world. In 1957, Dr. Hume, at Medical College of Virginia, performed an identical twin transplant without the complications suffered by R.H. and others whose renal failure was due to glomerulonephritis. Unfortunately, although some of the concerns voiced before the first case proved illusory, those patients whose renal failure was due to glomerulonephritis (instead of infection or obstruction), an autoimmune disease, developed the same disease in the transplanted kidney. Mr. R.H. died eight years after the transplant from a myocardial infarction and had developed glomerulonephritis before he died. Eventually, the drugs developed for suppression of rejection of transplants from non-identical donors would be used in twin donor cases.

ATTEMPTS TO INDUCE TOLERANCE

Attempts at suppression of the immune response had begun with attempts to induce tolerance by injecting the recipient of the graft with material from the donor and these had uniformly failed. Whole body irradiation was tried in an attempt to reduce the pool of immune cells, but this risked loss of resistance to other foreign cells and overwhelming infection. Then, bone marrow transplantation was used, combined with whole body irradiation, to produce a chimera, like the blood donor in England. This technique has now been adapted to the treatment of cancer, especially some advanced cancers and leukemia. In the first case, advanced non-hematological cancer, the patient's own marrow can be used if it is not involved in the cancer; in the case of leukemia, another donor must be used and this is exactly what the early transplant teams were doing.

The animal experiments had not been very successful when Mrs. G.L. arrived in April of 1958. She had been operated on for severe bleeding from an abnormal kidney and, after it had been removed, it was found to be her only kidney. Dialysis restored her to good condition but chronic dialysis was still not possible in 1958. She was given whole body radiation, enough to destroy her marrow, and then given an infusion of marrow cells from eleven donors in an attempt to induce tolerance. A kidney from a child, removed as part of a hydrocephalus shunt procedure, was transplanted into her thigh. Mrs. G.L. was also infused with marrow cells from the donor. The bone marrow transplants did not seem to take and her white count was very low. The kidney functioned well, but she began bleeding from a low platelet count and died of hemorrhagic complications after one month. At autopsy, there was no sign of rejection of the kidney; the radiation had worked to prevent rejection but the patient could not survive it. There must be another way. Five more cases were treated this way in the next two years and finally the last case was successful. A smaller dose of radiation was used and the donor was a fraternal twin of the patient. Ten years later the kidney was functioning with only a single episode of possible rejection, treated with cortisone. Finally, drug therapy overcame the rejection phenomenon, but the story is long and complex.[475]

Recently, Dr. Tom Starzl, pioneer of transplantation (especially liver-to be discussed), has studied a series of early kidney transplant patients and concluded that tolerance can be induced in adult humans by careful use of immunological suppression. The key is to avoid complete suppression of the cohort of T-lymphocytes present at the time of transplantation. A low titer of these immunologically competent cells can become tolerant of the graft if tissue typing is close enough. Complete suppression, as is commonly used in transplants, results in regeneration of an entire new clone of T-lymphocytes and a need for lifetime suppression of rejection. Dr. Starzl has a series of transplant recipients who are alive with functioning transplants up to thirty-five years post transplant. Most of these patients are not taking immunosuppressive drugs and some have had no episodes of rejection in many years. Analysis of this unusual series of cases may lead to new approaches in transplant immunology.[476]

DIALYSIS AND CHRONIC RENAL FAILURE

The development of renal dialysis progressed slowly until 1960 when Belding Scribner, an internist and nephrologist in Seattle, invented a device to attach renal failure patients to the dialysis machine. Chronic renal failure patients require two or three dialysis treatments a week to survive and have any hope of normal life. Attachment to the dialysis machine requires an arterial catheter and a venous catheter, both large enough to permit the necessary flow rate for the machine. Scribner developed a silicone rubber catheter which had a small plastic tip that inserted into the vessel. The tips came in various sizes so they could be matched to the artery or vein caliber. The "Scribner shunt," as it came to be called, included two rubber tubes, two tips for the vessels, and a connector to attach the two catheters together creating an arterio-venous fistula. The high flow in the shunt (because of the AV fistula), when it was not connected to the dialysis machine, kept it from clotting. This solved the problem of connecting to the machine. When the patient came in for dialysis, the connector was removed and the two catheters were attached to the machine, arterial side to the intake and venous catheter to the return line.

The other major problem was a shortage of dialysis machines. In the summer of 1961 Seattle's "Life or Death Committee," an anonymous committee of seven (including one surgeon for technical advice) began meeting to evaluate applicants for the Swedish Hospital chronic dialysis program. Not all could be accepted since there were not enough machines. The committee chose the most deserving patients to be saved; the others would die. *Life* magazine ran an article on this committee about that time, preserving their anonymity.[477] At the time, mid-1962, only ten patients could be maintained on the artificial kidney for the entire city of Seattle and Seattle was the only city with a chronic dialysis program.[478] Eventually, the number of machines increased and Medicare, after 1965, began to pay for the treatment making it more available. Alternatives were devised that did not require circulation of the blood through the machine (using the peritoneal cavity as a dialysis system), but hemodialysis remains the main-stay until transplantation can be performed. Some patients, especially older ones, are not considered candidates for transplantation and they remain on dialysis for life.

In 1966, a group of vascular surgeons in Israel described a new method of creating a fistula to attach the patient to the dialysis machine.[479] An artery and vein at the wrist are connected, creating a true arterio-venous fistula. High flow through the fistula will cause the veins of the forearm to enlarge and the dialysis nurses can then insert large bore needles into the veins (two at a time) for dialysis and remove them when the patient goes home. This solved several of the weaknesses of the Scribner shunt. The patient had to keep the site of the Scribner shunt dry to avoid infection since the silicone rubber tubes acted as foreign material. The shunts were also subject to clotting in spite of the flow rate. The "Cimino fistula," as it is called, solved these problems and lasts much longer than the Scribner shunt. It is a little more difficult to construct and some patients have poor veins which never dilate enough to be used. Also, the patient has to have needles, big needles, stuck in their arm three times a week. Children, in particular, preferred the Scribner shunt. Other alter-natives have been developed and Scribner shunts are rarely used in recent years.

TISSUE TYPING

Tissue typing became an important part of transplantation technology as it became more and more apparent that some donors and recipients were better "matches" than others. Blood types were the first to be tested in the 1930s. Paul Terasaki, at UCLA in Los Angeles, spent a post-doctoral fellowship with Peter Medawar in 1958. They tried to prove that lymphocytes were the cells carrying the graft-versus-host reaction in chickens. Eventually Terasaki and others identified a series of antigens called, from the acronym Human Leukemia Antigen, HL-A 1, HL-A2, etc. By 1966, they had HL-A types on 196 kidney transplants. They found that short term rejection was not strongly related to HL-A mismatches but, after two years, chronic rejection problems correlated with the HL-A types and mismatches. The types were those on the surface of the lymphocyte, not the red cell. The class of match was described as "class A," "class B," etc., producing some confusion with blood types. Extensive tissue typing has improved long term success rates in transplantation.

TRANSPLANTING OTHER ORGANS

Liver transplantation is considerably more difficult than kidney for several reasons. First, there is no artificial liver to keep potential candidates alive while a donor is found. By 1960, dog experiments had shown the feasibility of the procedure. Rejection of the transplanted liver involves the portal triads, areas of the organ where tiny bile ducts and vessels are clustered together as they pass through the sheets of liver cells. The rejection process resembles diseases called cholangiolytic hepatitis and sclerosing cholangitis, suggesting that these diseases are autoimmune in origin. Early questions involved the liver diseases suitable for treatment with transplantation. Cirrhosis, usually a consequence of alcohol abuse, is common, but there was some question about the morality of replacing the liver in such an individual who might resume the self-destructive lifestyle. Similar questions arise with the more recent situation of hepatitis C, often related to IV drug abuse. Some cases of hepatitis attack the transplanted liver further complicating the matter. Cancer was an early indication, but immunosuppression produced a high rate of recurrence, even in patients with no evidence of persistent cancer at the time. In 1963, the drug treatment of rejection had progressed to the point that a trial series of liver transplantation was considered appropriate.

The first six attempts, by Dr. Tom Starzl, all failed for various reasons. Donor liver preservation proved to be a more difficult problem than with the kidney and this resulted in several of the early failures. Clotting also proved to be a more difficult problem than anticipated. It was necessary to shunt blood from the lower body around the liver area while the transplant was being performed. Several of the early deaths resulted from clots forming in the shunts used to divert the venous flow; fatal pulmonary embolus claimed three of the patients in the first series. Clinical attempts were suspended until 1967 when they were resumed. By 1969 there were ten living patients out of a total of sixty-nine attempts worldwide. By October 1970 there were only twelve survivors of 133 attempts. The early toll was high.

Heart transplantation would be shown to be simpler although more dramatic than liver and kidney and it began with a bang in 1967. Dr. Christian Bernard had studied in the U.S., at the University of Minnesota with Lillehei, before returning to Cape Town South Africa to practice cardiac surgery. He had published very little on the subject of transplantation. His first heart transplant case, Louis Washkansky, did not do well (he lived only eighteen days) but the world-wide publicity made his name famous everywhere. The second case, in December 1967, did have a prolonged course and eventually the patient died of coronary disease in the transplanted heart rather than rejection. It would later be found that chronic rejection in heart transplants resembles atherosclerosis rather than the findings seen in other transplanted organs. One year later the one hundreth heart transplant in the world was performed, an indication of the frenzy stimulated by the interest in Barnard's feat. By 1969, the mortality rate was still eighty percent but these were patients facing death anyway and enthusiasm continued. During the next thirty years improved tissue matching and better immunosuppression would reverse this ratio for all organs and mechanical heart assist devices would provide some backup for the failing hearts. Chronic renal dialysis would continue to provide a reasonable life for many renal failure patients although transplantation offered a better quality.

469 A. Carrel and C.C. Guthrie, "Successful Transplantation of both kidneys from a dog into a bitch with removal of both normal kidneys from the latter," *Science* 23:394-395 (1906).

470 C.S. Williamson, "Further studies on the transplantation of the kidney," *Journal of Urology,* 16: 231-253 (1926).

471 MFA Woodruff, B. Lennox "Reciprocal skin grafts in a pair of twins showing blood chimerism," *Lancet*; 2:476. (1959).

472 Oliver Cope, et al, "Management of the Cocoanut Grove Burns," *Annals of Surgery* 117:801-965 (1943).

473 WJ Kolff, and H Th Berk, Jr., "The artificial kidney: a dialyser with a great area," *Acta Medica Scandanavia,* 117:121-134 (1944).

474 WJ Kolff, *New Ways of Treating Uremia: The Artificial Kidney, Peritoneal Lavage and Intestinal Lavage,* London, W&M Churchill (1947).

475 Schwartz, R. and Dameshek, W.: "Drug-Induced Immunological Tolerance," *Nature.* 183: 1682 (1959).

476 Thomas E. Starzl, Rolf M. Zinkernagel, "TIMELINE: Transplantation tolerance from a historical perspective," *Nature Reviews Immunology* 1: 233 - 239 Perspective (01 Dec 2001).

477 Shana Alexander, "They decide who lives; who dies," *Life* Magazine November 9pp 103-123 (1962).

478 "Who is Worth Saving?" *Newsweek* Magazine June 11, pp 62-63 (1962).

479 MJ Brescia, JE Cimino, K Appell, BJ Hurwich, BH Scribner, "Chronic hemodialysis using venipuncture and a surgically created arteriovenous fistula 1966," *Journal of the American Society of Nephrologists,* 10:193-199 (1999).

22
Psychiatry

IN THE THIRTEENTH CENTURY, THE PRIORY OF ST. MARY OF BETHLEHEM, in London, opened a hospice for the care of the sick. By 1403, it contained six insane men, among other inmates. Eventually, the hospital, or asylum (meaning a refuge from the world), was given over to the care of the insane completely. In 1547, the City of London took over custody of the asylum whose name, by that time, was corrupted to "Bedlam." In 1733, William Hogarth, in his series of drawings titled "The Rake's Progress," depicted a scene in Bedlam. In the nineteenth century, it became less important as newer asylums, and some private facilities often called "madhouses," opened. Care consisted of little more than custody, as no effective treatment for mental illness had been discovered. In 1826, the total number of patients confined in such facilities was about five thousand, sixty-four percent in private madhouses.

A recent movie, *The Madness of King George*, depicts typical eighteenth century therapy for insanity, albeit modified to accommodate the royal patient. When King George recovered his wits, probably because of a remission in his porphyria, his physician, Francis Willis, a "mad doctor," was rewarded with a large estate in northeast England, which continues today as a hotel, called "Raven Hall," on Robin Hood's Bay. Phillipe Pinel, in his *Treatise on Insanity*, quotes Willis frequently and accepts him as an authority.[480] In France, King Louis XIV established two large hospices in 1656. Bicêtre was established for the care of men and Saltpêtriere was for women. Over the next century, they became asylums for the custody of the insane and were widely described as scenes of horror with patients in chains and subjected to flogging. Lest this be thought of as mistreatment of the poor, King George received similar treatment and his recovery (temporary) was attributed to this regime. Even here, the number of insane confined in these institutions was small compared to the population and the probable incidence of psychosis. In Germany, such institutions were referred to as "Tollhäuser" (fools' houses), because of the bizarre behavior of inmates and spectators were admitted and allowed to watch them. In America, towns built small houses for confinement of insane persons at town expense. Families often constructed cells for confinement of an insane relative in their own home and, in 1840, Dorothea Dix, a New England social reformer, found many such individuals confined in cells or chained to stakes. Some were in almshouses, but many were kept by relatives. A few asylums were constructed in the colonies and, in 1808, the New York Hospital constructed a separate building and designated it the "Lunatic Asylum."

The concept of therapy, rather than custodianship, is attributed to William Battie in England and Phillipe Pinel in France. In 1758, Battie wrote his *Treatise on Madness*, which attributed therapeutic value to the asylum itself. He advocated isolation of the patient from family or friends, and emphasized the curability of madness. In 1793, in revolutionary France, Charlotte Corday assassinated Jean Paul Marat (avenging Lavoisier inadvertently), that event the subject of another recent movie. This act set off the Terror, but the Jacobin government assigned care for her insanity to Phillipe Pinel who took over Bicêtre hospice. He is credited with removing the chains from inmates of that institution and, in 1795, doing the same for inmates of Salpêtriere. He replaced chains with straitjackets where necessary. In 1801, he published a book that advocated psychological treatment of the insane in groups. He used warm baths and occupational activity in his treatment. A student of Pinel, Jean-Etienne Esquirol, continued this approach and recommended a "therapeutic community" that included patients and physicians living together.

The Germans, typically, advocated an approach that included military drilling, and tight daily schedules of activities. The sense of limits and control that resulted from this regimen was actually similar to behavioral methods of modern times. The term used to describe pre-twentieth century psychiatrists was "alienists," those who treated "mental alienation." The therapeutic asylum remained the standard until modern anti-psychotic drugs appeared after World War Two. Unfortunately, the numbers of patients in asylums increased to the point that the reformers' dreams of therapeutic confinement became overwhelmed by the need for custodial care. The reason for the increase in numbers is controversial. Some of this increase may have resulted from a transfer of responsibility from families to the state. There may also have been an actual increase in mental illness in the nineteenth century.

One condition that did seem to increase was neurosyphilis. Treatment of General Paresis of the Insane is discussed a little later, but there is no question that it became more common. One problem in the interpretation of statistics is that tertiary syphilis produces its psychiatric symptoms after a symptom free interval of many years. The patient may not recall, or may deny in spite of his own suspicions, the initial presentation of the primary lesion leading to an impression of insanity unrelated to syphilis. A common symptom of tertiary syphilis is mania with grandiose delusions. Physical signs included tabes dorsalis, a degeneration of the spinal cord, with a characteristic high stepping gait and abdominal pain, called "lancinating pain." The end result before penicillin (or at least salvarsan), in any case was paralysis and death. The typical history, by which it is possible to estimate the incidence of neurosyphilis, is a middle-aged businessman (mostly men, city dwellers and prosperous enough to afford prostitutes in an era with no premarital sex with "nice" girls) who develops grandiose delusions, then dies paralyzed. By the middle of the nineteenth century, the incidence of tertiary syphilis in the population, based on these criteria plus records of diagnoses, was about six percent, an enormous number, millions.

Another cause of mental illness, increasing in the same period, was alcoholism. The distillation of gin began the problem in the seventeenth century and, for a time (before alcohol taxes), gin was cheaper than food in England. By the end of the nineteenth century, alcohol (delirium tremens) was responsible for about thirty-nine percent of admissions to Charite Hospital in Berlin, twenty-seven percent of admissions in Paris and fifteen to twenty percent of male admissions in the Royal Edinburgh Asylum. It is more difficult to analyze the incidence of schizophrenia, since the descriptions are not clear. Pinel, in France, and Haslam, in England, give the first recognizable examples, both in 1809. Young people are described as previously of "prompt capacity and lively disposition" whose "sensibility appears to be considerable blunted; they do not bear the same affection towards their parents and relations. As their apathy increases, they are negligent of their dress, and inattentive to personal cleanliness." The description, although attributed by the author to drink, is probably an early description of schizophrenia.[481] There are those who believe schizophrenia to be a new disease but it is impossible to resolve the argument from historical records.

The early psychiatrists all believed that the cause of mental illness was biological, and psychiatry and neurology were closely linked. Eventually this concept would lead psychiatry into several cul-de-sacs, including phrenology, the study of bumps on the skull. Another interest was heredity and families with a high incidence of melancholy (depression) were identified, no doubt accurately, as there is some truth to this theory. Beginning with Virchow, German pathologists became interested in brain changes in mental illness. Wilhelm Griesenger produced *Pathologie und*

Therapie der psychischen Krankheiten, ("Pathology and Therapy of Psychiatric Diseases") in 1845, establishing the core tradition of university psychiatry in Germany. While he conceded that recognizable brain lesions do not accompany all psychiatric diseases, he proposed that all mental disease is progressive, beginning with depression and progressing to more disruptive conditions with time.

Carl Wernicke graduated from Breslau in 1870 and, in 1874, demonstrated that a stroke in a specific section of the brain produced a syndrome in which the patient did not understand speech and spoke only an incomprehensible jargon. This area, the supramarginal and angular gyri of the parietal lobe, became known as "Wernicke's area" and the condition, Wernicke's Aphasia. He spent the rest of his life trying to identify other areas of the brain responsible for insanity. Wernicke-Korsakoff syndrome is a severe neurological disorder involving both behavior changes (and often mistaken for psychosis) and paralysis (classically of the eye muscles). Thiamine deficiency is the cause and it is usually seen in alcoholics. One of my medical students recognized a case recently that had been missed by the residents. His contributions to neurology overshadow his influence on psychiatry; he discovered cerebral dominance and described the symptoms of brain injuries setting the stage for Broca's work and the localization of speech centers.

In France, Jean-Marie Charcot, the physician who described the symptoms of biliary sepsis caused by common bile duct stones,[482] became interested in neurological disease and discovered amyotrophic lateral sclerosis (Lou Gehrig 's disease). The disease was originally called "Charcot's Disease" until the famous baseball player's affliction became known in 1939. Charcot's interest in neurology, in which he also described the consequences of loss of sensation in the lower limbs, Charcot joints,[483] led him to psychiatry. Because of his enormous influence in France in the mid-century, he produced a whole syndrome that probably never existed. He became convinced that "hysteria" was a major problem. He set out "iron rules" for what he called "grand hysteria." Most of these cases were probably a result of the powers of suggestion from stern physician to gullible patient. His theories were debunked at the turn of the century and the result was damage to his reputation. Another theory of etiology, especially of the suspected increasing incidence of insanity, which resulted in much harm, was that of "degeneration" in which families became progressively burdened with psychosis because of heredity. Emile Zola picked up on this theme in his novel *Germinal* in 1885. The notion of degeneration became an impetus to eugenics and finally emerged as a nightmare in the doctrines of the Nazis in the 1920s and 30s. In America, the trial, in 1881, of Charles Guiteau, the assassin of President Garfield, brought up the subject of degeneration as the defense testified that he was a victim of hereditary insanity. The result was pressure for eugenics and immigration control to keep out "degenerates."

PSYCHOLOGY

In 1850, Hermann von Helmholz discovered that nerves conduct electrical impulses and even determined their speed of transmission, twenty-five to forty meters per second. Galvani had demonstrated muscle response to electrical stimulation of nerves but had not studied the nerve conduction phenomenon. The next year, von Helmholz went on to construct the first ophthalmoscope and to study the physics of vision. He remained chiefly interested in physics and this work would be continued by his student Heinrich Hertz, who measured electrical conduction in air and in metals (and determined the speed of light). Wilhelm Wundt became his assistant in 1858 and it was he who continued the experiments on nerve conduction learning about reflexes.[484] Wundt, using nerve conduction speeds, began to map brain functions based upon reaction times. In 1875, he was appointed to a chair in philosophy in Leipzig, but he was no philosopher. He is considered the father of experimental psychology and in 1874, he published the work that established psychology as a field separate from philosophy.[485] In resistance to the biological theory of mental illness, a German physician named Emil Kraepelin became interested in psychology and spent time observing patient behavior instead of looking through a microscope (his eyes were bad). In 1882, he moved to Leipzig to study under Wundt and conducted experiments on the effect of drugs on nerve conduction and on patient mental reaction. He used morphine, cocaine, alcohol, caffeine, and other drugs that had been purified by the burgeoning chemical industry. In 1890, he moved again to Heidelberg to accept a professorship where he began to keep detailed records on his patients to follow the progress of their illness. In 1892, summarizing his experiments, he coined a new term, "pharmacopsychology."

With him at Heidelberg were two neurohistologists who were to become famous: Franz Nissl, who learned to stain the nucleus and other structures of nerve cells, and Aloys Alzheimer, who discovered the disease named after him in 1906. Nissl was an odd duck, a bachelor who worked from 7PM to dawn in his laboratory every night. In 1899, Kraepelin would describe "manic-depressive illness," the first of the products of his study of the course of mental disease. He and his residents would fill out a file card they called a "diagnosis card" on each patient as they were admitted to the clinic. The cards were constantly updated and eventually began to make sense with patterns emerging. In the 1893 edition of his textbook, he described "dementia praecox," producing the first complete picture of schizophrenia, the disease first described by Pinel. By 1899, his classification of diseases had rejected the biological model and assumed the form used by the Diagnostic and Statistical Manual of Mental Disorders of the American Psychiatric Association a few years later. For the first time, he was able to group functional psychiatric illness into two great categories, manic-depressive illness and schizophrenia, and to predict prognosis on that basis. If it was manic-depressive, the patient would probably get better. If dementia praecox (the term schizophrenia would be coined in 1908 by Eugen Bleuler), they would not. He had also categorized the organic psychoses (like syphilis) as well. His prognosis for dementia praecox was probably too grim, the patients do not all become demented as syphilitics are demented. Nissl and Alzheimer helped to end the sway of the biological psychiatrists; what they could see in the microscope was neurology, what they could not see was psychiatry. His ideas about the effect of drugs on mental disease would be largely ignored until the 1950s. Adolf Meyer was an American psychiatrist who adopted Kraepelin's model enthusiastically and took it to Johns Hopkins in 1910. He became the leading American psychiatrist and then, as his interest in psychoanalysis superseded his interest in the Kraepelin models, the greatest supporter of Freud in America.

FREUD

Sigmund Freud was born in 1856 to a merchant, Jacob Freud, and his third wife Malia. When Sigmund was four the family moved to Vienna. They were a middle-class Jewish family and Jews constituted almost all of Vienna's middle class at the time. In 1890, one third of students at the Vienna University, one half of the medical school faculty, and two thirds of the physicians in Vienna were of Jewish origin. Sigmund graduated from medical school in 1881 into this intensely Jewish middle-class community. His initial interest in ophthalmology, which led to his investigation of cocaine, waned and he studied neurology. He spent the next five years training as a neurologist and observed for a time at Charcot's clinic in Paris in 1885, just as Charcot was most obsessed with hysteria. In his early practice of neurology, he used the methods of the time including hypnosis, water cure, and electrotherapy.

In 1886, he gave a lecture on hysteria to the Society of Physicians of

Vienna, which was poorly received, but Josef Breuer, a busy family doctor, began referring hysterical Jewish girls to Freud for treatment. In 1895, Breuer and Freud published a book together, *Studies on Hysteria*. His first patient, named "Annie O." in the book, did not respond well but his enthusiasm was undiminished. Freud became very interested in the sexual element of the stories of these girls. During therapy, one of his early patients, Elizabeth von R., who had found her sister dead, recalled that she had previously wanted her sister's husband. She was feeling guilt because, with her sister dead, "Now he is free again and I can be his wife." Freud believed that this conflict had produced hysterical paralysis in his patient. He began to believe that hysteria and anxiety in other patients could be explained by early experience with sexual trauma and by adult experience with masturbation, sexual abstinence, and *coitus interruptus*, a common method of birth control at the time. At first, he believed that their fathers had molested these girls and the repressed memories of this seduction were producing their problems. After 1897, he began to focus on childhood fantasies of incest, rather than actual sexual trauma as the cause of neurosis in his adult female patients. He confessed to Wilhelm Fleiss, "I no longer believe in my neurotica," his seduction theory. Now, he believed that the stories of seduction were fantasies, arising in the erotic wishes of infants. This was the origin of his concept of infantile sexuality and the Oedipus complex. Some of these theories may have been stimulated by his own ruminations on his relationship with his father who had just died. He began to spend more time talking about sex with his patients, most of them young Jewish women in very conservative middle-class families. Pressure for revelation of sexual fantasies was characteristic of early psychoanalysis.

Another Viennese psychiatrist complained that Freud's patients knew in advance what he would ask them. That psychiatrist, Emil Raimann, added that, in working-class, non-Jewish, families in Vienna, there was plenty of sexual contact and even incest, but no hysteria.[486] In the cloistered families of Freud's patients, there was little chance of sexual contact but plenty of hysteria. In 1902, Freud started a discussion group to develop this new "movement." Dissenters were accused of "resistance" as though doubt was evidence of psychological pathology. Many early supporters and colleagues became skeptical of the focus on infantile sexuality that, by its very nature, made any objective analysis impossible.

Franz Alexander, a Berlin analyst, moved to Chicago and established a center of psychosomatic medicine. He expressed the belief of the advocates that: "You knew positively that... repressed sexual impulses were the main source of neurosis of the Victorian and post-Victorian Westerner, and above all, that sexuality was there from the beginning of life, and its objects in the infant were incestuous; you were right and the world was wrong." Freud described himself as an adventurer: "I am actually not at all a man of science, not an observer, not an experimenter, not a thinker. I am by temperament nothing but a conquistador, an adventurer if you want it translated…"[487] Many of Freud's followers depended on him for referrals and objective analysis of his methods was lacking. This was an issue for psychoanalysis that would shadow it until modern times. The other problem was, even if psychoanalysis could explain people's feelings and unconscious longings, could it cure anyone of mental illness? Freud confided to a colleague: "I often console myself with the idea that, even though we achieve so little therapeutically, at least we understand why more cannot be achieved."[488]

In spite of these handicaps, weak or no science and little evidence of success in therapy, his ideas took psychiatry on a ride for fifty years. The reason was probably the enthusiasm of the middle class for self-knowledge, the search for insight. American intellectual and social speech and thought is filled with Freudian concepts. Alfred Adler, an early immigrant, introduced the "inferiority complex" in his 1912 book *Uber den nervosan Charackter* ("The Nervous Character"). Freud had abandoned hypnosis in 1890, but public understanding of this new, powerful therapeutic method often included it. The movie "Spellbound," in 1945, gives a popular picture of a psychoanalyst (Ingrid Bergman) curing a war veteran (Gregory Peck) and incidentally solving a crime with hypnosis. The terminology of psychoanalysis has entered the language and is likely to remain in spite of the failure of analysis to cure anyone of mental illness. Early (1890 to 1920) analytic sessions were more likely to involve vigorous questioning about masturbation and *coitus interruptus* than the later portrayal of a silent analyst listening to a patient describe dreams or do word associations.

Carl Jung, an early favorite of Freud's, broke with him in 1912 over the sexual origin of neuroses. Jung, and his associates and students in Switzerland, introduced the concepts of personality type, introvert and extrovert, plus the other pairs of opposites so popular with radio psychologists today: animus and anima, male and female sides of the personality, etc. He also proposed a "collective unconscious" filled with archetypes, like the "earth mother," and symbolism. All of this is interesting and may even explain some aspects of personality. Does it have anything to do with psychosis?

Asylum psychiatry was already on the defensive over questions of crowding and unhygienic sanitation conditions. The older asylum doctors watched, with frustration and anger, the younger men abandon the thousands, if not millions, of psychotic patients in asylums for young neurotic women who were not mentally ill. Their life's work was being relegated to the past. Some of the young adopted the methods of Freud to improve doctor-patient communication, but others saw a popular trend (and paying patients) and rushed to join the bandwagon. Psychoanalysis had replaced the water cure and electrotherapy as a fad. European spas were quick to advertise the new "cathartic cure" before World War I. The war changed Freud's theories once again as he now argued the influence of two great forces, the life and death instincts, *Eros* and *Thanatos*. The irrational nature of the war and its causes emphasized these issues and increased the apparent relevance of Freud's concept. Eventually psychoanalysis invaded the asylum itself as young doctors tried new methods to reach the psychotic mind. By 1926, private practice of psychiatry in Europe was nearly synonymous with analysis, at least office practice.

The 1930s brought the Nazis who snuffed out the role of analysis in Germany and Austria and, largely, the lives of the mostly Jewish practitioners. Not only the practitioners suffered from the Nazis, mental patients were sent to the camps and gassed, even in countries occupied by the Germans. Rolv Gjessing, a Norwegian psychiatrist, became a hero for protecting his asylum patients from Nazi liquidation. He studied catatonia among Laplanders and became one of the first to recognize circadian rhythm and the effect of light on mood. He refused to report his success in German and, by maintaining his honor, relinquished the chance for a Nobel Prize.[489] In 1945, psychiatry was dead, literally and figuratively, in Germany.

In America, the "mental hygiene" movement and the concept of "mental health" brought the middle class onto the psychoanalytic couch. In the postwar era, America became the center of psychoanalysis for the world. Freud toured the United States in 1909, although he hated America and most Americans.[490] In May 1911, the American Psychoanalytic Association was founded in New York, where it would continue until 1932, when it was reorganized as a national association. In America, from the beginning, psychoanalysts had to be physicians, not the case in Europe since analysis had little to do with medicine. By 1935, *Fortune* magazine, of all places, was explaining, "The suppression of the sexual instinct in childhood pushed certain experiences and desires deep into the unconscious, where they reappear in the adult as neuroses." The piece was titled "The Nervous Breakdown." Psychoanalysis had taken over psychiatry. The movement was aided by the emigration of prominent Jewish analysts to America to escape the Nazis. Of 4,000 physicians from Germany and Austria who immigrated to the US between 1933 and 1944, about 250 were psychiatrists. One of those émigrés was Martin Grotjahn whose son, Michael, attended medical school with the author. Language barriers were difficult to overcome and one lecturer may not have understood why his use of the term "penis envoy" (sic) brought down the house during a lecture at the Menninger Clinic. The prestige of the émigrés, not to mention their energy and bravery, setting out for the New World on a minute's notice, made them very influential no matter their language skills. They also brought orthodoxy that failed to adapt to new information on the nature of brain function and chemistry. Ultimately, this would bring down psychoanalysis as a serious branch of psychiatry. In the 1960s, there were twenty training institutes and twenty-nine local psychoanalytic societies in the US. In 1948, young psychoanalysts ousted Eugene Kahn as chairman of the Yale University department of psychiatry. He had studied the genetics of schizophrenia but, as a biologically-oriented psychiatrist, he was now out of date. In the 1950s, the analysts ruled American psychiatry as they had never ruled in Europe. They wrote the textbooks and trained the residents. By 1966, one third of American psychiatrists had received psychoanalytic training and two thirds said that they used "the dynamic approach," code words for analysis, in therapy.

The problem was how were analysts to account for psychosis? In 1935, Frieda Fromm-Reichmann, ex-wife of analyst Eric Fromm, arrived from Germany. She coined the term "schizophrenogenic mother,"[191] that burdened the mothers of schizophrenic boys for a generation. She wrote, "The schizophrenic is painfully distrustful and resentful of other people due to the severe warp and early rejection he encountered in important people of his infancy and childhood, as a rule, mainly in a schizophrenogenic mother." This was the high point of psychoanalysis in psychiatry. By 1958, psychoanalysts were taking over mental hospitals. In 1956, Karl Menninger said, "The old Kraepelinian terms (the classification of mental illness) have largely disappeared." All mental illness could be explained by infantile sexuality. In fact, mental illness did not exist. Menninger added, "It is now accepted that most people have some degree of mental illness at some time." Classifications, and such matters as genetics and the natural history of manic depressive illness, were superfluous, or so Americans thought. The Europeans were aghast. The trouble was, the new method did not work. The analysts liked patients who were young, intelligent, educated, and able to pay. They had less interest in the poor, uneducated psychotic. They also displayed incredible arrogance. In 1964, a survey of psychiatrists was published (in *Fact* magazine) in which 1,189 of 2,400 surveyed concluded that Senator Barry Goldwater was "psychologically unfit to be President." None had examined him, or even met him.[492]

In 1962, I spent a summer with George Harrington, professor of psychiatry at UCLA and founder of what would become "Reality Therapy," a behavioral method of treating psychotic patients. He described his experience as a young Kansas medical student, working in a state mental hospital his first summer of medical school. His father was an analyst at Menninger and George was actually qualified as an analyst at age seventeen. He attempted to use analysis on the patients he encountered in the state hospital (all the psychiatrists had taken off on vacation the day their medical student relief had arrived). One elderly lady had psychotic depression and he got nowhere with her in a month of trying. Then the staff psychiatrists arrived back from vacation and sent Harrington's patient for shock therapy, which according to analytic theory, should have demolished her psyche. Instead, she demonstrated a lucid interval of several days, common in psychotics with shock therapy, especially depressives. His faith in analysis was shaken and would not survive many such experiences.

OTHER THERAPY

In 1887, Julius Wagner-Jauregg, a Viennese professor of psychiatry, wrote an article on the possible role of high fever in the treatment of psychosis. During his training, in 1883 at the Vienna Asylum, a female patient developed erysipelas, a severe streptococcal infection, and Wagner-Jauregg noticed that her psychosis went into remission during the illness. He speculated on the role of fever and suggested that it be tried in neurosyphilis. Fever was still poorly understood and its role in infection was variously thought to be part of the disease or part of the body's defense against infection. Wagner-Jauregg was in the latter school of thought. In 1890, Koch announced his new vaccine for tuberculosis, tuberculin, and Wagner-Jauregg injected the vaccine into several neurosyphilis patients in order to induce a febrile reaction. The theoretical basis for this treatment was a belief that heat would inhibit the spirochete. By 1909, he was obtaining remissions in neurosyphilis patients with tuberculin but suspended his study because of a concern with toxicity of the substance. In 1917, he obtained blood from a malaria patient intending to inject the blood into neurosyphilis patients. His plan was to infect the psychotic patients with malaria, then, once he had obtained the effects of fever on the psychosis, treat the malaria with quinine. On June 14, 1917, he injected his first patient, an actor, named T.M., who had advanced neurosyphilis, with malaria-infected blood. The patient sustained nine attacks of malarial fever over the next few months. After the sixth attack, his psychosis and convulsions ceased and he appeared to recover completely. After the ninth febrile episode, he was given quinine. On December 5, 1917, T.M. was discharged apparently well.

A year later, Wagner-Jauregg presented the results of nine such cases, the first successful treatment of neurosyphilis. Salvarsan, Paul Erlich's chemotherapy for syphilis, was useful in primary and secondary stages but had been unsuccessful in the late stage of neurosyphilis. Now, all stages could be treated with a fair chance of success. In 1927, Wagner-Jauregg was awarded the Nobel Prize for the "fever cure" of neurosyphilis. The method resulted in about fifty percent success, but was difficult and expensive. Of course, it was tried on every other form of mental illness without success. The coming of penicillin in 1943, finally ended (or should have) the scourge of syphilis, but the fever cure had contributed when nothing else worked. Patients who had spent years in asylums and were thought hopelessly psychotic, responded to the fever cure with remission.

Functional psychoses, schizophrenia constituting the majority of cases, did not respond to the fever cure and neurosyphilis was the only example of psychosis with an infectious cause. During the nineteenth century, various drugs, mostly sedatives, were used with little success. Henbane, a plant alkaloid that produces hallucinations, was used. Morphine and opium were tried. Hyoscyamine was isolated from henbane, in 1833, and, in 1868, was being used as a sedative. Hyoscine, another henbane alkaloid, and mandragora, extracted from mandrake root, have been used for millennia for "nerves" and, in the 1970s were found to be anti-cholinergics. They can produce hallucinations and were a common ingredient of "witches brew."[493] By the 1880s, they were in use for sedation of asylum inmates. In 1880, scopolamine, the active ingredient in hyoscyamine, was isolated and used to sedate manic patients thereafter. It continues in use as a medication for motion sickness today (in skin patches). The other popular sedative of the nineteenth century was chloral hydrate and there were many chloral hydrate addicts until newer drugs replaced it after World War Two. Virginia Woolf, famous writer and character in another recent movie, named in the title of the play and movie *Who's Afraid of Virginia Woolf*, was a heavy user of chloral hydrate in the 1920s. It became notorious as the "knockout drops" and "Mickey Finn" of gangster movies.

Another well known sedative was the salt of bromine, potassium bromide. It was discovered in 1826 in the ashes of seaweed. Initially, attempts were made to use bromine as a substitute for iodine but toxicity prevented this practice. Then the French discovered that bromine salts produced sedation. In 1857, a London physician used potassium bromide in the treatment of "hysterical epilepsy." By 1891, it was in widespread use and Paris asylums were using thousands of kilos per year. In 1879 Dr. Neil Macleod, an Edinburgh graduate, treated a patient in a manic state by putting her into a bromide sleep. He had used this technique, a large dose of bromide, to treat recovering narcotic addicts going through withdrawal. She went into a two-year remission, and then had a relapse of mania. He treated her with another bromide sleep of twenty-three days and, again, she recovered. He reported a number of such cases and the concept of drug cure of mental illness took hold although bromine was too toxic for wide use.

In 1903, Emil Fischer, the German chemist, modified a class of drugs discovered in 1864 and called barbiturates (after the inventor's girlfriend Barbara). His new drug was called "diethyl barbituric acid," or barbital. It proved to be an effective sedative. The Bayer Company named the new drug Veronal and it quickly became popular. The drug was used in mania for sedation and for sleeplessness in depression. In 1912, Bayer marketed Luminal, the brand name for phenobarbital, still in use for epilepsy. In 1915, a young physician named Giuseppe Epifanio first used phenobarbital for sleep therapy in psychosis, using the experience of Macleod as his model. By 1920, the same method was in use to treat schizophrenia. At first, there seemed to be an improvement allowing attempts at conventional psychotherapy. Unfortunately, there was a series of deaths from pneumonia, a serious risk of prolonged sleep. By the 1930s, however, there seemed to be a real breakthrough with induced sleep periods of twelve to sixteen hours per day. The psychoanalysts were, of course, scathing in their criticism of the technique and dismissed any benefit. In the 1950s, the method went off the rails at the hands of a Canadian psychiatrist named Ewen Cameron. He combined sleep therapy with a form of "brainwashing" using tapes to repeat subliminal messages to the sleeping patient. It was later learned that his research was supported by the CIA, anxious to learn more about "brain washing," the conditioning methods used on U.S. POWs in Korea. In 1955, he added shock therapy to the regimen, calling it "depatterning," a concept of rearranging brain wiring to break down the psychosis pattern. Eventually, he began using the method without patient consent and had to leave Montreal in disgrace.

SHOCK THERAPY

INSULIN

In the late 1920s, a young psychiatrist named Manfred Sakel, who was working as an assistant physician in a private sanatorium, noticed improvement in the condition of several patients being treated for morphine withdrawal. They were diabetic patients who had been given the new hormone insulin, just discovered in 1922. After going into hypoglycemic coma, a real problem when insulin therapy was still in a steep learning curve, they were no longer "restless and agitated." They had become "tranquil and accessible." He reported this finding in 1933 and speculated on the role of insulin coma in the treatment of psychosis. The same year Sakel, who was Jewish, returned to Vienna to escape the Nazis and accepted a post at the university psychiatric clinic with Wagner-Jauregg's successor. They began to treat schizophrenic patients with insulin coma and were astonished at the results. In 1934, Sakel reported a seventy percent rate of remission in fifty schizophrenics with insulin coma. In 1936, Sakel emigrated to the US and took up private practice in New York. His methods were not adopted in Austria, soon to be in turmoil with the *Anschluss*, but in the US and Switzerland, insulin coma became very popular. British psychiatrists, unenthusiastic about sleep therapy, adopted insulin coma quickly. By 1939, insulin coma was the first choice of treatment for depression and schizophrenia in Britain.

Joseph Wortis introduced it to the US. He was a young psychiatrist who interrupted his own analysis with Sigmund Freud after seeing insulin coma therapy in Vienna and he returned to Bellevue in New York to start an insulin unit. The therapy involved giving enough insulin to produce severe hypoglycemia, then reviving the patient with a glucose infusion into the stomach after twenty minutes. The mortality rate was about one percent. In some hospitals, longer comas were used, up to two hours. This was repeated and, after about twenty comas, prolonged "lucid intervals" would be seen, sometimes lasting for days. Convulsions did occur but were avoided, if possible. Eventually insulin coma had about the same rate of success as sleep therapy but with less risk.[494]

CONVULSIVE THERAPY

Soon after the first use of insulin coma, real convulsive therapy was attempted using a drug named metrazol. Ladislas von Meduna, a Budapest neuropathologist, became convinced from autopsy studies that the brains of schizophrenics with epilepsy showed differences from those without epilepsy. In 1929, others had reported a reduction in the seizure activity of epileptics who developed schizophrenia and some even believed the two conditions to be mutually exclusive.[495] Meduna wondered if the converse could also be true. Would epileptic fits affect schizophrenia? Camphor was a drug known to produce seizures. In January of 1934, Meduna administered camphor to a schizophrenic. The first patient, L.Z., heard voices and had a delusion that "people often wave at me." He had spent the entire year of 1933 under his bedcovers and the past four years in the asylum. During a two-week period, von Meduna gave L.Z. five injections of camphor. By February 10, the patient was getting out of bed, interested in his surroundings and eating. He had been hospitalized for four years. The published account did not include the additional information that the patient felt so well, he escaped from the hospital and went to his home, where he found his wife with her lover. He beat both of them severely and announced that he was returning to the hospital where he could live in "peace and honesty."[496] The patient was still well when Meduna left Europe five years later.

In January 1935, Meduna had treated twenty-six patients with ten showing dramatic improvement. Camphor had several side effects, including nausea and pain at the site of injection. Other drugs were tried, principally metrazol, until electroconvulsive therapy replaced the use of drugs.

Before 1938, Ugo Cerletti, professor of psychiatry in Rome, studied epilepsy and performed experiments producing electricity-induced convulsions in dogs. In 1936, he assigned his assistants to study the new insulin coma and metrazol convulsion therapies. The dog experiments finally produced a safe method of inducing convulsions without cardiac rhythm disturbances from the electrical current. Further experiments were carried out on pigs in a Rome slaughterhouse after they learned that the pigs were stunned with electrical current before being killed. With great trepidation, they treated their first patient, a young engineer found wandering in a railroad station. They began with a dose of eighty volts for a tenth of a second with the electrodes applied to his head (as they had learned from their dog experiments). The patient had a spasm but suffered no ill effects. They increased the voltage until he had a grand mal seizure. He awakened with a lucid interval. After ten treatments, he was discharged from the clinic with a complete remission. His wife reported that, after three months, he began to hallucinate again but he did not require hospitalization.

Electroconvulsive therapy was not a cure for schizophrenia but it did seem to improve the patient's functional state. By 1940, ECT, as it was called, was in use at Columbia University in New York. The patients did not fear ECT, as they had metrazol (because of the nausea and pain at the injection site), although doctors and nurses were nervous about it until they gained experience. It was a marked improvement over what had been the dismal prognosis for asylum patients before. Catatonia, a condition long believed to be a form of schizophrenia, is cured by ECT.[497] The psychoanalysts resisted the new technology although they did accept its use in depression since it reduced the suicide rate (from about twenty-five percent). They continued to resist the concept that it altered brain biology and insisted on some psychological mechanism such as punishment or pseudo suicide as the source of the effect. If the brain's neurons were the cause of psychosis, how could psychoanalysis accomplish anything? ECT and psychoanalysis were on a collision course. Resistance to ECT also came from real complications like fractures from the convulsions. The result was the introduction of curare, which paralyzes muscles, into medicine in 1940 as a means of preventing fractures during ECT. Curare, with a long lasting effect, was dangerous in its own right. In 1949, succinylcholine was introduced in anesthesia as a short acting paralytic agent to facilitate endotrachial intubation. It was then adopted by psychiatry, in 1952, combined with the new very short acting barbiturate Brevital, to prevent fractures during ECT seizures. By 1959, ECT was the treatment of choice for major depression. In the 1960s, the anti-psychiatry movement fixed upon ECT as an evil practice used by wicked psychiatrists to punish patients. Allegations of brain damage were made but never proven. Eventually, the anti-ECT movement acquired the trappings of a religious crusade.

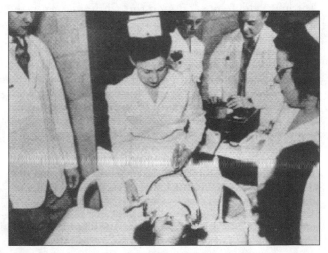

Figure 18 – Electroconvulsive therapy

Lobotomy

Trepanation of the skull, the creation of a burr hole (so named because a drill bit with a burr tip is used to create it), was attempted in the 1890s for relief of the symptoms of neurosyphilis. Drainage of cerebrospinal fluid did not improve the condition of the patients. Johann Mikulicz attempted to treat focal epilepsy by removing a portion of the cortex in the 1890s, but did not report his experience, presumably bad. In 1927, Egas Moniz, a Lisbon neurologist, described cerebral angiography, an accomplishment that brought nomination for the Nobel Prize but he was not selected. In 1935, at the Second International Congress of Neurology in London, Moniz attended a session on the results of ablation of the frontal lobes of a chimpanzee. He asked the presenters, neurologists from Yale, if they had any opinion on the effect of such a procedure on anxiety in humans.

During the following year, Muniz prompted a neurosurgeon, Almeida Lima, to perform partial prefrontal lobotomy on twenty patients in his asylum. His report of this experience describes "cure" of seven of them and six who were ameliorated. Unfortunately, he provided little detail on the results and, worse, his report prompted Walter Freeman, a Washington, DC neurologist to adopt his idea enthusiastically. In 1936, Dr. Freeman, and neurosurgeon James Watts, reported their first case and in 1946, they devised an approach through the roof of the orbit, the eye socket. They ended the partnership in 1947, and Freeman carried on alone, advocating this mutilating procedure and traveling around the country. There were two types of procedure involved: Moniz used two burr holes, through which he suctioned the white matter in the center of the two frontal lobes; Freeman advocated a transverse sweep of an instrument like an ice pick (he actually carried an ice pick around with him) inserted from below the brain via the roof of the orbit. In 1949, the peak year, 5,074 operations were performed in the US. Between 1936 and 1951, 18,608 patients were operated on (including Rosemary Kennedy, John F. Kennedy's sister).

The appearance of the psychotropic drugs in 1954 ended the lobotomy phase of psychiatric practice, but not before Moniz finally got his Nobel Prize in 1949. There may have been a few back-ward patients, too agitated for any of the primitive drugs to be effective, who were helped but, aside from this tiny subset, there is little excuse for the widespread adoption of this mutilating procedure. As a first year medical student, I examined patients who had received prefrontal lobotomies. In the few cases I had personal contact with, none of the patients was capable of life

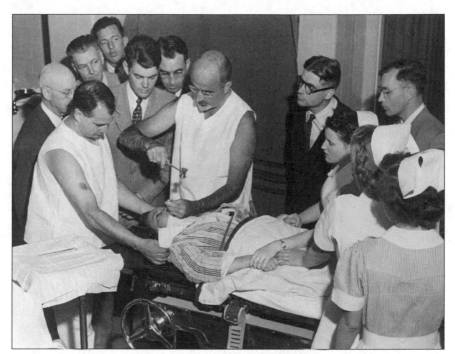

Figure 19 – Freeman performing lobotomy in 1949.

outside of an institution. My small personal experience with electrocon-vulsive therapy, ECT, was completely different and these patients, actively psychotic the morning of the treatment, had lucid intervals, with no evidence of psychosis, lasting for hours to a few days after the ECT.

PSYCHOTROPIC DRUGS

The second era of brain biology began with the identification of the first neurotransmitter, acetylcholine. Otto Loewi discovered it in 1926, after five years' work. His discovery came to him as the result of a dream in 1921. He removed the heart from a frog, placed it in a dish of culture medium and then added the "juice" from the vagus nerve, which he called *vagusstoff*. The heart slowed its beating after addition of the vagus juice. If he blocked the fluid from reaching the heart, vagus stimulation produced no slowing. He had proven the existence of chemical transmission of nerve impulses. Adolf Baeyer had synthesized acetylcholine in 1865. Now, Loewi had shown it to be a natural compound.[498] In the 1930s, acetylcholine was actually given to schizophrenic patients in hopes that it might improve their condition, but there was no effect. Asylum psychiatrists conducted what seem now to have been bizarre and, possibly, cruel experiments in hopes of finding something that worked. In 1949, John Eccles demonstrated that acetylcholine was important in central nervous system functions. A few years later, Curtis and Watkins, working in Eccles' lab, showed that glutamate was also a neurotransmitter.[499] More were coming but it would be twenty years before their work was accepted.

In 1951, Henri Laborit, a French Navy surgeon, began experimenting with a new drug that "potentiated" anesthetics. He had begun his work in 1949, while stationed at a naval hospital in Bizerte, Tunisia. He studied synthetic antihistamines as a way of blocking the sympathetic nervous system in shock. There was a theory at the time that histamine release caused, or exacerbated, shock. Histamine release will decrease blood pressure, but it has no role in shock, except perhaps in anaphylactic allergic reactions. Antihistamines had been discovered in 1933, but none had shown any effect on psychotic patients. The original antihistamines included Benadryl, synthesized in 1942 and soon noted to produce sedation. Antihistamines are considered over-the-counter drugs of minor significance today, but Danial Bovet received the 1957 Nobel Prize for his discoveries in neuropharmacology, including his work on anti-histamines.

In 1883, the first phenothiazine compound was synthesized from methylene blue, but the early molecules were too toxic for human use. The Rhône- Poulenc drug company had produced some new members of the phenothiazine family, in a search for new anti-malarial compounds, and Laborit noticed that one produced a marked indifference, not sedation, in one of his patients. He called this state "ataraxic." He later asked an army psychiatrist to watch some of these "tense, anxious Mediterranean type patients" while Laborit administered anesthetic and performed surgery. "After surgery, he agreed with me that the patients were remarkably calm," reported Laborit. The thought of trying the drug on psychotics did not occur to the psychiatrist. One of these first compounds was Phenergan, still used to potentiate narcotics and for preoperative sedation.

Later in 1951, Laborit was transferred to a physiology laboratory to continue his work on shock. The phenothiazines had not been as effective in blocking autonomic impulses as he would like and he asked the drug company for other variations that might be more effective for his purposes. The company produced a new phenothiazine, 4560 RP, which Paul Charpentier, the company chemist called chlorpromazine. Laborit began using the drug on surgical patients and noticed a greater "ataraxic" effect. In November 1951, he gave an intravenous dose to a female psychiatrist at the institute to test the drug for toxicity. She fainted and the psychiatry department would have nothing further to do with it. In early 1952, he reported his surgical experience with the new drug and mentioned, out of the blue, "These findings allow one to anticipate certain indications for the use of this compound in psychiatry." The surgeon was dragging psychiatry toward the greatest development in mental health history. He had convinced his psychiatrist colleagues at the military hospital (Val-de-Grace) to try the drug although they mixed it in with a series of other treatments, including ECT. At least it had not harmed the patients, but little was learned. In March 1952, two senior psychiatrists at the St. Anne mental hospital, one of whom (Deniker) was Laborit's brother-in-law, began using chlorpromazine on psychotic patients. In May, they briefly described their results, omitting any mention of Laborit. The psychiatrists, Delay and Deniker, have been credited with the discovery of the phenothiazine drugs and Laborit has been ignored until recently.

In 1952, a young woman intern at Ontario General Hospital noticed an anesthesiologist using chlorpromazine with anesthesia and later, when she began her psychiatry residency in 1953, she received permission to use the drug with twenty-five psychotic patients. She was a first year resident. In November 1953, still a first year resident, she reported "the remarkable effects of this drug" at a Toronto psychiatry meeting. Heinz Lehmann, at Verdun Hospital in Montreal, received samples of chlorpromazine from a drug company representative and used them to treat seventy-one patients. The results were astonishing. After a few weeks, many of the patients were symptom free. A few months later, however, he began to notice peculiar effects in some patients. "They walked with a peculiarly stiff gait (they had that peculiar mask-like face) and we said 'that looks like Parkinsonism,' but it did not seem possible because at that time there was no such thing as drug-induced Parkinsonism." They named the effects "extrapyramidal symptoms." The pyramidal tracts in the spinal cord conduct nerve impulses responsible for voluntary control of muscles. Involuntary movements, therefore, must be "extrapyramidal." The side effects seemed minor compared to the benefit derived from the effect on the psychosis, but they would become a major problem in getting patients to take their medicine when not hospitalized. Lehmann presented his results to psychiatry meetings and the revolution followed. The young woman resident, Ruth Koeppe-Kajandar, was also forgotten. All this work had taken place in French-speaking institutions of Canada or in France. The United States was going to be the toughest market, because the psychiatry profession was so dominated by the psychoanalysts.

Smith Kline & French was a small American drug company that had been mostly a patent medicine maker although it had also supplied the US Army with quinine during the Mexican War. It signed a licensing agreement with Rhône-Poulenc thinking that it was getting an anti-nausea drug. They had no research budget and marketed the new drug, which they called "Thorazine," as an anti-emetic (it is a very effective anti-emetic). No one in the US knew about the anti-psychotic effects. The medical director of Smith Kline & French happened to be William Long, a psychiatrist. He tried it on five psychiatric patients, the first of whom was a manic nun. The results were dramatic; the sister reverted to nun-like behavior. In 1953, the *New England Journal of Medicine* published the first American study, by Willis Bower. The result was a battle between the asylum psychiatrists and the psychoanalysts over the treatment of psychosis. The analysts lost the battle and the war. One of the first psychiatrists to use the new drug, Al Kurland, was so impressed that he mortgaged his house to buy stock in Smith, Kline and French.[500]

George Harrington was a young psychiatrist, having just finished his residency at Menninger Clinic, when the results of chlorpromazine treatment were first published. He had been in a severe auto accident and was laid up, at the time, in traction for a fractured femur. He was to walk with a limp the rest of his life. Here he was laid up, wanting to get started with his career and someone has discovered a pill that cures mental illness! As soon as he was out of the hospital and saw the extrapyramidal side effects of Thorazine, he knew that it was not going to be the end of psychiatry. He could still have a career. Still, the difference was amazing. "The wild, screaming, unapproachable patients [became] a thing of the past," wrote one staff physician. The effect was similar to that of penicillin on general medicine. It was not the absolute cure of psychosis but it abolished the cardinal symptoms and allowed therapy and something approaching normal life for patients. Henry Rollin, an English psychiatrist wrote that chlorpromazine "tore through the civilized world like a whirlwind and engulfed the whole treatment spectrum of psychiatric disorders." A cornucopia of new drugs followed, not all an unalloyed benefit.[501]

LITHIUM

A young physician named John Cade was studying mania, looking for some toxic product in the urine of patients (much as glucose appears in the urine of diabetics). He injected urine from manic patients into the bellies of guinea pigs. The guinea pigs died, but so did the controls injected with "normal" urine. He began trying to analyze urine components looking for something like urea or uric acid that separated the manic patients from normals. He mixed uric acid with lithium to make it soluble, an old observation about uric acid (lithium had even been tried as a treatment for gout in the nineteenth century). Carl Lange had even tried lithium as a treatment for manic-depressive disorders in the nineteenth century.[502] Its use was abandoned about 1900, because the uric acid diathesis theory of depression, which was the basis of its use, was discarded. The fact that it worked was not enough without the theory, a problem that would reappear from time to time. As part of his study, Cade injected a control group of guinea pigs with lithium alone and noticed that it sedated them. On a whim, the sort of whim that makes history, he injected some manic patients with lithium. First, he tried lithium citrate and lithium carbonate on himself to test for toxicity. Then he injected ten manic patients, six schizophrenics and three chronic psychotic depressives with lithium. It had no impact on the psychotic depressives, it calmed the schizophrenics a bit and it had a dramatic effect on the manic patients. Fortunately, he had tested it on mild manics, as it is not effective in severe mania. In late 1949, he reported his results.[503] The time was not good and no one noticed his paper.

In 1952 Mogens Schou, a young Danish psychiatrist doing research, was looking for a subject to study. The department chairman, Erik Stromgren, suggested that he conduct a double blind study of lithium using Cade's article as a basis. Schou had manic-depressive disease in his family and was interested. His trial confirmed Cade's work but still the profession ignored the implications.[504] Schou's study has been called the first randomized clinical trial in psychiatry and included both major elements, random assignment of patients and a placebo control group. The fact that his paper (the original version) was not in English may have detracted from its impact although it is now recognized as a major work. The psychoanalysts were still in charge of the journals and the departments of psychiatry in America. The first American study was carried out in 1960, and the Food and Drug Administration finally relented and approved the use of lithium in 1970. Why the delay? First, lithium is not patentable and there was no drug company (like the ones pushing chlorpromazine) trying to market the drug. Second, the drug was another nail in the coffin of psychoanalysis and the professors were all analysts. Thirdly, lithium had been banned in the US because of complications from its use as a salt substitute in 1949. Many young psychiatrists finally began to use lithium without FDA approval in a show of civil disobedience and this stimulated the eventual approval.

DEPRESSION

Chlorpromazine had little effect on severe depression and other antihistamines were studied. In 1954, the staff of Münsterlingen asylum asked the

Geigy pharmaceutical company for a sample of an antihistamine that they had tried as a sleeping pill. It had few hypnotic (sleeping pill) effects but they wanted to try it on psychotics. Roland Kuhn was a psychiatrist with some chemistry experience and, while an enthusiast for psychoanalysis early on, he had introduced electro-encephalo-grams (EEGs or "brain wave" studies) to Switzerland. His enthusiasm for analysis had faded after a disappointing experience with a young depressed woman patient. At first, his analytic therapy had seemed to bring her out of her depression, and then she returned in an obvious manic phase. He had mistaken the swing in mood of a "bipolar" (the modern term for this cyclic illness) patient for a cure. The discovery of chlorpromazine had given him hope. Now he was looking for help with depression. They tried a drug called G 22150; it failed to help depression. Kuhn then asked for another drug with a side chain identical to chlorpromazine, drawing on his chemical background. They tried the new "designer drug" on schizophrenics but it made them agitated. Kuhn discussed this new, unexpected effect with the Geigy chemists. Then in 1955, they gave the drug to a group of depression patients. The response was "absolutely incredible, so exciting." Kuhn, and the Geigy scientists, had discovered the first drug to relieve depression. The patients themselves spoke of "a miracle cure." Kuhn announced the new drug at the Second International Congress of Psychiatry in Zurich, in September 1957. He named the new drug imipramine (Tofranil) and classified it as a "tricyclic antidepressant." Chlorpromazine has an almost identical structure, differing in only two atoms. Other tricyclic antidepressants became common, with Merck producing amitryptiline (Elavil) in 1961.

The discovery of isoniazide's effect on tuberculosis in 1951 produced another family of anti-depressant drugs when side effects of the new drug were studied. Somewhat like the story of the oral diabetes drugs, the discovery was unexpected. Isoniazide, and its close relative iproniazide, are derivatives of hydrazine, a chemical rocket fuel used by the Germans in the V2 rocket in World War II. Both have potent effects on tuberculosis, especially in retarding the development of resistance to streptomycin, the primary antibiotic. Soon mental changes were noted in patients receiving the new drugs. The patients, in addition to improvement in the tubercular lesions, seemed to have mood changes unrelated to the status of their disease. A newspaper account described patients "dancing in the wards with holes in their lungs."[505] Iproniazide was found to inhibit the enzyme monoamine oxidase (MAO), a critical enzyme in dopamine and adrenalin metabolism. Soon, both drugs were tried on depressed patients with resulting mental stimulation and weight gain, both improvements. The mental effects of iproniazide were powerful enough that it fell from favor in the treatment of tuberculosis but isoniazide (which is not an MAO inhibitor) is still in use. Nate Kline, a Columbia University psychiatrist, received a Lasker Award in 1964 for the discovery of the MAO inhibitor family of drugs in spite of some controversy over credit for the work.

Eventually iproniazide was found to have a number of significant side effects, including the notorious "cheese effect," and other MAO inhibitors have replaced it. A number of cases of jaundice had already prompted the replacement of iproniazide with other drugs like tranyl-cypromine, a non-hydrazine based MAO inhibitor. Then, in 1961, a fatal subarachnoid (brain) hemorrhage was reported in a patient taking tranyl-cypromine for depression; seven more cases were reported by 1963. Primary care physicians prescribing the drug also noted a high incidence of headaches in their patients. A British pharmacist wrote a letter to the medical journal, *Lancet,* describing headaches suffered by his wife after she ate cheese. Initially, there was amusement at the pharmacist's letter but soon other reports prompted investigation and elevated levels of tyra-mine, absorbed from cheese, beans, and even beer, were discovered in patients taking the drug. MAO inhibitors have dangerous interactions with other compounds, including the tricyclic anti-depressants, and fatal blood pressure collapse occurred in some patients during general anes-thesia. The drugs themselves fell out of favor but research on the chem-ical family eventually produced the serotonin reuptake inhibitors. A flood of new drugs appeared over the next decade, mostly derivatives of the older families. By 1980, American physicians were writing ten million prescriptions per year for antidepressants.

NEUROPHYSIOLOGY AND NEW TREATMENTS

After World War Two, with discoveries in the biology of mental illness, the rate of progress increased. In 1934, Stanley Cobb founded the department of psychiatry at the Massachusetts General Hospital. Cobb was a neurolo-gist and continued the MGH tradition of cross-trained specialists. In 1965, every member of the gynecology department (there was no obstetrics at MGH) was board certified in thoracic surgery, for example. Alan Gregg, medical director of the Rockefeller Foundation supported Cobb's research with Rockefeller money. The result was the discovery of Dilantin, the first drug effective in epilepsy. In 1946, Cobb helped found the Society of Biological Psychiatry. Claude Bernard had suggested using poisons to study brain function in the 1860s. Kraepelin coined the term pharmacopsycholo-gy in the 1880s. The discovery of LSD (lysergic acid diethylamine) in 1943 stimulated some of this research, as it seemed to produce an experimental psychosis. Betty Twarog discovered serotonin in 1952 and identified it as a neurotransmitter. The next year, she and Irvine Page, of the Cleveland Clinic, identified it in the mammalian brain. The LSD molecule was similar to serotonin and this produced speculation about a role of serotonin and related compounds in the etiology of schizophrenia. The drug industry funded a good deal of the research looking for new drugs, especially after 1953. In 1957, Arvid Carlsson, at the University of Lund, Sweden, discovered that dopamine was also a neurotransmitter. In 1963, Carlsson gave chlorpromazine to mice and showed that dopamine levels changed. This brought up the subject of dopamine and schizophrenia. Did dopamine cause schizophrenia? Amphetamines, which potentiate dopamine, make schizophrenia worse.

In 1953, another discovery complicated the lives of psychoanalysts. Aserinsky and Kleitman discovered REM sleep[506] Using EEG methods they found that dreaming was accompanied by rapid eye movements (hence REM) and that this activity occurs in short periods of fifteen minutes separated by hour long intervals without REM. Others learned that this activity is found in all animals. What was going on? Probably not what the analysts, who spent hours analyzing their patients' dreams, thought.

It soon became clear that serotonin was implicated in depression. This came from research on reserpine, the active ingredient in *Rauwolfia*, the compound known in ancient Indian medicine and named for the European discoverer (Leonhard Rauwolf) in 1558. Bernard Brodie, at the National Heart Institute, was interested in hypertension and reserpine was the first effective drug for the treatment of hypertension. When President Roosevelt died of a hypertension-related stroke in 1945, the only effective treatment for high blood pressure (outside of India) was bed rest. Missy LeHand, Roosevelt's private secretary was treated for hypertension by being put at bed rest for several weeks, in the early 1940s, not very practical therapy for a U.S. President in the midst of a war. When reserpine was given to animals, serotonin vanished from the tissue, including the brain.[507] Depression was a known side effect of reserpine therapy. When I was a teenager, my dentist was being treated for hypertension with reserpine. He began to warn his patients that he would occasionally burst into tears while he was drilling teeth. In 1960, when English scientists gave imipramine to depressed patients, their blood levels of serotonin dropped precipitously. This began the study of what came to be called the "reuptake mechanism." Arvid Carlsson unraveled the mystery of where the serotonin was going in 1968, and demonstrated that the tricyclic anti-depressants prevented neurons from taking back the serotonin they had released into the nerve synapse. If the serotonin remained in the synapse, depression was reduced. This was the beginning of the "serotonin hypothesis" of depression.[508,509]

The mechanism of nerve transmission was being uncovered in this research. Maybe dopamine was also involved in carrying the nerve impulses in the brain. Paul Erlich used the concept of "receptor" in thinking about why organic dyes stained some structures (bacteria, white blood cells) and not others. The concept of a specific receptor gained validity from studies of organic molecules that show biologic activity in one isomere (spatial arrangement of a crystal or molecule) such as the rotation of polarized light by the two isomers of tartaric acid discovered by Pasteur. Atropine has two isomers, a D-form and an L-form. They have different effects. Only a specific receptor for the molecule would be so discriminating. Carlsson found that reserpine depleted both serotonin and norepinephrine from the nerve endings. Reserpine makes rabbits sleepy and both compounds are depleted. Giving the sedated rabbits norepinephrine does not restore them to normal. Giving serotonin does no good either. When Carlsson gave rabbits L-dopa, a precursor of both dopamine and norepinephrine, they quickly recovered. D-dopa has no effect. He concluded that dopamine may be the neurotransmitter depleted by reserpine and further research showed this to be true. He also noted that reserpine can cause a state similar to Parkinson's disease.[510] In 1974, Solomon Snyder of Johns Hopkins, discovered that chlorpromazine attaches itself to the dopamine receptor on the neuron and prevents dopamine from acting. It is a dopamine blocker. That blockage of dopamine effect is the cause of the extrapyramidal side effects that are so debilitating for patients on phenothiazines. This led, eventually, to an understanding of the mechanisms of Parkinson's disease, which is (partly) a dopamine deficiency disease. Later, dopamine producing cells in the brain (the "substantia nigra") would be found to be deficient in Parkinson's' patients. Carlsson's early work on this subject brought him the Nobel Prize in 2000. In 1967, George Cotzias used L-dopa in the treatment of Parkinson's disease with relief of some symptoms.[511]

Modifying the action of neurotransmitters at the receptor site was the mechanism by which the neuroleptic drugs (like chlorpromazine and presumably the others) worked. For a while, the concept of "one transmitter, one disease" stimulated research. The catecholamines, like adrenalin, seemed related to mood disorders. This was the "amine theory" of depression. Serotonin was added to the list of amines and dopamine was linked to psychosis. By the 1980s, this concept had collapsed. New drugs like clozapine had little effect on dopamine metabolism, did affect serotonin and were effective in schizophrenia for reasons that could not be explained by theory. They were called "atypical" drugs because they did not fit the current model. By the mid 1990s, over forty neurotransmitters were identified and at least six dopamine receptors, labeled D1, D2, etc. were discovered. The "typical" anti-psychotic drugs like chlorpromazine were D2 receptor blockers. Then two types of D2 receptors, D2a and D2b, were identified as the plot thickened. As evidence accumulated that the "atypical" drugs blocked other sites, the understanding of brain chemistry became more complex. At the same time, the evidence for schizophrenia as an organic brain disease was increasing.

In Japan, methamphetamines were widely used after the War. The Japanese army had used methamphetamines to prevent fatigue (US Air Force pilots have used them as well, and an accidental bombing in Afghanistan may have resulted). By the 1950s, Japanese psychiatrists were seeing patients who had developed acute paranoia because of methamphetamine overuse. In 1955, methamphetamine paranoia was proposed as a model for schizophrenia.[512] In 1958, Paul Janssen synthesized an amphetamine-blocking compound, named haloperidol. The first patient to be given this new drug was a Belgian doctor's son who had developed an acute psychosis. The initial dose was ten milligrams, later determined to be too high, but soon, on a daily dose of one milligram, he was discharged to his home. He returned to college, married, became a successful architect with children and, seven years later, his doctors stopped the drug. Acute psychotic episodes sometimes are followed by recovery and no one knew if the continued treatment was necessary. His physician father participated in the decision. Three weeks after the drug was discontinued, he was readmitted acutely psychotic. Renewed therapy resulted in remission, but he never had as good a response as the initial one had been. Haloperidol became a widely used anti-psychotic drug and recent studies have focused on treating young patients at the first sign of psychosis. There are even attempts to treat young patients who are not yet psychotic, but who show signs of high risk, in an attempt to prevent schizophrenia.[513]

Disorganization of neurons is found in schizophrenic brains and the changes seem to be due to embryological development. Epidemiology finally disproved the Freudian concept of the etiology of schizophrenia. Children adopted into families with an increased incidence of schizophrenia are no more likely to develop the disease than the general population. Conversely, children of a schizophrenic parent, who are adopted by normal families, have the same incidence of schizophrenia as those raised by the natural parents. This clearly establishes the genetic nature of the disease.[514] The "schizophrenogenic mother" was finally shown to be a cruel myth of psychoanalysis. Neurochemistry is trying to identify abnormalities in brain receptors and blood flow studies in sets of identical twins, in which one twin is schizophrenic, show consistent prefrontal cortex abnormalities in the schizophrenic twin. The normal twin does not have these findings. Positron Emission Tomography has been applied to obsessive-compulsive behavior, a classic case for a psychoanalytic mechanism. A feedback loop from frontal lobe to basal ganglia has been identified and suggests a biological cause.[515] The use of psychoactive drugs abolishes the PET scan loop.[516] Stereotactic surgery has cured a number of cases.[517] Psychoanalysis no longer has any scientific basis (if it ever had any to begin with) to explain mental illness (psychosis). Its vocabulary continues in common usage, especially in the conversation of non-medical people, in explanations of "normal" human behavior and it may have some role here.

THE LAW OF UNINTENDED CONSEQUENCES

THE DEINSTITUTIONALIZATION OF THE MENTALLY ILL

In the 1960s and 1970s, social changes and a general skepticism toward authority eroded the doctor-patient relationship. Doctors, themselves, bear much responsibility for this and that will be discussed in the next chapter. The effect on psychiatry was more severe and long lasting. The adoption of drug treatment for mental illness, even mild cases, eroded the only real benefit of the psychoanalytic methods. The close relationship between doctor and patient that was the chief virtue of the psychoanalytic model was reduced and the new chemical treatment of psychosis actually brought alienation (no pun intended) between psychiatry and the public. An anti-psychiatry movement gained strength from several developments in society. Michael Foucalt, a prominent French leftist writer, produced *Madness and Civilization,* a book which argued that the notion of mental illness was a social and cultural invention of the eighteenth century. Thomas Szasz, a Chicago-trained psychoanalyst, wrote *The Myth of Mental Illness* in 1960 and argued, like Foucalt, that the psychiatric theory of mental illness was "scientifically worthless and socially harmful."[518]

In 1961, sociologist Erving Goffman, who had served a fellowship at the National Institute of Mental Health (NIMH from the movie *The Secret of NIMH,* another blast [albeit an entertaining one] at psychiatric research), attacked the whole concept of the asylum. Goffman asserted the, by then popular, belief that there were no mental illnesses which justify involuntary confinement. These scholarly works set the stage for the fatal blow to the asylum system. In 1962 a novel appeared, written by Ken Kesey, titled *One Flew Over the Cuckoo's Nest*. The hero of the story, Randle McMurphy, was described as "just a wanderer and logging bum" who wanted only to "play poker and stay single and live where and how he wants to." The message of the novel was that psychiatric patients are not ill, they are just different. The movie, made from the novel in 1975, won five Academy Awards. A generation of university students learned the lesson: mental illness is a myth. There were opposing views. Joanne Greenberg, author (under the pseudonym Hannah Green) of *I Never Promised You a Rose Garden,* an account of actual mental illness, hated the Kesey book and said, "Craziness is the opposite [of imagination]: it is a fort that's a prison." She was one voice in a hurricane of contrary opinion.

The mental hospitals before 1960 had deteriorated and a 1948 book, *The Shame of the States,* by Albert Deutsch-a journalist, depicted all the horrors of overcrowding and underfunding of state hospitals. Still, this preceded the new drugs and things were unavoidably grim when the best treatment available was ECT and insulin coma. In 1949, an autobiographical novel by Mary Jane Ward was made into another devastating movie, *The Snake Pit,* starring Olivia DeHaviland. These accounts of asylum conditions preceded the anti-psychiatry movement but set the stage. Of course, there was no excuse for the poor hygienic conditions in asylums or the indifference of the staff. Worse was to come, however, at the hands of the reformers.

The final blow to the asylum was the new chemical treatment with chlorpromazine and its derivatives. In 1954, the Food and Drug Administration licensed chlorpromazine and the effect on psychotic patients was so dramatic that the pressure to empty the asylums became irresistible. Patients could live in community settings until the psychosis would just "burn itself out." A "Social Psychiatry" movement, which became prominent at the same time and which advocated group therapy and "therapeutic communities," increased the pressure to empty asylums. In 1955, the total population of state and county mental hospitals was 559,000. By 1970, it had declined to 338,000 and in 1988, it was down to 107,000, an eighty percent decrease in thirty years. The pressure to deinstitutionalize came from the anti-psychiatry movement assisted by well-meaning psychiatrists of the "therapeutic communities" school. "Community Mental Health Centers" were established in 1963 legislation (The Short-Doyle Act in California) but were never adequately funded to care for the acutely psychotic patients dumped on the streets.

In Los Angeles in 2000, sixty percent of the homeless population is psychotic; sixty percent are alcohol or narcotic addicts, and half of each group is both. Thus, ninety percent of the homeless population is homeless due to major mental disease (psychosis or addiction). The remaining ten percent, who are homeless for "situational" reasons, are transient members of the street population, living in their cars or using shelters for short-term problems.[519] The chronic "street people," living in refrigerator boxes and sleeping bags for years, are largely the individuals who would have been patients in the closed state hospitals or in state-supervised group homes. No matter what the disadvantages of the old asylums, it is difficult to sustain the argument that the mentally ill are better off now.

Psychotic patients in unsupervised settings do not regularly take the anti-psychotic medications that set off this drastic change in the care setting. One of the basic characteristics of psychosis is lack of insight, the inability to recognize the illness. I have talked to chronic schizophrenics who are taking their medication and they remember what it felt like to be "crazy." When they are not taking the medication that insight is gone. Part of the resistance to use of the medication is due to the extrapyramidal side effects, so even some patients with insight will stop the medicine because of facial twitching and muscle spasms. Eventually a new industry of private psychiatric hospitals arose to replace the state institutions for those who could pay. For those who could not pay, there are the streets. In 1994, 1.6 million Americans were admitted to psychiatric institutions; forty-three percent were in a general hospital, thirty-five percent in a state or county hospital, and eleven percent in a private mental hospital.

Psychiatry acquired another enemy with the rise of a movement called Scientology. In 1950, a science fiction writer named L. Ron Hubbard wrote a book titled *Dianetics* and proposed an alternative to psychiatry. In 1954, Scientology became a "church" and acquired a consultant, Thomas Szaz, the author of *The Myth of Mental Illness*. They focused particularly on ECT and, in conjunction with "patient's rights groups," succeeded in having ECT outlawed by twenty-six states, beginning with Utah in 1967. An appeals court stopped a similar California law in 1974. In the 1980s, several scientific studies (including a personal account by a well-known psychologist of his own battle with depression) supported the use of ECT in severely depressed patients and it has been rehabilitated for a few indications. The public perception remains heavily influenced by the negative view in the press, often abetted by the singled minded antagonism by Scientology.

Another problem for psychiatry has been a schism between medical psychiatry and clinical psychology, which denigrates the MD psychiatrists' use of drug therapy. Psychologists are not licensed to prescribe drugs and, while the psychology profession was largely founded to fill a role in psychological testing, the psychologists have replaced the psychoanalysts as psychotherapists, using "talk therapy." The psychologists feel a competition with the psychiatrists and a few have adopted some peculiar approaches, such as the "recovered memories" treatment of eating disorders and substance abuse, which alleges parental incest as the basis of the patient's present problems. Another has been the growth, now ended, of hysterical allegations of bizarre child abuse in day-care centers. A few psychologists "specialized" in extracting evidence from small children of improbable sexual experiences including surgical procedures which left no scars and, in the McMartin Preschool case in Los Angeles, of tunnels and "secret rooms" that could not be found when the school was demolished looking for them. The result was not the harmless endless dream analysis of the analysts' sessions, but legal attacks on hapless parents and day care center operators, some of whom are still in prison. "Recovered memories" have largely been debunked as another example of suggestion by therapists, but the damage done exceeded that of the seventeenth century Salem witch trials, which the episode most resembled. Psychotherapy, the talk therapy popularized by psychoanalysis, is useful in helping adults to deal with life stress. It has little or no role in treating psychosis. The serious mental illnesses are increasingly seen as biological disorders.

Psychiatry continues under attack as a cursory examination of the Amazon.com or other book selling sites or bookstores will show. Thomas Szaz, for example, continues to write successful books attacking psychiatry and the entire concept of mental illness. A search for "psychiatry" in such sites and in large bookstores will turn up a long list of titles hostile to scientific treatment of mental illness. In spite of this trend, research in neurochemistry and neurophysiology is rapidly expanding the knowledge of how the brain works. The understanding of psychosis will surely follow although successful permanent cure may be more elusive.

480   Phillipe Pinel, *A Treatise on Insanity,* pages 49-51, Facsimile Edition of 1806 English Translation. New York Academy of Medicine. The History of Medicine Series, Hafner Publishing Company, New York (1962).

481   John Haslam, *Observations on Madness and Melancholy,* London, Callow (1809).

482   Charcot's Triad- fever [Charcot's intermittent biliary fever], jaundice and shaking chills.

483   Joints damaged by repetitive injury with degeneration of the cartilage and articular surface. They are seen in diabetes and in patients with loss of sensation.

484   Wilhelm Wundt, *Contributions to the Theory of Sense Perception* (1858-62).

485   Wilhelm Wundt, *Principles of Physiological Psychology* (1874).

486 Emil Raimann, *"Die hysterischen Geistesstorungen,"* quoted in Edward Shorter, "A History of Psychiatry," John Wiley & Sons (1997).

487 Jeffrey Masson, ed. *"The Complete Letters of Sigmund Freud to Wilhelm Fleiss. 1887-1904,"* Harvard University Press, p 378 (1985).

488 Gerhard Fichtner, ed. *Sigmund Freud/Ludwig Binswanger: Briefwechsel*, 1908-1938, p 81 (Frankfurt/M. Fischer, 1992).

489 David Healy, *Psychopharmacology*, Oxford Press, page 70 (2002).

490 Freud ed. *The Letters of Sigmund Freud and Arnold Zweig*, Harcourt, Brace, p. 122 (1970).

491 Frieda Fromm-Reichmann, *Selected Papers*, ed. by Dexter M. Bullard. Foreword by Edith V. Weigert, Chicago and London: The University of Chicago Press. Second Impression (1960).

492 Stanley A. Renshon, *The Psychological Assessment of Presidential Candidates*, New York University Press (1996). This book describes the incident, which resulted in the "Goldwater Rule" of the American Psychiatric Association. The rule bans such "long distance" analysis.

493 David Healy, page 58-60 (2002).

494 Brian Ackner, "Insulin Treatment of Schizophrenia: A Controlled Study," *Lancet*, ii, pp 607-611 (Mar 23, 1957).

495 M. Fink, "Meduna and the origins of convulsive therapy," *American Journal of Psychiatry* 141:1034-1041 (1984).

496 Ladislas von Meduna, "Autobiography of L. J. Meduna," *Convulsive Therapy* 1 (1985).

497 M. Fink, "Neglected Disciplines in Psychopharmacology:Electroshock Therapy and Quantitative EEF," in Healy, *The Psychopharmacologists*, volume 3, London: Chapman and Hall (1996).

498 The story of Loewi's dream is in David Healy, page 200 (2002).

499 D.R. Curtis, J.W. Phillis and J.C. Watkins, "Actions of amino-acids on the isolated hemisected spinal cord of the toad," *British Journal of Pharmacology* 16:262 (1961).

500 A Kurland, "Chlorpromazine in the treatment of schizophrenia," *Journal of Nervous and Mental Disease,* 121:321 (1955). The story of him buying the stock is told by David Healy in Psychopharmacology, page 98.

501 See David Healy, *Psychopharmacology* for a complete description of the consequences of chlorpromazine and the anti-psychotic drugs.

502 Carl Lange, *Om periodiske Depressionstilstande og deres Patagonese*, Jacob Lunds Forlag, Copenhagen (1886).

503 John F Cade, "lithium salts in treatment of psychotic excitement," *Medical Journal of Australia,* 2:349-352 (1949).

504 Mogens Schou, "Biology and Pharmacology of the Lithium Ion," *Pharmacology Review,* 9:17-58 (1957).

505 *New York Times*, July 5, 1952, p 1:2 (1952).

506 E. Aserinsky and N Kleitman, "Regularly occurring periods of eye motility and concomitant phenomena during sleep," *Science* 118:273-274 (1953).

507 A. Pletscher, P.A. Shore and B.B. Brodie, "Serotonin release as a possible mechanism of reserpine action," *Science* 122:374 (1955).

508   Arvid Carlsson, et al. "The Effect of Imipramine of Central 5-Htdroxytryptamine Neurons," *Journal of Pharmacy and Pharmacology,* 20:150-151 (1968).

509   Arvid Carlsson, et al., "Effects of Some Antidepressant Drugs on the Depletion of Intraneuronal Catecholamine Stores," *European Journal of Pharmacology,* 5: 367-373 (1969).

510   A. Carlsson, "The occurrence, distribution and physiological role of catecholamines in the nervous system," *Pharmacological Reviews* 11:490-493 (1959).

511   G.C. Cotzias, M.H. Van Woert and I.M. Schiffer, "Aromatic amino acids and modification of Parkinsonism," *New England Journal of Medicine* 276:374-379 (1967).

512   S. Tatetsu, A. Goto, and T. Fugiwara, Kakuseizaichuudoku ("Psychostimulant Toxicosis"), *Igaku-shoin: Tokyo* (1956). Quoted in Healy (2002).

513   Yung AR, Phillips LJ, Yuen HP, Francey SM, McFarlane CA, Hallgren M, McGorry PD. "Psychosis prediction: 12-month follow up of a high-risk ("prodromal") group," *Schizophrenia Research* 60(1):21-32 (2003 Mar 1).

514   Michael H. Ebert, Peter T. Loosen and Barry Nurcombe, *Current Diagnosis & Treatment in Psychiatry,* Lange Medical Books. (2000).

515   Baxter LR Jr., "Positron emission tomography studies of cerebral glucose metabolism in obsessive compulsive disorder," *Journal of Clinical Psychiatry* Oct;55 Suppl:54-9 (1994).

516   Saxena S, Brody AL, Maidment KM, Dunkin JJ, Colgan M, Alborzian S, Phelps ME, Baxter LR Jr. "Localized orbitofrontal and subcortical metabolic changes and predictors of response to paroxetine treatment in obsessive-compulsive disorder," *Neuropsychopharmacology* Dec;21(6):683-93 (1999).

517   Sachdev P, Trollor J, Walker A, Wen W, Fulham M, Smith JS, Matheson J., "Bilateral orbitomedial leucotomy for obsessive-compulsive disorder: a single-case study using positron emission tomography," *Australian New Zealand Journal of Psychiatry.* Oct;35(5):684-90. (2001).

518   Thomas S Szasz, *The Myth of Mental Illness,* Harper and Row, New York (1974).

519   The statistics here have been provided by directors of shelters and acute treatment centers in downtown Los Angeles over the past four years.

23

The Economics of Medicine

P RIOR TO WORLD WAR II MEDICINE PROVIDED A MIDDLE CLASS LIFE, AT best, for physicians in America. Most had trouble collecting their fees and were sometimes paid with chickens or other barter arrangements. William Halsted once charged the wife of a railroad president $18,000 for a cholecystectomy, prompting outrage from the wealthy husband. Halsted replied that she had insisted on having the professor perform the surgery and that was his fee. Few others had such control of their fate. A family friend, a very successful orthopedic surgeon in Chicago in the 1940s, died leaving his wife with a huge, uncollectible accounts receivable list. For years, she had deeply resented seeing patients at social gatherings knowing that they owed her husband large amounts of money that he would never see. The city hospitals employed physicians to care for the poor, a practice beginning in the eighteenth century with the rise of hospitals, but private doctors in England and America were on their own until after World War II.

BISMARK AND SOCIAL INSURANCE

Otto von Bismarck established the first compulsory sickness insurance, in Germany in 1883. The motives for this very conservative man to establish this social program are the subject of debate. Germany had been united since 1871, a consequence of the successful Franco-Prussian War (started by France). There had been considerable social upheaval in Europe since 1848, when a revolution and accompanying rioting brought Napoleon III to the French Presidency, then to the throne as Emperor. Similar disturbances in Germany had forced Virchow, a political liberal, to leave Berlin in 1848. In Bismarck's *Memoirs* he gives one explanation; "The democrats will play vainly their flute while the people will perceive that the princes are preoccupied with their well-being." The fact that the first welfare system was established in Germany, and in a single stage, has also been attributed to the new unified state and its prosperity. Bismarck had outlawed the German Social Democratic Party after their 1875 union of Marxists and socialists. In 1881, a new law created obligatory insurance for work accidents. The sickness plan followed three years later with contributions by both employers (thirty-three percent) and workers (sixty-seven percent) being required. In 1884, work accidents were included in the same plan and in 1889 the first state sponsored pension scheme began (for which Bismark established a retirement age of 65). The funds were administered by the states (the Lander), and contributions were mandatory based on the employment of the workers. There were sickness funds based on employer and also on the city of residence so workers could choose between several. Those with incomes above a minimum level, set quite high, were allowed to pay for their own health care. Everyone else was obliged to join a fund. Rapid industrialization brought the social unrest but it also brought the prosperity that could pay for the plan. Belgium and Holland followed soon with plans based on the guild system, which was extensive in both countries. Austria adopted the German system very quickly (1888) as an answer to Marxist complaints about the economic problems of the poor.

Sweden and Norway

The Scandanavian countries were later in adopting the Industrial Revolution. These societies had a long tradition of communal living and care of the sick was the responsibility of the church until the sixteenth century when the state, as part of the Reformation, appropriated its property. With the property came the responsibility for the care of the poor and sick. During the eighteenth century, the King of Sweden decreed that the local parish must "sustain its sick and support its poor." The first Swedish hospital, Serafimer Hospital, was built in 1752 in Stockholm. By 1800, there were twenty-one hospitals in Sweden and the counties assumed responsibility for the sick while the parishes continued to care for the poor. Formal County Councils were established in 1862, and taxes supported the system. There has never been a significant private health care system in Sweden and in 1969, there were only two private hospitals in the country. Social solidarity has always been a major concern of Swedish society and "rich" regions have supported "poor" regions since the medieval period. In 1913, a mandatory insurance program was instituted, beginning with the old age pension. Health insurance was added to the program in 1955 and the trade unions were involved in the insurance program since Sweden has always had a very high percentage of workers enrolled in unions. This program has resulted in high taxes but is supported by a population that is unusually homogeneous.[520]

Norway has a similar history of mutual assistance and the added influence of geography, which results in a large part of the population living in small, isolated villages. The government has provided health care for its citizens for 400 years. In 1857, after a series of epidemics (leprosy in particular), the "Norwegian General Health Act" was proposed and, in 1860, passed. The local community was given the responsibility for local health care and the power to levy taxes for implementation. With the increasing sophistication of medicine, the government passed obligatory health insurance, for those below a certain income, in 1911. Health care is a right. Lodges and labor unions provided private insurance programs until 1953 when ninety percent of the population was covered. In 1956, automatic health insurance was provided for the entire population. This does not pay the entire cost; there is some patient responsibility. Hospital care is free for all, however. Maternity benefits even cover the taxi ride to the hospital. Transportation benefits are an important part of the program since much of the population is at some distance from hospitals.[521]

THE NATIONAL HEALTH SERVICE

France never adopted the Bismarck system, although some industries like railroads had their own health and pension plans. England eventually adopted another model following World War II. "The Beveridge Report," by Sir William Beveridge in 1942, advocated a new principle. Where the German system covered workers through employment and mandatory contributions, the English plan would provide state payment for medical services for everyone, worker or not. Certainly, the ravages of the war, especially among the poor who bore the brunt of the Blitz in London, prompted a new approach. Before the war, there had been some effort on health care of poor children but the English never had a good public hospital system as existed in most of the United States.

Application of the Poor Laws[522] had stimulated some provision of health services and, by 1939, many of the most affluent and progressive local authorities (towns and rural districts) were providing something close to comprehensive services.

The Dawson Report in the 1920s, proposed a national comprehensive program of health centers and a National Health Insurance scheme provided some coverage. The NHI, as it was called, was established in 1911 and provided minimal care for the poor who contributed weekly income deductions. Those too poor to contribute were not eligible. The Local Government Act of 1929 attempted a rationalization of the system but, before the War, England had the least effective system for health services of any developed country. In particular, the Dawson Report lamented the rivalry between the voluntary hospital system, many of whose members were teaching hospitals, and the public hospital system. There were 1,000 voluntary (private) hospitals and 3,000 public hospitals, which were run by local health authorities.

The War led to the Emergency Medical Service (EMS) program, a civil defense system that brought all hospitals under a single national administration. "The *Luftwaffe* achieved in two months what had defeated politicians and planners for at least two decades," says a recent history of the National Health Service.[523] The anticipated devastation from aerial bombing that stimulated this emergency program mercifully failed to materialize. In 1941, as the worst of the Battle of Britain was ebbing, the Political and Economic Planning (PEP) group, a social science lobby, advocated immediate conversion of the EMS system into a National Hospital Service.[524] Promises were made in response to this initiative and the Beveridge Report followed. The government issued a White Paper in 1944, *A National Health Service*, which the medical associations and the voluntary hospital association heavily criticized.

The election of the Labour government in 1945 brought Aneurin Bevan, a radical member of Labour (often described as a "leftist political maverick"), to the position of Minister of Health. Bevan's proposal was for a nationalized and regionalized (for administration) hospital service. On March 21 1946, Bevan introduced the National Health Service Bill to Parliament and, on November 6, it passed with minimal amendment. The new program had a three-fold administration plan. Hospitals, public health agencies and independent contractors (general practitioners) would each have their own administration. For hospitals, fourteen Regional Hospital Boards (representing fourteen natural hospital "catchment areas") would delegate local administration to District Committees while the Regional Board would control strategic planning and budgets. Major teaching hospitals would be grouped in the regional system but would preserve most of their independence and their own Governing Boards (except for Scotland, which integrated them into the regional system from the start). Local authorities (called Local Health Authorities-LHAs) remained in control of district nursing, school health and ambulance services.

The British Medical Association (largely dominated by GPs as is the American Medical Association) objected strongly to any attempt to place the GPs on salary or to prevent the purchase and sale of practices. The BMA became the chief opponent of the new program after a member survey it conducted recorded an eighty-eight percent disapproval rate. The voluntary hospitals were allowed to retain private beds and, relieved to be free of the local control, acquiesced to the plan. Consultants, the medical specialists, had long been in favor of regionalization. They had cared for charity patients without payment in return for access to private beds for paying patients in the same hospitals. The NHS offered them the opportunity to accept full-time contracts at a satisfactory salary or part-time contracts at a small discount, which would allow them to see private paying patients in the NHS hospitals. They accepted this with alacrity and the Colleges became peacemakers in the remaining disputes. Bevan announced that he had "filled their mouths with gold," referring to the generous terms of the contracts. Eventually a compromise was accepted. Sale of GP practices (the sticking point was the value of "goodwill") was a demand of older physicians but younger BMA members were less interested in this issue since they would be buying, not selling. The abolition of practice sale was upheld (creating a crisis for older GPs who had counted on this for pensions). The GPs insisted on a capitation arrangement in which the doctor receives a monthly payment for each patient on his "list" but no government salary. Finally, on July 5, 1948 the "Appointed Day" came when the NHS would begin operation. The great change from previous experience was the absence of "direct charges" and access to all services, without charge, for the entire population. The employees and contractors of the new service totaled 500,000 making the NHS the third largest employer in Britain. Hospital staffs totaled 360,000, of whom 150,000 were nurses and midwives.

It was not long before the same phenomenon I have described in the instance of diabetes treatment with insulin and the provision of chronic renal dialysis appeared. Demand far outstripped predictions. For the 1948/49 period, estimated cost was £268 million; the actual expenditure was £373 million. For 1949/50, estimated cost was £352 million, actual was £449 million. Finally, in 1950/51, estimates caught up and the actual cost was almost exactly equal to the estimate. Of course, the wartime predictions of the cost of the proposed service were far too low, £145 million, about one-half of the later estimate and only thirty-nine percent of the actual cost for the first year. The cost overruns created embarrassment and eventually Bevan resigned from his post as Minister of Health in 1951. The initial overspending had long-term consequences as some cost sharing (drugs, dental, eyeglasses and hearing aids, among others) was introduced and the NHS budget was frozen for years at about £400 million, leading to eventual problems with delayed modernization and queues for services. From 1950 to 1964, NHS spending increased at a rate of 2.5 percent in constant units and the service consumed about 4.1 percent of GDP in 1950/51. This share slowly declined in the 1950s although it rose again to the same level by 1964. The departure of Bevan from the Ministry in 1951 also led to its breakup into a Ministry of Town and Country Planning and a rump Ministry of Health that no longer merited Cabinet membership. This diminished status resulted in a high turnover of ministers and a decline in the quality of Civil Service officers. The growth of high technology medicine would aggravate problems with underfunding but control of expenditures was spectacular compared to later US experience.

In the 1970s, with a Labour government in power, unionized NHS hospital employees began to refuse to care for private patients in NHS hospitals. These patients had been allowed private rooms, telephones and care by specialists who were in such demand that ordinary NHS members had to wait for months to see them or to have them perform surgery. Now private patients would no longer be admitted to NHS hospitals unless they took their place in line and in the ward with everyone else. Harley Street (the London street where the outstanding specialists had their offices) was affected as many specialists moved their medical practices to Belgium. Private patients were welcome in Belgian hospitals and the doctors moved across the channel. A small scandal ensued when it became known that the Labour health minister, a woman, had gone to Belgium for gynecologic surgery.

Finally, in 1979, the Conservative Party returned to power with Margaret Thatcher and changes were made in the NHS. In addition, the Conservative government allowed the construction of private hospitals in Britain for the first time since the founding of the NHS. Medical specialists returned from Belgium, Harley Street regained its cachet and private medical care was available again. By 1995, about twenty-five percent of the residents of southeast England (the most affluent region) had private, American-style health insurance and were seeking care in private hospitals similar to those seen in suburban communities in the US. The NHS, itself, adopted a new system called "fund-holding" in which GPs or GP groups could function something like American HMOs, contracting with district hospitals, negotiating price for specific operations and sending patients to competing hospitals if service was not satisfactory. A medical practice website in London, looking very much like an American group practice internet site says: *"We are a fundholding practice. This allows us the freedom to choose the quickest and most effective hospital services for our patients. Since we became fundholding we have seen a dramatic reduction in waiting times for outpatient attendances and pathology results."* The practice is called the Westminster and Pimlico Practice, London, England and has a web site. Since the election of the Labour government of Tony Blair in 1997, some changes have taken place as Primary Care Trusts, with larger patient populations, have replaced fundholding as an option for primary care practice within the NHS.

AMERICAN MEDICINE

The US, in 1900, was much decentralized and the central government, with the exception of the extraordinary period of the Civil War, had always been weak. There were hospitals for merchant seamen and the Marine Hospital Service was expanded into the US Public Health Service in 1912. Socialism had little impact in the US and most health care was local and private. There were some union health programs; the Granite Cutters Union established the first union health plan in 1877. After 1896, insurance policies, covering specific diseases or injuries, appeared. Life insurance was an exception to this trend and many US citizens had "Industrial Life" policies, which would pay for a funeral. In 1911, Americans bought 183 million dollars of such burial insurance, an amount equal to the cost of the entire German social insurance system. American railroads provided health coverage for their own workers and families; the father of the famous Mayo brothers built the Mayo Clinic with a contract to provide care for employees of the Chicago and Northwestern Railroad. I was born in Chicago in the Illinois Central Hospital, established for employees of that railroad but open to anyone. The Santa Fe Hospital, which stood in East Los Angeles until twenty years ago, was staffed by physicians who had contracts with the railroad to care for its employees.

In California, in the 1930s, the richest physician in the state was the Medical Director of the Southern Pacific Railroad. The status symbol for local doctors was a position as a railroad physician, which included a free pass for Southern Pacific trains. In 1915, the American Medical Association met with the American Association for Labor Legislation, a group that had been pressing for a European-style workers health program since 1912. The negotiations broke down over the unions' insistence on per capita fees, much like the German model, while doctors, who had had bad experience with such schemes involving fraternal lodges and industrial firms, refused. The break up of the Progressive Party in the 1916 election doomed the prospects for a national plan of compulsory insurance. The unions were not interested in a universal plan but wanted something like the German program, which covered workers (about twenty-seven percent of the German population).

The entry of the U.S. into the War in 1917 ended most of these efforts. Many doctors, who had been interested in social insurance of some kind, went into military service and the entire concept was deemed, "a dangerous device invented in Germany." A health insurance referendum in California in November 1918, just as the War ended, was defeated three to one.

The Depression brought an era that should have been more amenable to social insurance. The priorities had changed, however; unemployment and old-age insurance had taken precedence over health care. The excellent city and county hospitals provided adequate, and sometimes superior, care in many cities. In Los Angeles, older physicians have told me, the County Hospital became a serious competitor for health care delivery in the Depression and private physicians denigrated the County Hospital to their patients, and potential patients, out of fear of economic loss, not out of concern with any deficiencies at the hospital. Los Angeles had spent ten years building what was probably the most scientifically advanced hospital in the United States and it opened on December 12, 1933, just as the Depression arrived. Its bed capacity was 3,500 patients for a city of 1,250,000. Even the founder of the American Association for Social Security advised the administration in 1934 to be politically realistic and to go slow on health insurance although he was later critical of the limited scope of the Social Security bill.[525] The American College of Surgeons endorsed compulsory health insurance in 1934, but the AMA was now bitterly opposed, even though the Depression severely impacted physician's incomes. The average income of California physicians fell from $6,700 in 1929 to $3,600 in 1933. In 1935, the California Medical Association proposed a mandatory statewide health insurance program. This prompted furious opposition by the AMA and Morris Fishbein, editor of *JAMA* and virtual dictator of the AMA, sent representatives to California to discourage the association from such a radical course. The association persisted but the Legislature turned it down as being too favorable to doctors (which of course it was).[526] In the 1938 Gallup poll sixty-eight percent of low-income respondents reported that they had put off medical care because of cost and the payment of bills by patients who had seen a doctor dropped until the delinquency rate for physicians' bills was sixty-six percent. In farm states, a new federal program began to pay for medical services and by 1937 a quarter of the population of the Dakotas was covered.

"THE BLUES"

In 1929, Baylor University Hospital established a health plan for 1,500 schoolteachers in Dallas. The hospital would provide twenty-one days of inpatient care for a flat fee of six dollars per year in dues. When the plan became a success, the hospital extended it to other groups of subscribers and soon there were several thousand members in Dallas. Other hospitals in Dallas, feeling the pressure of competition, developed similar programs. When the Depression dawned, hospital revenues fell and, in 1932, a book,

The Crisis in Hospital Finance, warned that hospitals could not rely on patients to pay their bills. Some form of insurance was needed to secure the hospitals' expenses. In Sacramento, California and in Essex County, New Jersey hospitals began to offer service contracts to groups of employed people that would pay for hospital care. The American Hospital Association approved these arrangements and they began to spread across the country. They did not provide for any physician services and, unlike insurance companies, they had no capital reserve to pay losses. The hospitals agreed to provide services rather than ask for payment from some third party. In New York, the state insurance commissioner insisted that these plans were insurance and were subject to rules requiring financial reserves. A law exempting the plans, now beginning to be called "Blue Cross," from insurance rules passed in New York in 1934. The hospital underwriting ensured that they would control Blue Cross for many years.

With time, the plans became community-wide programs that included all the hospitals in the area, in effect a monopoly. The AHA encouraged this trend, which would eventually become a problem once high technology came to medicine. By 1935, twenty-nine states had passed laws permitting "hospital service plans," Blue Cross. The plans divided the territory among themselves so there was no competition between them. Insurance actuaries warned the hospitals that they were "insuring" risks that could not be accurately estimated; they were blank checks. In spite of this concern about future liability, commercial insurance companies also began writing health insurance plans for employers, in 1934. In 1937, the New York Blue Cross Plan had 350,000 subscribers. Blue Cross had tax exemptions but the insurance companies had more money. In 1939, as the Second World War began, Blue Cross had six million members in thirty-nine plans and there were 3.7 million subscribers to private (commercial) health insurance plans.

PREPAID GROUP PLANS

Doctors did not want to be paid by hospitals, and this would be an issue with hospital-based specialties like pathology and radiology for many years, but the hospital insurance, by covering the usually larger hospital bill, improved the doctor's chance of being paid by the patient. Doctors had some bad experiences with company health programs that employed physicians and succeeded in passing legislation in California that prohibited "corporate practice of medicine." The law banned an entity that did not have a medical license from billing another party for a physician's services. Only four states passed such laws. Companies were still allowed to employ doctors and pay a salary; they just could not charge anyone else for his, or her, services in California. Mining companies, railroads and lumber companies could and did employ doctors to care for their workers. British author A.J.Cronin, in his book, *The Citadel*, has described some of the conflicts of interest inherent in these company health plans. The book is about a doctor in a Welsh mining town in the 1920s and also gives a picture of pre-NHS medical practice in Britain.

By the mid-thirties, about 400 businesses, with approximately two million employees, had established health care programs. In Washington State, several county medical societies established prepaid plans to provide physician's services in parallel with hospital plans. These were later used as models for the California Physicians' Service program. In California, in 1929, the Los Angles Department of Water and Power contracted with physicians Donald Ross and H. Clifford Loos (whose daughter Anita later wrote a play called "Gentlemen Prefer Blonds") to provide complete health care, including hospital care, for 2,000 employees and their families. By 1935, the Ross-Loos Clinic provided care for 12,000 workers and 25,000 family members, mostly government employees. The subscriber paid two dollars per month for comprehensive care (although hospital care was not covered for dependents at first). Ross and Loos started their own insurance company to provide hospital coverage, the Independence Insurance Company, and both ventures prospered making Ross and Loos wealthy men.

Similar plans, usually for government programs in remote areas, appeared. Sidney Garfield, a Los Angeles surgeon, organized a clinic for men working on the Los Angeles Aqueduct in the Mojave Desert in 1933. In 1938, he set up a similar program for Henry J. Kaiser whose company was building the Grand Coulee Dam in Washington State. Similar efforts prompted retaliation by the American Medical Association, which was opposed to these programs. Doctors employed by the pre-paid plans were not eligible for membership in the medical associations and many medical schools would not accept them on their faculties. In 1943, the AMA lost an anti-trust case arising from opposition to the Group Health Association of Washington, DC, a cooperative owned by members.

BLUE SHIELD

In 1939 (actually beginning in 1934 when the medical association decided to do something about doctors' coverage- see above) the California Medical Association formed the "California Physicians Service," later called "Blue Shield," as an alternative to the California governor's advocacy of compulsory insurance for all workers with less than $3,000 per year incomes. The governor's plan would have covered ninety percent of the population at the time. The medical association used a program already established in Washington state and Oregon as the model although the fee schedule turned out to be inadequate for California, a much larger state. The first program offered complete care for a monthly payment of $2.50 per person. This was considered too expensive for most Californians and the membership growth was slow. It was fortunate for the doctors as it turned out that the plan was inadequately funded. The money collected each month was paid out to the doctors on a fee-for-service basis and the patient was not obligated to pay any additional amount. Supposedly only those with incomes below $3,000 per year were to be "members," with no obligation for additional payment, but doctors were loathe to ask about income and everyone was covered.

The doctors soon learned that they were getting about twenty-five cents on the dollar but, with the Depression still in place, it was better than nothing.[527] The Michigan Medical Association began a similar program the same year. Some of this was encouraged by Blue Cross, which was barred from paying physicians' bills. The commercial insurance plans were paying the doctors' bills and Blue Cross was interested in encouraging an alternative so the two "Blues" could combine to compete with the commercials. California Physicians' Service set up a fee schedule using a "unit value" system. Procedures were valued in arbitrary "units," determined by a committee of physicians from different specialties, which were to be multiplied by a "conversion factor" that could vary based on the location of the doctor's office. The units were established, for surgeons as an example, in "hernia units." An operation judged to be as difficult and time consuming as a hernia repair, would be valued at one "hernia unit." Another operation, say a gallbladder surgery, might be worth two "hernia units." Then the surgeons sat down with the medical doctors and decided how many office visits equaled one hernia unit. Eventually a whole schedule was set up and any doctor could use it to set his fees. There was no provision to control utilization, other than the patients' ability to pay. After some initial false starts, the fee schedule arrived at a level of $2.25 per "Relative Value Scale" (RVS) unit in 1945. Blue Shield remained a junior partner for some time; by 1945, Blue Cross had nineteen million subscribers, while Blue Shield had only one million. The Hill-Burton Act of 1946 began to build hospitals for the post-war world, and the volume of hospital care would skyrocket once those new facilities came on-line.

UNION HEALTH PLANS

After 1945, the provider-organized plans lost influence as unions became more powerful. During the war, wages and prices had been controlled. In order to attract workers many employers had included health benefits with wages since wage increases were controlled and the combination amounted to a wage increase beyond what was otherwise allowed. In 1942 the War Labor Board allowed fringe benefits of up to five percent of wages and this brought the number of members in hospital plans up, from seven million in 1941, to twenty-six million by the end of the war. Blue Cross still had two-thirds of the insured but that would not last. In 1946, only 600,000 workers were members of union health plans. In 1948, the CIO, the less skilled industrial workers union, made health benefits high priority. President Truman had plans for a national health plan like that enacted by the Labour government in England but the unions had doubts about his chances for success and went their own way. By 1954, twelve million workers and nineteen million dependents were enrolled in union health plans, which the unions began to manage themselves. Collective bargaining expanded the scope of coverage as well as the number of members and dependents covered.

Most union members remained in Blue Cross (as part of the union program) because the early commercial insurance companies tended to write "indemnity plans." This means the plan would pay a flat fee for a service and ignored the Relative Value Scale of the doctors or the hospital's bill. Indemnity plans tended to keep costs down and made premiums predictable. Actuaries can estimate the number of heart attacks or gall bladder attacks in a population quite accurately. The United Mine Workers were particularly aggressive in negotiating health benefits. In 1948, the mineworkers struck the coal companies over pension benefits. Eventually, the union and the industry settled the strikes and the union gained control over the health and pension plans. By the 1950s, the union owned ten hospitals in mining communities and employed a number of doctors. Most doctors, however, were still paid on a fee-for-service basis and the unions' experience with this system provides an early look at the problems that were to overwhelm medicine thirty years later. Collective bargaining tended to convert indemnity plans, with premiums set by actuaries and cost controls, into the Blue Shield-type with fees set by the doctors.

The doctors of Butler, Pennsylvania were accustomed to setting their fees by the patient's ability to pay, a traditional practice going back thousands of years. The going rate for maternity care, including delivering the baby, had been $50 for a number of years. The United Rubber Workers' Union health plan began to pay a $50 benefit for maternity services and discovered that the doctors raised their fees to $75. The union then raised the indemnity payment to $75 and, lo and behold, the doctor fee rose to $125. In less than a year, the standard charge for the same service had increased by the exact amount of the insurance payment. Economists call this difference in price a "rent" and the actions of the doctors in Butler, "rent-seeking behavior." To the doctors, their services were worth the $50 cash their patients had been able to pay for years out of their own pockets. Now, a new entity, the union health plan, appears and is willing to pay the doctor a fee, a "rent" that is in addition to the standard transaction between doctor and patient. The cash transaction between the doctor and patient ($50 for a delivery) remained essentially the same. This phenomenon, the rent-seeking by the physician (and the hospital), would eventually doom fee-for-service medicine.

THE CANADIAN EXPERIMENT

Prior to 1957, the Canadian health care system was essentially identical to the American one. In that year, the Canadian House of Commons passed legislation to encourage provinces to form health insurance plans for hospital services. Saskatchewan had anticipated the national trend in 1947 by establishing a provincial hospital insurance system that provided universal coverage. The 1957 law encouraged the other provinces to follow Saskatchewan's example and by 1961, all ten had done so. The program was popular, especially given the small population and huge areas involved in providing services. In 1962, Saskatchewan again set the trend by offering insurance to pay for physician fees. In 1968, the central government added this provision to its incentive program and, by 1972, all provincial and territorial plans included doctors' services.

In 1979, a review of the Canadian system, by Justice Emmett Hall, concluded that the health system ranked among the best in the world, but he expressed concern that user fees from hospitals and balance billing by doctors were creating a "two-tiered system" in Canada. In Britain, this was called "jumping the queue." In both cases those able to pay extra received preference, had shorter waiting times and amenities like private rooms and telephones in their hospital rooms. In 1984, Parliament passed the Canadian Health Act, which banned extra billing by doctors and user fees from hospitals. At the time, health care spending per capita was similar in Canada and the US. In 1960, Canada was spending 5.4 percent of Gross Domestic Product on health care and the US was spending 5.2 percent. The NHS in England was spending only 3.9 percent and the countries spending over four percent of GDP included Germany, Australia, France, New Zealand, and Sweden, in addition to Canada and the US. By 1990, Canadian health care spending was 9.2 percent of GDP and US was 12.6 percent. No other country spent more than 8.9 percent and the NHS share was only 6.0 percent. The ban on extra billing by physicians was vigorously protested, including a physician strike that ended only after the government adopted punitive measures against the doctors. A mass exodus of Canadian physicians, especially highly trained specialists ensued. The remaining physicians were allowed to bill for services on a fixed fee-for-service basis, paid from a government fee schedule. The fee schedule gradually declined as the central government reduced cost sharing with the provinces over the next decade. Hospital budgets are global and are negotiated with provincial health ministries, much as is done in the NHS. Hospital admissions fell by thirty-three percent between 1986 and 1996, a trend which has continued and which is also seen in the US as outpatient care is emphasized.

The initial federal program included fifty-fifty cost sharing between the central government and the provinces as an inducement for them to adopt the universal coverage plan. By 1977, the central government was becoming concerned at rising medical costs and the fifty-fifty sharing was reduced. Since 1977, the federal share of payments has declined, leaving the provinces to absorb the increases. In 1980, the federal share of the total health care budget of 14.1 billion Canadian dollars was 44.6 percent. In 1990, the total cost to the provinces was $39.2 billion Canadian and the federal share was down to 36.7 percent. Canada had serious budget problems in the 1980s; because of excessive government expenditures in all fields, (only Italy had a higher debt to GDP ratio of developed countries). The effect of reduced spending on health, in addition to a "brain drain" of physicians to the US, was a declining public satisfaction with the health plan. In 1991, a government survey returned a sixty-one percent level of satisfaction with health care but by 1999, only twenty-four percent were satisfied. No one wanted to go back to a system like that of the US, but thousands of patients were seeking care south of the border and some, the more affluent, even carried American health insurance in addition to the Canadian Medicare card. The policy of restricting supply, as a method of controlling costs, has been subject to unfavorable publicity. One hospital was providing CAT scans on sick pets to veterinarians after regular hours in spite of lengthy waiting lists for patients to obtain CAT scans. The hospital was able to charge for the pet scans (pun intended) while they obtained no additional revenue for patient services after regular working hours.

The number of applications to medical schools dropped in the 1990s and admissions to nursing schools dropped from 12,621 to 5,063, according to the Canadian Nursing Association, in spite of perceived nurse shortages in Canada and the US.[528] The enrollment of first year medical students was 1,887 in 1983 and dropped to 1,581 by 1998. Provincial health ministers cut funding for medical education by ten percent and emigration is estimated at a steady rate of 400 per year. Retirement has also affected the number of active physicians and the rate of retirement increased forty percent in the 1990s compared to the 1980s. The Canadian Medical Association believes that there is a physician shortage of about 750 physicians per year over medical graduates but government ministers have suggested accepting more foreign-trained doctors over training native Canadians if a shortage does exist. During the 1990s, hospitals declined from 1,128 to 877 and beds from 175,376 to 122,006. The government has used a mechanism similar to the American base-closing commission, used to deflect political backlash, in the US example, over closing unneeded military facilities in the wake of the end of the Cold War. The bases needed closing, but were twenty-two percent of Canadian hospitals unneeded? Given the rural nature of the country and the huge geographic area to be serviced, that may be questionable. A recent article by John Iglehart describes the current problems with the Canadian system.[529] The experience may serve as a cautionary tale for reformers of the US health care system who want to use the Canadian program as a model.

THE COMING OF THE HMOS

Prepaid medical care, in which the physicians and hospitals are paid a standard amount to provide care for a group (it will only work with a group; otherwise only the sick would join), began to grow after the war. The railroads and mining companies had joined the trend to service plans and free choice instead of the company doctor and clinic. The railroad unions regarded the company hospitals as vestiges of paternalism. An exception to the trend was the formation of Group Health of Puget Sound, and another cooperative, Group Health of Washington, DC, both of which were owned by the members. The Kaiser Company set up foundations to provide health care for workers in the war industries and shipyards they established on the West Coast, using the model of the Garfield Clinic at the Grand Coulee Dam in the 1930s. In 1942, Henry J. Kaiser set up Permanente Foundations in the Seattle area, in Portland, Oregon, and in Oakland and Fontana, California. Kaiser Foundation ran the hospitals and the Permanente Medical Group employed the physicians on a salary. At the end of the war, 200,000 people were enrolled but, with the end of the war and the decline of war industry, the foundations must be closed or opened to the public. Kaiser was pleased with his experience in pre-paid care and decided to try to reform medicine. He opened the system to the public. The medical associations were bitterly opposed to the group plans; not totally (but mostly) from self interest.

ETHICAL ISSUES

With the rapid growth of surgery in the early twentieth century, surgeons came under pressure from general practitioners to rebate part of the fee paid by their patients who had had operations. This was called "fee-splitting" and was considered unethical. The general practitioner might be tempted to refer his patients to the surgeon who paid the best kickback and this occurred, especially in Chicago and the Midwest. In 1900, two members of the Chicago Medical Society, in a hoax designed to demonstrate the level of fee-splitting in Chicago, sent out a questionnaire. It was sent to all the prominent surgeons in Chicago and purported to be from a country doctor asking the surgeons what percentage of their fee they would pay the country doctor for referring a patient. The answers, with names attached, were published in a Chicago newspaper. In the ensuing scandal, the Society expelled the two members who had circulated the questionnaire and no took no action against the fee-splitters. John B. Murphy, widely rumored by jealous colleagues to pay kickbacks, peremptorily refused the purported offer from the "country doctor."[530]

When I began practice in 1972, some GPs were still performing their own surgery, only calling a surgeon for complicated cases or if they got into trouble. Some surgeons performed the operation, but the GP, who assisted, was listed as the surgeon and collected the fee. This was called "ghost surgery" and was common in some small towns. Some surgeons hired general practitioners to provide primary care and refer all those requiring surgery to the surgeon. Surgeons established the large groups, like Mayo Clinic and Cleveland Clinic (although the Mayos began as general practitioners in the 1880s) and other, less ethical surgeons, adopted the model for less honorable reasons. The American College of Surgeons was established in 1912 to fight the practice of fee splitting and ghost surgery as well as to improve the educational resources available to surgeons. The Kaiser Permanente system was seen as a form of fee-splitting although this was really a stretch of the principle. It is true that, at a time when well-trained surgeons could easily develop a busy practice, not many good surgeons were interested in a salaried job at Kaiser. Still, some excellent surgeons liked the idea of spending their time doing surgery and caring for patients instead of worrying about entertaining primary care doctors and hoping they would send their patients to them. Kaiser provided a good, solid workman-like quality of medical care. Many two-earner families, in the 1970s, had Kaiser as one member's health plan and Blue Cross as the other. The idea was that they would use "private care" for routine matters, like well childcare, because they did not want to wait in line at a clinic but, if disaster struck, Kaiser would pay for everything.

MEDICARE

In 1960, the Kerr-Mills Act passed the Congress establishing a program for the "aged poor." Liberal politicians opposed means testing for benefits and states, with the exception of the large industrial states, did not take advantage of the funds. When I was a medical student in 1964, the orthopedic service of the Los Angeles County Hospital admitted so many elderly patients with broken hips that interns were doing some of the procedures, inserting a "pin" or "nail" to stabilize the fracture. In 1964, after the Kennedy assassination, Lyndon Johnson made Medicare one of the priorities of his "Great Society" program. The AMA, belatedly realizing that its resistance to government medicine was not strong enough to stop the legislation, proposed an alternative called "Eldercare," which was means tested and contained other controls on utilization. Twenty-five years later the government would try to come back to something like the Eldercare proposal but it was too late. A survey sponsored by the AMA in 1964 found that seventy-two percent of respondents thought that Medicare should also cover doctors' fees. The result was a compromise: Part A of Medicare was the original plan which paid hospital bills, Part B was the Republican plan of partial subsidy (similar to Eldercare) of doctors' bills, and the third section, called Medicaid, was an expanded program for the poor based on Kerr-Mills. The result, which became law in 1965, was a vast expansion of health care delivery. In 1966, when I was an intern, the elderly were virtually gone from the County Hospital; the private doctors had enthusiastically joined the Medicare program and, like the specialists of the British National Health Service in 1948, the government had "filled their mouths with gold." The reckoning would come in twenty-five years; in the meantime, the coming years would be a golden age for medicine. Doctors who had driven Buicks were now ordering Mercedes.

The coming of high technology medicine would strain the resources of the health care industry and health insurance severely. The commercial insurers, by covering employment-based groups, were selecting a healthier segment of the population. Blue Cross and Blue Shield became the health plans for individuals and suffered from "adverse selection," the tendency of people with chronic illness to seek better coverage. Doctors, in a slow but certain trek to the edge of the precipice, succeeded in forcing "Usual, Customary and Reasonable" fee structures on most insurance plans and Medicare. This meant that the benefits paid would reflect the usual charges in the community, not an underwriter's fee schedule based on premium income. Patients benefited because they would not be left holding the bag of unpaid bills. Still, "UCR," as it was called, put fee inflation into high gear since the doctors were setting their own fees. It got worse. Insurance companies, suspicious of hospital lump sum bills for "daily room rates," began to insist on minutely itemized hospital bills and then found themselves unable to deny payment for all those $10 syringes and aspirin tablets. Medical inflation was out of control. The advent of coronary bypass surgery and total joint replacement in 1967 to 1973 broke the bank.

In 1973, John Wennberg MD, an epidemiologist, and Allan Gittlesohn PhD, a biostatistician, published an analysis of health care practices in Vermont.[531] They had expected to find underservice since Vermont is a relatively poor rural state. What they found instead was a vast variation in the rate of common surgical procedures. The rate of tonsillectomy, a common pediatric surgical procedure, varied from sixty percent of the children in some communities to only seven percent in others. There seemed to be no systematic method for deciding which children needed the operation and there was no evidence of any medical consequence for either the high or low utilization group. Thus, the choice of treatment was based on local physician preference and communities seemed to follow patterns that were not based on medical evidence. Further study of the phenomenon of "small area variation" followed, and it was found to apply to benign conditions such as surgery for benign prostatic hypertrophy. Doctors were making choices and spending health care dollars without good evidence for the benefit to patients from those choices. Diagnoses like cancer, hip fracture, and heart attacks, life threatening conditions, produced hospital admission rates with little variation across the country. The variation was seen in more benign conditions, especially those in which there was no clear consensus about what the best treatment was: like hysterectomy for benign disease or benign prostate surgery (TURP). Eventually the study of variation and "small area analysis" evolved into "Outcomes Research" in an attempt to understand whether patients were helped or harmed by treatment. Efforts to measure these outcomes and choose effective treatment, and to correct the variation, became "Evidence Based Medicine." Evidence Based Medicine uses clinical research, especially randomized clinical trials, to select treatment programs with proven benefit. Both disciplines have met considerable resistance, initially from physicians and, more recently, from managed care organizations which fear that attempts to improve quality will cost more money.

By 1986, the effects of medical inflation brought more major changes. In 1970, Paul Ellwood, a Minneapolis physician who was director of the American Rehabilitation Foundation, proposed the concept of a "Health Maintenance Organization," which would devote resources to promoting the health of its members instead of curing the ills that were preventable but whose prevention was neglected by a system that dealt only with sickness. His rehabilitation medicine background made the concept of "health maintenance" an easy one and he found a willing audience in Washington, although not for the reasons he thought. Senator Ted Kennedy had been advocating a national health plan, a single federal program that provided free care for all. The Nixon Administration was looking for an alternative; Senator Kennedy was a potential presidential nominee for the Democrats. In 1971, President Nixon called on Congress to "change the incentives in health care" with HMOs. New York had begun to regulate the capital expenditures of hospitals in 1964 and, by 1972, twenty states did likewise with a program called "certificate of need." In 1971, the Nixon administration instituted wage and price controls, including doctors' fees. In 1973, these controls were ended except for doctors' fees. Another regulatory scheme was "Professional Standards Review Organizations," or PSROs, which were promoted by Congress as quality improvement mechanisms. Doctors noted that all the measurements concerned costs and "quality" seemed to equal "cost" in the standards.

In 1973, new legislation required all businesses with at least twenty-five employees to offer HMO alternatives to conventional insurance. Finally, in 1986, a research study by the State of New Jersey and Yale University, which attempted to set fixed prices for hospital services for 476 "Diagnosis Related Groups," became the basis for new Medicare regulations.[532] The concept behind DRGs was that the cost of hospital care could be standardized for the most common conditions, determined by diagnosis on discharge. The Medicare payment to the hospital was a fixed amount and was based on the discharge diagnosis (one of 476), no matter how long the patient was hospitalized or what the cost to the hospital had been for his or her care. Some patients would always be at risk for complications or unusual problems and they were called "outliers," those whose care was out of the usual pattern. Additional payment was available for some of these. This change immediately reversed the incentives for the hospitals and physicians noticed the change within days of the new regulation. Where hospital departments had actually marketed new services to patients, some without the physician's consent, now the hospital was pushing the patient out "sicker and quicker," as the saying went. Doctors received computer printouts every month with the length of stay of each of their patients, along with a list of the charges and the Medicare payment. Doctors who were "money losers" for the hospital got the message. They could be asked to leave. Some specialties were particularly hard hit. Critical care specialists were cut out of Medicare payments. Only one physician could bill each day, even for patients in ICU. Critical care and infectious disease specialists found their incomes crashing and went on salary or, if the hospital could not afford them, left the area for larger cities.

THE FOR-PROFIT HMO

Several years later, for-profit HMOs appeared on the New York Stock Exchange and the final death spiral of medical economics began. Paul Ellwood, of course, had the Kaiser model in mind when he proposed the "Health Maintenance Organization" and he assumed that future developments would all be in the non-profit mold.[533] He was wrong and he has expressed dismay, in recent years, at the developments in the HMO model. The Reagan and Bush Administrations were convinced of the superiority of the private, capitalist model with some justification (The VA system had a series of scandals about that time). It had not occurred to most people familiar with health care that a for-profit model would work. For the next ten years, enormous sums would be collected from corporate employee health plans and stock market investors and distributed to HMO shareholders in stock dividends. This transfer of wealth is rivaled only by the more recent phenomenon of the "Dot-Com" industry where stockholder investment was transferred to customers buying books, pet supplies, and groceries over the Internet. Business owners and managers had no sympathy for doctors and hospitals whom they viewed as having profited from years of excessive fees and payments. The HMO model with its focus on prepayment and capitation (a fixed amount per member per month) payments to hospitals and doctors proved to be an excellent vehicle for rationing of access to care and controlling costs. The "health maintenance," that was the theoretical justification for the adoption of the HMO model, especially for the Medicare program, was given lip service only. Kaiser and Group Health of Puget Sound had long enrolled subscribers who tended to remain members for years, even after retirement from their employers. Preventive medicine was part of the program in these systems and Kaiser, for example, was a pioneer in routine mammography. The for-profit HMOs, unlike Kaiser and the other non-profits, quickly realized that it was unnecessary to establish an expensive infrastructure like that built up over decades by the non-profits. They also concluded that members tended to change jobs and move from place to place, changing doctors and HMOs. Preventive medicine took years to "pay off" and, if the subscriber was gone in three years (the industry average), the HMO got no "return on investment" from that expenditure. Traditional HMOs had been organized in two models; "staff model," in which the physicians were salaried employees of the HMO, and "group model," in which the physicians were members of large groups and the group paid their salaries. Kaiser was a group model with all physicians members of the Permanente Medical Group. Group Health was a staff model and employed all the physicians directly.

The for-profit HMOs came up with a third model. They created "medical groups without walls" by subcontracting all health care delivery to doctors and hospitals. The doctors organized Independent Practice Associations, often created by entrepreneurial physicians who then signed up their local colleagues. The "IPAs" were essentially unregulated and there were many abuses by the officers and small boards of directors that had almost unlimited power over colleagues who only wanted to care for patients and be left alone. The providers, as doctors and hospitals came to be known, were often willing to sign contracts at inadequate reimbursement rates because they were unable to organize negotiating cartels. The Federal Government had outlawed any "collusion" by doctors in such negotiations and brought antitrust suits against those who tried to form groups, so the disparity in economic power favored the HMOs. The IPAs were allowed to negotiate because they were signing "at-risk" contracts, meaning contracts to provide services at a fixed price (much like the original Blue Cross hospital contracts). Soon, the HMOs became little more than brokers, signing contracts with employers to provide comprehensive care and then subcontracting all the actual services with providers, IPAs and hospitals. The HMO deducted a healthy percentage of the gross premium for "administration," which included salaries and bonuses in the millions for executives plus shareholder dividends. Traditional HMOs like Family Health Plan, a California staff model HMO, proved unable to compete because of their fixed costs and were bought up by the for profits for peanuts. The doctors in FHP were fired and the subscribers reassigned to the HMO's IPA groups who paid their own expenses and salaries. By 1998, most California medical groups and IPAs were insolvent. Kaiser and the other traditional HMOs were at a disadvantage because of the fixed costs for hospitals and clinics they owned and the salaries of doctors and nurses, the latter heavily unionized. As they cut costs to compete with the low cost for-profits, quality began to slip and preventive medicine became a losing proposition. Eventually, a national health plan began to look better than the existing system and the American College of Surgeons testified before Congress in 1998 supporting another look at a government single-payer program.

THE ERISA EXEMPTION

In recent years, a new issue, related to HMO care, has arisen. First, there is no longer any employer sponsored "health insurance." The concept of insurance includes investment of capital and payment of benefits from investment income. This is still true of life insurance and, to some extent of malpractice insurance. Health insurance is another matter. Health care costs have risen so rapidly that no true insurance scheme could keep up. What has replaced true insurance is the concept of an "administrative service organization." What this means is, the employer is paying the health benefits on a month-to-month basis with the insur-ance company acting as a claims agent and administrator. The employer has established an "employee benefit plan" and that plan pays the claims. The employer is self-insuring. The doctor's office or hospital submits the claim to the insurance company but it is acting as the employer's agent. In 1974, a law was passed by Congress to protect employees' pension plans. It was called the Employee Retirement Income Security Act, also called ERISA. One provision of the act affects health benefits: the employer is exempt from state law concerning these benefit plans. This was enacted to protect the large employer from med-dling by fifty different states in its pension plan, but it has severely impacted patient rights with HMOs. When an HMO denies care to a patient, it is immune to malpractice suits. The doctor may be sued, but the HMO cannot be sued in state court, the jurisdiction of malpractice and tort laws. Federal courts will not permit suits for damages other than the amount of the denied benefit. No economic damages or compensa-tion for pain and suffering is awarded. Government employees are allowed to sue HMOs since they are not covered by ERISA. Employees of private companies have been trying to get health benefits excluded from this provision for several years and a Patients' Bill of Rights was introduced by Congressman Charles Norwood, a dentist, about five years ago. The HMO and insurance industry has so far blocked its passage.

A MATTER OF INCENTIVES

A common thread runs through the recent economic history of medicine. There is a principle in economics called the "tragedy of the commons."[534] In fifteenth century England, most towns owned the grazing land within the town boundaries in common. It was in everyone's interest to share the common and maintain it. Overgrazing, especially by sheep which pull up grass by the roots, would diminish the usefulness for all. Still, if one person acquired more sheep than his neighbors and grazed them on the town common, he could accumulate wealth at his neighbor's expense. Abuse of such common areas led to their neglect, then to private property and the assignment of responsibility by the legal system. The same phenomenon has occurred in fishing, since no one owns the Grand Banks off Nova Scotia, and over-fishing has nearly wiped out breeding stocks of cod and other high-value fish. The private property solution will be more difficult in this instance. The invention of insurance (in the American Colonies fire insurance was organized by Benjamin Franklin) led to another problem called "the moral hazard of insurance."[535] If everyone pays the same premium for fire insurance, the man who neglects to take precautions in his own property increases the risk of loss for all who are insured with the same company. If I file an unjustified claim, I increase the costs for everyone, but I have reduced my own cost by the amount I collect from that claim. Insuring motorists probably increases the frequency of auto accidents, to use another example. It is as if I had grazed more than my share of sheep on the town common. The moral hazard of insurance prompted the fee increases of the doctors in Butler, Pennsylvania. The fact that the insurance paid their usual fee tempted them to increase it to include the cash co-payment they knew the patient was willing to pay. The insurance became a "rent," defined by Webster's as "income derived from ownership of property," in this case ownership of a medical license. Eventually the fee-for-service system was abused by too many physicians, and hospital administrators were no more immune to temptation than their professional staff members. Human nature was such that they justified their actions and felt no moral barrier to increase income since someone seemed to willing to pay for it. This does not imply that all physicians charged unreasonable fees or were dishonest. The fees themselves contributed less to the problem than the temptation to deliver unnecessary care and excessive hospitalization, both expensive. This is what John Wennberg MD has called "provider induced demand."[536] Hospital admission rates for conditions without clear indications (heart attacks and hip fractures always require hospital care; pneumonia and anemia do not) for proper treatment are more associated with the number of available beds than with the condition of the patients. If more empty beds are available, more people are admitted to the hospital. Patients were every bit as eager to take advantage of the third party payers. It was common for patients to request admission to the hospital for routine exams like barium enemas because "the insurance will pay." The attitude was, "I have already paid for it so why can't I get my money's worth?" The problem was that the premiums were calculated by actuaries on the basis of the expected risk of acute illness. When routine care was included the premiums were inadequate and had to go up. The existence of insurance and the political influence to change the law, to gain a larger share of the economic pie, accelerated a trend of rising costs already due to an aging population and an explosion of new medical technology. When I was a medical student, coronary care units did not exist, coronary bypass and total joint replacement did not exist and chronic renal dialysis was just becoming possible. Those four items, together with an aging population that has increasing health problems, added many billions to the annual medical expenditure and put increasing pressure on the economics of health care. Something had to give.

The problem with HMOs is that the incentives are reversed, but the temptation is the same. While it was once possible to earn more income from providing services that were either unnecessary or of doubtful value, it is now possible to increase income by withholding services that are of significant value and by creating obstacles to service with rules and bureaucratic procedures. There is some question which is worse. There is little question that the patient and the doctor have both lost power in the new health care system. At one time in the 1980s economists projected that by 2020 half of the federal budget would be consumed by health care. Projections, of course, are just that: they are based on assumptions that cannot be accurate over forty years. Things change. How they changed is the subject of this chapter. I have no idea what the future holds although most medical students are sensibly convinced that by the time they finish their training the problems will be somehow fixed.

Medical Malpractice

Professional malpractice suits began, at least in theory, with Sir William Blackstone's *Commentaries on the Laws of England*, published in 1768. This work restated the English Common Law in print and began the modern practice of law. In a section titled *mala praxis*, Latin for "malpractice," he listed "Injuries ...by the neglect or unskillful [sic] management of physician, surgeon or apothecary...because it breaks the trust which the party had placed in his physician, and tends to the patient's destruction."[537] In spite of the theoretical foundation established by Blackstone, medical malpractice suits were unknown in America until about 1840. By 1850, however, medical malpractice litigation was well established, probably because of a number of societal changes, but no doubt influenced by the development of modern medicine chronicled in the rest of this book. Another important factor was the absence of medical societies and guilds, which governed and lent some credibility to physicians in Europe. In America, there were few regulations at the state or local level and the marketplace was wide open. This applied to the law, as well as to medicine, and Abraham Lincoln brought suit on behalf of a client against a medical imposter in 1851.[538] His client, Edward Jones, had questioned the credentials of his physician, Joseph S. Maus, who claimed to be a graduate of Jefferson Medical College in Philadelphia. Lincoln was well acquainted with the medical profession in Illinois, having a number of physician close associates, as well as two brothers-in-law who were doctors.

Jefferson Medical College had been founded in 1824 and the rules of attendance were rather lax. From 1844 to 1849, the school accepted 465 applicants per year and graduated 166. Only three states required more than a diploma for medical practice and most had no requirement at all. Lincoln, himself, had attended no law school. In the end, he wisely negotiated a settlement between his client and the physician. Each paid his own share of court costs, a total of $3.20. Six years later, he tried another malpractice case that involved a chicken bone.[539]

From 1840 to 1860 the number of medical malpractice suits jumped 950 percent during a period when the population increased by eighty-five percent. This ten-fold increase accompanied increasing standardization of medical practice and the availability of medical texts with which the doctors' activities could be compared. The first great wave of malpractice suits involved orthopedic cases in which a fracture was mistreated resulting in deformity.[540] Many of these suits followed the introduction of antisepsis and, ironically, resulted from compound fractures, which would have resulted in amputation twenty years before. In 1878, Eugene Sanger wrote a report on malpractice suits in Maine stating that lawyers "follow us as the shark does the emigrant ship."[541] The schism between doctors and lawyers, which still exists to some degree, began here. Within a year of the introduction of the x-ray to medicine, the new diagnostic technique was used in a medical malpractice suit (see the chapter on New Science). This encapsulates one of the arguments for a theory of the increase in malpractice litigation: the "medical innovation" theory. Doctors resented having the goalposts shifted with each new advance in science.

The introduction of licensing laws and higher standards after the founding of the AMA in 1847 produced another paradox: higher standards must be met or the patient will sue. Some untrained practitioners were driven from the profession but those continuing to provide medical care were held to the new standards. Finally, in the 1890s medical malpractice insurance was introduced, particularly by "Medical Protective of Indiana," the largest of the insurance companies until the 1930s.

The legal profession introduced an innovation not found in English Common Law, the contingency fee. In 1887, the AMA commented unfavorably on a case in Massachesetts in which the plaintiff attorney proposed to the court that, if the verdict should be in favor of the defendant, the plaintiff would pay the cost of the trial. The assumption of the costs by the plaintiff's attorney in the event of an unfavorable verdict seemed to offer a "key to the courthouse" for poor potential plaintiffs. The AMA was uncertain of the effect of this innovation on malpractice litigation but expressed concern that it might increase the ability of the plaintiff side to "extort money from the defendant sufficient to secure a good fee for the prosecuting counsel."[542] The practice continues in spite of opposition from the usual roster of defendants. The contingency fee did tend to skew the type of case litigated since those with a large payout, regardless of the degree of culpability by the physician, offered the best chance for the lawyer to recover his fees and enough to absorb the cost of defeat in others. Cases with small damages but more serious levels of physician malpractice are often lost in the system.

The use of lay juries to decide esoteric issues of medical practice has lent an air of the lottery to medical malpractice litigation although modern, better-educated juries seem to be better able to decide the facts than those of a generation or two ago. As early as the 1850s the medical profession began seeking the use of expert panels or special expert juries for these cases but without success. Lawyers have fought this innovation successfully, invoking the image of the "Star Chamber" of Elizabethan England. The adversarial court system and lay juries have been the standard since the 1840s. The use of tort law in medical malpractice has not always been the obvious tactic it seems now. Late in the nineteenth century, some courts leaned to contract law as the preferred theory, concluding that the physician and patient had a contract and failure to fulfill the agreement was the preferred legal theory rather than the concept of the physician injuring the patient.[543] This concept threatened the professional status of physicians (it seemed), who did not want to be compared to tradesmen. The medical profession chose to deny the contractual relationship between equals that contract law suggested. The decision was costly since tort law is much less structured and lends itself to jury interpretation. Some have sought the return of the contract law principle in dealing with HMOs in recent years.

The next great wave of litigation occurred in the 1920s when courts, in the absence of legal experts willing to testify against colleagues (the notorious "code of silence"), began to apply the doctrine of *res ipsa loquitur*. This means, "The fact speaks for itself" and works well for such misadventures as amputating the wrong leg. The burden of proof was thereby transferred to the physician who must convince a jury that the treatment was proper. Another characteristic of this "Progressive Era" was a weakening of the "local standards" defense. With transportation and communications vastly improved, it was becoming difficult to convince a jury that medical practice could vary between rural and city locations. Physicians were licensed by the state and expectations were rising. The local standards defense can still be seen, especially in the South, but successful defenses on this basis are rare now.

The California Medical Association provided defense against malpractice suits for a charge of $10 per year until 1923. It did not pay damages, but provided legal assistance. This practice ended that year and other insurance was necessary. There were few lawsuits in California during the 1930s, the majority being for complications of x-ray. The judgements were small, but a malpractice crisis resulted causing most malpractice insurance companies to leave the business. Lloyds of London began to write malpractice insurance in California, but had a disaster when a shipyard doctor in Long Beach let his patients play with a fluoroscopy machine while they were waiting to see him. Many were burned and Lloyds was "burned" the worst of all when a large number of lawsuits resulted.

World War II ended the 1930s malpractice problems when a severe doctor shortage brought a reluctance to question the quality of care rendered in the absence of alternatives. The younger, better-trained doctors were away in the service and the public was grateful for what was available. Following the end of the war, the rapid discovery of "miracle drugs," like penicillin, brought new expectations but prosperity kept malpractice insurance rates low. Consumer consciousness in the 1960s increased the pressure and the bear market of 1974 collapsed the earnings of insurance companies from the stock market. Malpractice insurance rates skyrocketed.

I began my private practice in 1972 and obtained coverage from a brokerage firm called the Nettleship Company, which provided malpractice insurance for members of the county medical associations. It was a broker, not an insurance company, and obtained coverage for its subscribers from companies like Chubb Pacific, also known as Pacific Indemnity Company. The premiums were kept low and the broker, expected to manage premium rates and risks by the underwriters, did not do much except collect the checks. A year after I began practice this whole system collapsed.

The Nettleship Company had been in business since the 1920s and the owners did not keep track of the building "tail" of claims since the war. If I perform surgery in 1972 and a complication results, it may be 1978 before that case is tried in court. Most insurance companies allot a "reserve" of income and capital to cover potential losses. During the 1960s, the reserves had been grossly inadequate. That resulted from several factors. There was a bull market in stocks from 1966 to 1974. Investments were appreciating at a rapid pace and assets allocated to reserves were increasing in value with the market. Secondly, the insurers were complacent and malpractice suits, expensive to defend, were being settled for the cost of a successful defense, regardless of the merits of the case. Little effort was made to assess the merits of the suits. Slowly, the volume of suits rose as lawyers learned that just filing a suit could result in a nice payday (Lawyers, of course, will dispute this). Thirdly, juries were willing to award higher dollar awards, perhaps because everyone was getting more prosperous; perhaps because of higher expectations from modern medicine.

In 1974, this whole system collapsed and my malpractice insurance premium went from $3,500 per year to $35,000 per year, a 1,000 percent increase. Furthermore, it soon became apparent that many insurance carriers were insolvent. Their reserves were inadequate (the bear market in 1974 deflated stock values) and some of the smaller companies went out of business, including the company with which my partner and I were insured. Traveler's Insurance Company continued to write policies for another year or two, but we could not afford the premium. We went "bare." We placed a sign in our waiting room informing all patients that we did not carry malpractice insurance, choosing instead to keep our fees low. Our practice continued to grow rapidly and, fortunately, I was not sued for seventeen years.

By 1978, doctor owned insurance "cooperatives" were formed and we joined one called "Cooperative of American Physicians," or CAP. For three years, my partner and I had no insurance and it had been nerve-wracking to have everything you owned at risk for a mistake. The cooperatives, called "bedpan mutuals" by the lawyers and insurance people, involved doctor control with selective acceptance of new applicants and vigorous defense of cases that were not clearly malpractice. The idea was to band together and accept only other physicians you trusted to practice good medicine. Legislation in 1975 allowed this alternative and the reforms, including a cap on "pain and suffering" damages to $250,000, resulted in a stable situation to the present. Our annual cost for insurance stayed below $10,000 and, when I retired in 1994, the mutual company refunded my $20,000 capital contribution from 1978. Unfortunately, few states have the enviable situation of California and another crisis is brewing across the country. The doctors and lawyers battle in the California Legislature every few years, but attempts to relax the cap on damages and and other provisions of the Medical Insurance Compensation Reform Act (MICRA) have always failed. Other states did not enact reforms and continue to have severe problems. The recent stock market decline has a lot to do with malpractice rate hikes, but some of these insurers did not do enough to screen applicants. Another factor in the current crisis is the inability of physicians to raise fees to pay higher premiums. Managed Care and Medicare have strict controls on medical prices although non-physician costs, particularly pharmaceuticals, have skyrocketed. Increasing attention to errors in hospitals and medical practice is long overdue, but managed care companies and the federal government, so far, seem uninterested. I have a theory that these agencies, which are paying the bills, fear that high quality will be more expensive.[544] The auto companies found this was not true when Japanese cars took away a large share of their market. I attend conferences on medical quality and the Toyota auto company is a frequent participant. Toyota has no plans to practice medicine, but they are widely acknowledged the world expert on high quality in manufacturing. Quality control in service industries, like medicine, is more complex but needs to be addressed. The Dartmouth Medical School has a health care quality improvement project that is studying methods of accomplishing this. Perhaps the impression that quality is too expensive will finally be dispelled.[545]

520   *The Swedish Health Service System*, American College of Health Administrators, 82nd Fellows Seminar (1980).

521   Karl Evang, *Health Services in Norway*, S. Hammerstad Boktrykkeri, Oslo (1969).

522   Sidney and Beatrice Webb, *Minority Report of the Poor Law Commissioners,* (1909).

523   Charles Webster, *the National Health Service; A Political History*, Oxford University Press (2002).

524   PEP, *Planning* No 177 (16 September 1941).

525   Abraham Epstein, "Social Security – Fiction or Fact?" *The American Mercury* 33; 129-38 (Oct. 1934).

526   Howard Hassard, "Fifty Years in Law and Medicine," an oral history, published by California Medical Association (1984).

527   Howard Hassard oral history.

528   E. Ryten, *A statistical picture of the past, present and future of registered nurses in Canada, Ottawa*, Canadian Nurses Association (1997).

529   John K. Iglehart, "Revisiting the Canadian Health Care System," *New England Journal of Medicine,* 342:2007-2012 (2000).

530   Helen Clapesattle, *The Doctors Mayo,* pp 345-346, University of Minnesota Press (1941). The author recounts the story in describing the growth of the Mayo Clinic at the same time.

531   John Wennberg and Allan Gittlesohn, "Small area variations in health care delivery," *Science*. Dec 14;182(117):1102-8(1973).

532   M Lesparre, "Washington in 1985: focus on saving Medicare." *Hospitals.* Jan 1;59(1):68-73 (1985).

533   "An Interview with Paul Ellwood Jr, MD," *MANAGED CARE* (November 1997).

534   Garrett Hardin, "The Tragedy of the Commons," *Science* 162:1243-48 (1968). A famous article that discusses this principle applied to modern life including pollution and population growth.

535   Timothy Lane and Steven Phillips, "IMF Financing and Moral Hazard," *Finance and Development,* 38, no. 2 (2001). Not exactly a medical source but a good discussion of the problem of moral hazard of insurance.

536   John E. Wennberg, Jean L. Freeman and William J. Culp, "Are hospital services rationed in New Haven or over-utilized in Boston?" *Lancet* May 23, 1987 PP 1185-1189 (1987).

537   James C. Mohr, "American Medical Malpractice Litigation in Historical perspective," *JAMA* 283:1731-36 (2000).

538   Allen .D. Spiegel and Florence Kavaler, "Abraham Lincoln's suit against a medical imposter who assaulted his client," *Journal of Community Health*, 26:383-401 (2001).

539   Allen .D Spiegel and Florence Kaveler, "Chicken bones, defense lawyer A. Lincoln and a malpractice case," *Lincoln Herald* 99:156-170 (1997).

540   James C. Mohr, p 1733.

541   Eugene F. Sanger, "Report of the Committee on Suits for Malpractice," *Transactions of the Maine Medical Association*,6:360-382 (1878).

542   "Miscellaneous," *JAMA* 9:839 (1887).

543   K.A. DeVille, *Medical Malpractice in Nineteenth-Century America: Origins and Legacy,* New York University Press , N.Y. (1990).

544   Nelson EC, Rust RT, Zahorik A, Rose RL, Batalden P, Siemanski BA., "Do patient perceptions of quality relate to hospital financial performance?" *Journal of Health Care Marketing.* Dec;12(4):6-13 (1992).

545   Batalden P, Splaine M., "What will it take to lead the continual improvement and innovation of health care in the twenty-first century?" *Quality Management in Health Care.* Fall;11(1):45-54 (2002).

Postscript

RECOMMENDED READING ON MEDICAL HISTORY

1. Roy Porter. *The Greatest Benefit to Mankind. A Medical History of Humanity,* W.W. Norton & Co. This is a major work by an author who has written multiple volumes of medical history. It goes into much more detail than I have and is particularly good on the period prior to the twentieth century. It is readable and should be the starting point for someone who wants more detail.

2. Paul Strathern. *Mendeleyev's Dream. The Quest for the Elements,* Thomas Dunne Books. This is a history of chemistry that includes a great deal on early medicine and the parallel development of chemistry and medicine. The author has written a long list of books on related subjects including Pythagoras, Archimedes, and Alan Turing, who invented the computer.

3. Michael Bliss. *William Osler A Life in Medicine,* Oxford University Press. This is a new biography that is more readable than the classic Cushing biography, which was awarded a Pulitzer Prize in 1926. The Cushing biography is also by Oxford University Press and is still in print.

4. Frederick F. Cartwright & Michael Biddis. *Disease & History,* Sutton Publishing, (2000). This book goes into more detail on plagues and infectious diseases although it also has a chapter on hemophilia. It is short and well written. This is a revised edition of a 1972 book.

5. Harold Ellis. *A History of Surgery,* Greenwich Medical Media. (2002). This is a compact history of surgery with many illustrations.

6. John F. Fulton. *Harvey Cushing. A Biography,* Blackwell Scientific. This book is out of print but if you can find it and are interested in surgery, it is a marvelous biography of an incredible man. When Osler died in 1920, his widow asked Cushing to write his biography. It took four years and was printed in two volumes. Cushing would operate all day and write the biography at night. It is almost inconceivable that one man could do all this and do it well.

7.   Jurgen Thorwald. *Century of the Surgeon* and *The Triumph of Surgery,* Pantheon Books. These books are out of print but can be found in libraries and through the Internet. The story is a fictionalized history of surgery, using the device of a German grandfather who happened to travel around the world in the nineteenth century and witness many of the developments in surgery, beginning with the first use of ether in 1846. The facts are all accurate and extensive references are included although most are in German, the original language of the books.

8.   Randy Shilts. *And the Band Played On,* St. Martin's Press (1987). This is the story of the AIDS epidemic's early years from the point of view of a man who died of the disease a few years after the book was published.

9.   Paul Starr. *The Social Transformation of American Medicine*, Basic Books (1982). This is the classic study of the economic history of medicine and should be read by every physician and medical student.

10.   George Anders. *Health Against Wealth*, Houghton-Mifflin (1996). This is an account of the development of HMOs written by a Wall Street Journal reporter who has done excellent research.

11.   James B Herrick, *Memories of Eighty Years*, University of Chicago Press, (1949). This is a very readable autobiography of one the greatest of American physicians, providing his personal account of the period from 1885, when he entered Rush Medical College, until the 1930s when he was president of a number of medical societies. He was one the three founding faculty members of the University of Chicago School of Medicine and continued in practice until the Second World War.

These books are particularly readable and are referenced in places in the text. There are journals of medical history and these are in most medical libraries. The index of these journals should be scanned looking for individual articles of interest.

ILLUSTRATIONS

1. Page 17 – Trephined skulls with evidence of healing. Nationalmuseet, Copenhagen, with permission.

2. Page 22 – Cylinder seal – The Louvre, Paris, with permission.

3. Page 52 – Illustration of reconstructed nose from Gentleman's Magazine, 1794.

4. Page 62 – Pulse chart by Pien Ch'iao from Wellcome Collection, Wellcome Trustees, London, with permission.

5. Page – 117 Heron's steam engine from Keyser, P. T. (1992). A New Look at Heron's Steam Engine. *Archive for History of Exact Sciences* 44(2):107-124, with permission.

6. Page 134 – Skeleton of O'Brien (O'Byrne), the Irish giant. From the Hunterian Museum, London, with permission.

7. Page 154 – Discovery of Chloroform from http://fis.org/doctorinternet/x-graphics/chloroform-party.GIF.

8. Page 224 – X-ray of Bertha Roentgen's hand from *Vienna Die Presse*, January 6, 1896.

9. Page 245 – Illustration from Hays, Wooley and Snyder, *Journal of Pediatrics* 1:240-252 (1966), with permission.

10. Page 302 – Odile Crick's drawing, with permission – *Nature* vol. 171, page 737.

11. Page 347 – Chart of tobacco consumption from Doll and Bradford-Hill, *British Medical Journal* Sept. 30,1050 pp 739-748, with permission.

12 Vivien Thomas, Helen Taussig and Steven Muller at honorary degree ceremony 1976, Courtesy of Johns Hopkins University, with permission.

13. Page 394 – Gibbon performing open heart surgery. From Jefferson Medical College History, with permission.

14 and 15.. Page 398 – Hufnagel valve from *The Proceedings of the American Academy of Cardiovascular Perfusion*, Volume 7. January 1986, with permission.

16. Page 400 – Xrays from Albert Starr's paper on valve replacement. From *Annals of Surgery* 160:596-613 (1964), with permission.

17. Page 415 – Photo of patient being treated for traumatic wet lung,

from *Surgery in World War II*. Thoracic Surgery volume II. Medical Department United States Army. Page 230, 1965, with permission.

18.   Page 457 – Electroconvulsive therapy from: *History of Shock Treatment*, by Leonard Roy Frank, 1978, with permission.

19.   Page 460 – Walter Freeman performing Prefrontal lobotomy. Source: UPI/Corbis, with permission.

GENERAL SOURCES

1.   Roy Porter, *The Greatest Benefit to Mankind*, W.W. Norton, 1997. This general history of medicine is excellent on ancient medicine up to the nineteenth century. Thereafter it is quite brief regarding modern surgery and other developments.

2.   Kenneth F. Kiple, *The Cambridge World History of Human Disease*, Cambridge University Press, (1993). Especially complete on infectious disease.

3.   W.F. Bynum and Roy Porter, *Companion Encyclopedia of the History of Medicine*, Routledge: London, (1993).

4.   Albert S. Lyons MD and R. Joseph Perucelli, II, MD, *Medicine. An Illustrated History*, Harry N Abrams, (1987).

5.   Ira M. Rutkow, MD, *American Surgery. An Illustrated History*, Lippincott-Raven (1998).

6.   Harold Ellis, *A History of Surgery*, Greenwich Medical Media (2000).

7.   James Le Fanu, *The Rise and Fall of Modern Medicine*, Carroll & Graf, (1999). This covers the modern period with comments about trends covered in the last chapter on medical economics.

8.   Erwin H. Ackerknecht, MD, *A Short History of Medicine*, The Ronald Press Company, NY (1955). Doctor Ackerknecht was educated in Germany, was assistant curator in anthropology at the American Museum of Natural History and was chairman of the Department of the History of Medicine at the University of Wisconsin. His view is unusual.

9.   The Nobel e-Museum maintained by the Nobel Foundation provides biographies and the addresses presented by laureates dating back to the first Nobel Prizes. This provides useful explanation of the research, and the lives, of Nobel Prize winners.

CHAPTER 1 – IN THE BEGINNING

1. Jared Diamond, *Guns, Germs and Steel,* W. W. Norton and Co., 1997. This popular anthropology book poses the theory of North-South axis of continents and the evolution of agriculture. It describes modern study of New Guinea tribes living in primitive conditions conducted by the author.

2. Charlotte Roberts and Keith Manchester, *The Archeology of Disease,* Cornell University Press, Ithaca, New York (1995). This describes in detail the diseases and state of health of ancient people, primarily from osteology.

3. Hans Zinsser, *Rats, Lice and History,* Bantam Books (1934). This classic, also used extensively as a source in sections on plagues and infectious diseases, covers the prehistoric period briefly.

4. Brenda Fowler, *Iceman,* Random House (2000). This recent book covers developments in the investigation of the man recovered from a glacier in the Tyrolean Alps in 1991.

CHAPTER 2 – EARLY GREEKS

1. Jurgen Thorwald, *Science and Secrets of Early Medicine,* Harcourt, Brace and World, (1962). This work covers Egyptian, Babylonian and other early civilizations and their medical practices.

2. Paul Strathern, *Mendeleyev's Dream: The Quest for the Elements,* Thomas Dunne Books, St. Martin's Press, (2000). Chapter one – "In the Beginning."

3. J.B. Bury, *The History of Greece to the Death of Alexander,* third edition, Macmillan (1951).

4. Roy Porter, ibid.

CHAPTER 3 – CLASSICAL GREECE AND ROME

1   Morris Kline, *Mathematical Thought from Ancient to Modern Times,* Oxford University Press, (1972), Volume 1. Greek mathematics and science of the classical period.

2. *The Genuine Works of Hippocrates,* translation by Francis Adams LLD for the Sydenham Society 1849, Classics of Medicine Library Edition.

3.   Paul Strathern. Chapter 2 – "The practice of alchemy."

4.   Frederick Cartwright & Michael Biddiss, *Disease and History,* Chapter 1 – "Disease in the Ancient World," Sutton Publishing, second edition 2000. The Roman Empire and the contribution of plagues to its fall.

5.   Jane Bellemore, Ian M. Plant and Lynne M. Cunningham, "Plague of Athens – Fungal Poison?," *The Journal of the History of Medicine* and Allied Sciences, 49:521-545 (1994). Discusses the Plague of Athens and postulates a rare fungal syndrome similar to ergotism.

6.   Graham Shipley, *The Greek World after Alexander*, Routledge, 2000.

7.   J.B.Bury, ibid.

CHAPTER 4 – INDIA AND CHINA

1.   Jurgen Thorwald. *Science and Secrets of Early Medicine*, Harcourt Brace and World (1962).

2.   R.B. Lenora, "Ayurvedic Medicine. The strange and Fascinating Tale of the Art and Science of Indian Medicine," *Clinical Pediatrics* 7:239-242 (1968). The author is an Ayurvedic physician, as well as a modern physician, and served in the Parliament of Ceylon.

3.   AF Hoernle, *Medicine of Ancient India*, Oxford University Press (1926).

4.   WF Bynum and Roy Porter, *Companion Encyclopedia of the History of Medicine,* Volume I Chapter 33 – "Indian Medicine," Routledge (1993).

5.   Lu Gwei-Djen and Joseph Needham, "Diseases of Antiquity in China," in Kenneth F. Kiple Ed., *The Cambridge World History of Human Disease,* Cambridge University Press (1993).

6.   Dominique Hoizey, *A History of Chinese Medicine*, translated by Paul Bailey, UBC Press, Vancouver (1993).

7.   Will Durant, *Our Oriental Heritage*, Simon and Schuster (1954) Rather subjective but a classic history of ancient civilizations.

8.   Roy Porter, *The Greatest Benefit to Mankind*, Chapter VI – "Indian Medicine," Chapter VII – "Chinese Medicine," W.W. Norton & Co. (1997).

9.   There are a number of Internet sites providing information on the Indus River civilization.

CHAPTER 5 – THE RISE OF ISLAM AND ARABIC MEDICINE

1. Paul Strathern, Chapter 2 – "The Practice of Alchemy"

2. Bernard Lewis, *The Middle East*, Simon and Shuster, 1995.

3. Roy Porter, Chapter IV – "Medicine and Faith."

CHAPTER 6 – THE MIDDLE AGES

1. Paul Strathern, Chapter 3 – "Genius and Gibberish."

2. Frederick Cartwright & Michael Biddias, – Chapter Two – "The Black Death."

3. Norman F. Cantor, *In the Wake of the Plague*, Perennial (2001).

4. Roy Porter, Chapter V – "The Medieval West."

5. Joel Mokyr, *The Lever of Riches*, Oxford University Press (1989) A history of technology in the Middle Ages.

CHAPTER 7 – THE BEGINNING OF MODERN SCIENCE

1. Paul Strathern – "Mendeleyev's Dream" Chapter 2.

2. Ambroise Paré, *The Apologie and Treatise of Ambroise Paré*, Edited by Geoffrey Keynes, University of Chicago Press, (1952).

3. Wallace B Hamby MD, *Ambroise Paré Surgeon of the Renaissance*, Warren H Green, Inc. (1967).

4. Frederick Cartwright & Michael Biddias, Chapter Three – Syphilis.

5. *Medicine's 10 Greatest Discoveries*, Meyer Friedman MD and Gerald W Friedland MD, Yale University Press, (1998) Chapter one.

6. Hans Zinsser, Chapter eleven.

7. Kenneth Kiple, "The Geography of Human Disease," in *The Cambridge World History of Human Disease*, Cambridge University Press, (1993) This huge work describes the evolution of infectious disease and its relationship to agriculture and climate change over the last 50,000 years.

8. Roy Porter, Chapter VIII – "Renaissance," Chapter IX – "The New Science."

9.   Henry M. Pachter, *Magic into Science*. The Story of Paracelsus, Henry Schuman (1951).

10.   Joel Mokyr, ibid.

CHAPTER 8 – THE ENLIGHTENMENT AND MEDICINE

1.   Meyer Friedman, – Chapter two – "William Harvey and the Circulation of Blood," Chapter three – "Antony Leeuwenhoek and Bacteria."

2.   Paul Streathern, – Chapter seven – "A Born-again Science."

3.   Frederick Cartwright & Michael Biddias, – Chapter Four – "Smallpox, or the Conqueror Conquered."

4.   Roy Porter, Chapter X – "Enlightenment."

5.   David H. Clark and Stephen P.H. Clark, *Newton's Tyranny*, W.H. Freeman & Co. (2001).

CHAPTER 9 –THE CENTURY OF THE SURGEON

1.   Frederick Cartwright & Michael Biddias, – Chapter five – "General Napoleon and General Typhus."

2.   J. Henry Dible, *"Napoleon's Surgeon,"* Heinemann (1970) A biography of Baron Dominic-Jean Larrey, one of the greatest military surgeons of all time.

3.   Robert E. Gosserin MD phD, "Exhuming Bonaparte," *Dartmouth Medicine*, Spring 2003, pp38-47, 61. A thorough discussion of the Emperor's last illness and a possible explanation of the arsenic.

4.   Frank Kells Boland MD, *The First Anesthetic*, University of Georgia Press (1950).

5.   Meyer Freidman and Gerald W Friedland, ibid – Chapter five – "Crawford Long and Surgical Anesthesia."

6.   Cecil Woodham-Smith, *Florence Nightingale*, McGraw (1951).

7.   Tim Coates Ed., *Florence Nightingale and the Crimea 1854-55*, The Stationery Office, (2000). This is a collection of letters and reports to the Crown from the time.

CHAPTER 10 – THE GERMANS

1. Karel Absolon, *The Surgeon's Surgeon*, Kabel Publishers, Rockville, MD (1999) This is the largest English language biography of Theodore Billroth.

2. Loyal Davis, *J.B. Murphy, Stormy Petrel of Surgery*, Putnam, 1938.

3. Jurgen Thorwald, *The Triumph of Surgery*, Pantheon Books (1960). Thorwald presents the German side of the dispute regarding the treatment of Crown Prince Frederick's laryngeal cancer.

4. R. Scott Stevenson, *Morell Mackenzie*, Henry Schuman, New York (1946). This biography presents Mackenzie's side of the story of Crown Prince Frederick although the facts differ little.

CHAPTER 11 – MEDICINE, BACTERIOLOGY AND INFECTIOUS DISEASE

1. Frederick Cartwright & Michael Biddias, – Chapter 6 – "Cholera and Sanitary reform."

2. Martha Marquardt, *Paul Erlich*, Henry Schuman, New York (1951).

3. Roy Porter, Chapter XIV "From Pasteur to Penicillin."

CHAPTER 12 – THE RISE OF MEDICINE

1. Roy Porter, pages 337-341 - Claude Bernard, pages 350-352 – 19th Century physicians.

2. Michael Bliss, *William Osler, A Life in Medicine*, Oxford University Press (1999).

3. Helen Clapesattle, *The Doctors Mayo*. University of Minnesota Press (1941).

CHAPTER 13 – THE NEW SCIENCE

1. Faraday and Maxwell – *Revolution in Science*, chapter 20, J. Bernard Cohen, Harvard University Press (1985)

2. Thomas K Simpson. *Maxwell on the Electromagnetic Field. A Guided Study*. Rutgers University Press (2001).

3. J. L. Heilbron, *Electricity in the 17th and 18th Centuries. A Study in Early Modern Physics*. Dover Publications (1979).

4.   Friedman and Friedland – "William Roentgen and the X-Ray Beam," *Medicine's Ten Greatest Discoveries*, Yale University Press (1998).

5.   Eve Curie, *Madame Curie,* English Translation,. Heinemann, London (1939).

6.   Guy Williams, *The Age of Miracles*, Chapter 15, "X-Rays and Their Application," Constable, London (1981).

7.   Charles R R Hayter, "The Clinic as Laboratory: The Case of Radiation Therapy, 1896-1920," *Bulletin of the History of Medicine* 72:663-688 (1998).

CHAPTER 14 – THE DEVELOPMENT OF MODERN SURGERY

1.   John E Fulton, *Harvey Cushing, A Biography*, Charles C Stone (1946).

2.   Grace Crile Ed., "*George Crile. An Autobiography*," J.B. Lippincott (1947).

3.   Ira M. Rutkow, MD, *American Surgery. An Illustrated History*, Lippincott-Raven (1998).

4.   Harold Ellis, *A History of Surgery*, Greenwich Medical Media Ltd. (2000).

5.   Owen H. Wangensteen MD and Sarah D. Wangensteen, *The Rise of Surgery*, University of Minnesota Press (1978).

CHAPTER 15 – BLOOD

1.   M. Whitten Wise and Patrick O'Leary, "The Origins of Blood Transfusion: Early History," *The American Surgeon,* 68:98-100 (2002).

2.   Guy Williams, *The Age of Miracles*, chapter ten, "Blood and Blood Transfusions," Constable, London (1981).

3.   Grace Crile, ibid.

4.   Kim Pelis, "Taking Credit: The Canadian Army Medical Corps and the British Conversion to Blood Transfusion in WWI," *Journal of the History of Medicine and Allied Sciences,* 56:238 (2001).

5.   Douglas Starr, *Blood. An Epic History of Medicine and Commerce*, Perrenial: Harper Collins (1998). A history of transfusion, hepatitis and AIDS.

CHAPTER 16 – THE STRUCTURE OF DNA

1. Friedman and Friedland, Chapter 10, "Maurice Wilkins and DNA."

2. James D Watson, *The Double Helix*, Scribner Classics (1968.)

3. Maxim D Frank-Kamenetskii, *Unraveling DNA*, VCH Publishers, New York (1993).

4. Ann Sayre, *Rosalind Franklin and DNA*, Norton (1975).

CHAPTER 17 – FLEMING, FLOREY AND PENICILLIN

1. Friedman and Friedland, Chapter 9, "Alexander Fleming and Antibiotics."

2. David Wilson, *In Search of Penicillin*, Alfred Knopf (1976).

3. Roy Porter, Chapter XIV "From Pasteur to Penicillin."

CHAPTER 18 – TWENTIETH CENTURY MEDICINE

1. William Osler – *The Principles and Practice of Medicine*, Appleton and Company, (1892), The Classics of Medicine Library.

2. Michael Bliss, *The Discovery of Insulin*, MacMillan Press, (1982) This is a detailed history of the discovery with a strong bias toward MacLeod's point of view.

3. Seale Harris MD, *Banting's Miracle*, J.M. Dent & Sons, (1946). This is a biography of Banting by a personal friend partial to his point of view.

4. Louis J Acierno, *The History of Cardiology*, Parthenon Publishing Group, (1994).

5. Allen B Weisse, *Heart to Heart*, Rutgers University Press (2002).

6. Leon Speroff, Robert Glass, Nathan Kase, *Clinical Gynecologic Endocrinology and Infertility,* Chapter 22 – "Oral Contraception The story of the synthesis of steroids from the Mexican yam."

7. John R Paul, *A History of Poliomyelitis*, Yale University Press (1971).

8. John Crewson, *Science Fictions*, Little, Brown and Company 2002. This is the account of the discovery of the HIV virus and the

controversy about Robert Gallo claiming credit for the French discovery.

9.   Randy Shilts, *And the Band Played On*, St Martins Press (1987). This is Randy Shilts', a newspaper reporter in San Francisco who subsequently died of AIDS, account of the early days of the epidemic.

10.   Edited by Fauci, et al, *Harrison's Principles of Internal Medicine*, McGraw-Hill (1998). The chapter on AIDS for current therapy and epidemiology.

11.   Edward Hooper, *The River,* Little, Brown and Company, (1999). A history of the AIDS epidemic with speculation on the origin of the virus and its transmission to the human species.

12.   William J Mallon, *Ernest Amory Codman: The End Result of a Life in Medicine,* Saunders (2000).

13.   "History of Orthopedics in North America," *Clinical Orthopedics and Related Research,* 374:2-187 (2000).

14.   David Le Vay, *The History of Orthopedics,* The Parthenon Publishing Group (1990).

CHAPTER 19 – CARDIAC SURGERY

1.   Steven L. Johnson, *The History of Cardiac Surgery, 1896 – 1955,* The Johns Hopkins Press (1970).

2.   Louis J Acierno, ibid.

3.   Harris B. Schumaker, Jr., *The Evolution of Cardiac Surgery*, Indiana University Press (1992).

4.   Allen B Weisse, ibid.

5.   René G. Favaloro, *The Challenging Dream of Heart Surgery*, Little Brown & Co (1994).

CHAPTER 20 – CRITICAL CARE MEDICINE

1.   Gordon L Snider "Historical Perspective on Mechanical Ventilation: from Simple Life Support to Ethical Dilemma," *American Review of Respiratory Diseases* 140:S2-S7 (1989).

2. Julie Fairman and Joan Lynaugh, *Critical Care Nursing. A History*, University of Pennsylvania Press (1998).

3. Grace Crile Ed., ibid.

4. Richard S Atkinson and Thomas B. Boulton, Eds. *The History of Anesthesia* Parthenon Publishing Group. (1989) This is an international symposium on the subject with many essays relating details of anesthesia development.

CHAPTER 21 – TRANSPLANTATION

1. Francis D. Moore, *Transplant; The Give and Take of Tissue Transplantation*, Simon and Schuster, (1972). This is an expanded version of his 1964 book, *Give and Take*.

2. Thomas E. Starzl, "The Saga of Liver Replacement, with Particular Reference to the Reciprocal Influence of Liver and Kidney Transplantation (1955-1967)," Charles G. Drake History of Surgery Lecture, *Journal of the American College of Surgeons* (2002).

CHAPTER 22 – PSYCHIATRY

1. Ernst L Freud editor, *The Letters of Sigmund Freud and Arnold Zweig*, Harcourt, Brace (1970).

2. Edward Shorter *A History of Psychiatry*, John Wiley and Sons, (1997)

3. Hannah S Decker Freud, *Dora and Vienna 1900*, The Free Press, Macmillan (1991).

4. William Glasser M.D., *Reality Therapy*, Harper and Row (1965). This book describes the Harrington method of treating psychotics in 1962 when I spent a summer with him. Glasser was one of his residents at UCLA before writing the book.

5. David Healey, *The Anti-depressant Era*, Harvard University Press, (1997) – This gives a good history of the development of psychopharmacology and the development of the pharmaceutical industry, especially those producing psychoactive drugs.

6. David Healy, *Psychopharmacology*, Harvard University Press (2002). This is a larger and more complete history of psychiatry and the use of psychotropic drugs including all forms of therapy.

Chapter 23 – Economics of Medicine

1. Paul Starr, *The Social Transformation of American Medicine*, Basic Books (1982). The history of American Medicine to about 1988.

2. Sir William Beveridge *Social Insurance and Allied Services - report*, (November 1942).

3. Charles Webster, *the National Heath Service. A Political History*, Oxford University Press (2002)

4. Paul Andre – *Health Against Wealth*, Houghton Mifflin Company (1996) A critical history of HMOs

5. Charles E Rosenberg, *The Care of Strangers, The Rise of America's Hospital System*, Basic Books (1987).

6. Bradford H Gray, *The Profit Motive and Patient Care*, Harvard University Press (1991). A critique of fee-for-service medicine.

7. Thomas H Ainsworth, *Live or Die*, Macmillan (1983).

8. Philip Jacobs, *The Economics of Health and Medical Care*, Aspen Publishers, (1991).

9. Michael Millenson, *Demanding Medical Excellence*, University of Chicago Press (1997) This book provides a good description of the recent interest in quality improvement methodology, additional material on the renewed interest in Amory Codman, and a more positive view of HMOs than my own.

Index of Terms

D

E

K

L

M

R

492

Index of Names

E

F

Q

R

Web Resources

www.historyofmedicine.org